P9-AGG-034

Milady's
VAN DEAN MANUAL

A Practical Course on the Fundamentals of Cosmetology

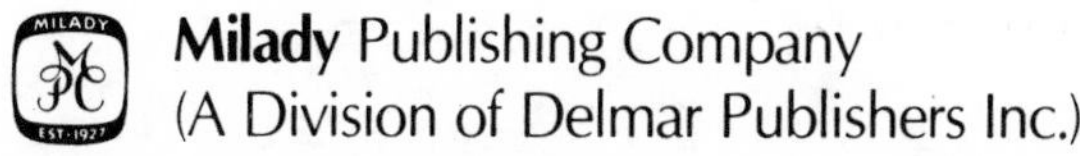

Milady Publishing Company
(A Division of Delmar Publishers Inc.)

EDITOR: Catherine Frangie

PRODUCTION MANAGER: Jan M. Lavin

ART DIRECTOR: John P. Fornieri

GRAPHIC ARTISTS: Pat Miret, Mark Stein, Pat Genova

ILLUSTRATIONS: Shiz Horii

MEDICAL ILLUSTRATIONS: Sheri Amsel

COVER: Courtesy of Belvedere Company

PHOTOGRAPHER: Steven Landis

PHOTOGRAPHER FOR PAGE 128: Eric Von Lockhart

STYLISTS: Vincent and Alfred Nardi,
Nardi Salon

MAKEUP ARTIST: Michael Constantini

ISBN 0-87350-516-6

Printed in the United States

10 9 8 7 6 5 4 3 2 1

This edition of the revised Milady's Van Dean Manual is dedicated to you, the future Cosmetology Professional

Preface

Hello and welcome to cosmetology! You are entering a very exciting profession! Studying cosmetology will be the beginning of a varied and rewarding career!

In the next few months you're going to be learning the art of helping people look their best and feel better about themselves by improving their physical appearance! Cosmetic changes like a haircut, a hair color change, a manicure, or a new hairstyle are important factors in the way people build self esteem and in the way that they interact with others.

As a cosmetologist you will build a trust with your clients. They'll ask you for your professional advice on everything from their hairstyle and make up to their skin care. Your clients will be sharing a prized possesion with you—their appearance and you'll be sharing your knowledge with them. As you build your relationship you'll teach your clients about the composition of hair, about the chemical processes that hair undergoes and how to use that information in making decisions about products like shampoos, conditioners and styling tools.

We're all partners in the beauty industry. We're working hard, together, to make our industry as rewarding and as professional as it can be.

A cosmetology license is only the beginning of your career options in the beauty industry! You can use your experience in the cosmetology field to go into sales, management, retail, distribution, publishing, travel and a host of other exciting career paths.

Cosmetology is so much more than just a job. It is a profession that will introduce you to innovative, exciting and creative people. And the key to that profession is your cosmetology license!

We all want to help you make it happen—your teachers, your school and us. We're all working together to educate you in cosmetology so that you can be the best professional that you can be! That's why we have redesigned this book, with you in mind. At Milady we've spent months contacting the top experts in the cosmetology industry. We asked them to read and comment on our text and then with their suggestions in mind we revised and rewrote our book. We've made this book the clearest, the most accurate, informative and exciting book on the market—for you.

For teachers we have designed lesson plans, theory and practical workbooks, audio cassettes, instructional videos and state board exam review books to complement their experience and to enhance your education.

Good luck in the program—we know that you can master it, and we're looking forward to having you as a fellow professional in the best industry in the world—Cosmetology!

Table of Contents

Chapter 1 **HYGIENE AND GOOD GROOMING** **1**
HYGIENIC RULES 2
HEALTHY THOUGHTS 2
A Well-Groomed Female Cosmetologist 3
A Well-Groomed Male Cosmetologist 4
MAINTAIN GOOD HEALTH 4

Chapter 2 **VISUAL POISE** **5**
GOOD POSTURE 5
Stand Correctly 6
Correct Sitting Technique 8
Correct Stooping Technique 9
Correct Lifting Technique 9
Foot Care 10

Chapter 3 **PERSONALITY DEVELOPMENT** **11**
DESIRABLE QUALITIES TO CULTIVATE 12
Voice and Conversation 13
How to Aquire Conversational Charisma 14
YOUR PERSONALITY CHART 15
Personality Quiz 15

Chapter 4 **PROFESSIONAL ETHICS** **17**
ETHICS 17
PROFESSIONAL ATTITUDE TOWARD CLIENTS 18

Chapter 5 **BACTERIOLOGY** **21**
BACTERIOLOGY 21
Bacteria 22
Types of Bacteria 22
Pronunciations of Terms 22
To Avoid the Spread of Disease 23
Classifications of Pathogenic Bacteria 24
Bacterial Growth and Reproduction 24
Bacterial Infections 25
IMMUNITY 26

Chapter 6 **STERILIZATION AND SANITATION** **27**
STERILIZATION AND SANITATION 27
Definitions Pertaining to Sanitation 28
Methods of Sterilization and Sanitation 28
CHEMICAL SANITIZING AGENTS 30
Sanitizing with Chemical Disinfectants 31

Sanitizing with Alcohol 31
SAFETY PRECAUTIONS 32
SANITIZING RULES 32
PUBLIC SANITATION 32
SUMMARY 34

Chapter 7 **DRAPING** **37**
PREPARATION FOR DRAPING 38
DRAPING FOR WET HAIR SERVICES 38
DRAPING FOR DRY HAIR SERVICES 39
DRAPING FOR THERMAL SERVICES 40
DRAPING FOR A COMB-OUT 40
DRAPING FOR FACIALS 40

Chapter 8 **SHAMPOOING AND RINSING** **41**
SHAMPOOS 41
Water 42
Selecting the Correct Shampoo 42
HAIR BRUSHING TECHNIQUE 43
Plain Shampoo 44
Cleanup 46
SHAMPOOING LIGHTENED HAIR 47
TYPES OF SHAMPOOS 47
Plain Shampoo 47
Soapless Oil Shampoos 47
Liquid Cream Shampoos 47
Cream or Paste Cream Shampoos 47
Acid-Balanced or Nonstrip Shampoos 47
Antidandruff or Medicated Shampoos 47
Liquid Dry and Powder Shampoos 48
Other Types of Shampoos 48
HAIR RINSES 48
Instant Conditioning Rinses 48
Color Rinses 48
Medicated Rinses 48
Stabilizing Rinses 48

Chapter 9 **SCALP AND HAIR CARE** **49**
SCALP CARE AND TREATMENTS 49
SCALP MANIPULATIONS 50
Anatomy 50
Scalp Manipulation Technique 50
TREATMENT FOR NORMAL HAIR AND SCALP 53
DANDRUFF 53
DRY HAIR AND SCALP TREATMENT 54
OILY HAIR AND SCALP TREATMENT 55
CORRECTIVE HAIR TREATMENT 56

TREATMENT FOR ALOPECIA 56
TREATMENTS FOR ALOPECIA AREATA 57
REMINDERS AND HINTS ON SCALP AND HAIR CARE 58

Chapter 10 **HAIR SHAPING 59**
IMPLEMENTS USED IN HAIR SHAPING 60
SECTIONING FOR HAIR SHAPING 62
HOLDING HAIR SHAPING IMPLEMENTS 63
Scissors 63
Thinning Shears 63
Comb and Scissors 63
HAIR THINNING 64
Hair Thinning Areas 64
Thinning with Thinning Shears 65
Thinning with Haircutting Scissors (Shears) 65
HAIR SHAPING WITH SCISSORS 66
Crown Section 67
Top Section 67
Completion 67
TAPERING (SHINGLING) 68
USING CLIPPERS 68
USING A RAZOR 69
Thinning with Razor 70
HAIR SHAPING WITH RAZOR 70
LEARN HOW TO HANDLE CHILDREN 70
SHAPING OVER-CURLY HAIR 73
DEFINITIONS PERTAINING TO HAIR SHAPING 75

Chapter 11 **SHAMPOOING AND RINSING 77**
PREPARATION 77
FINGER WAVING LOTION 78
HORIZONTAL FINGER WAVING 78
Shaping the Top Area 78
Shaping the Left Side of the Head 80
ALTERNATE METHOD OF FINGER WAVING 81
VERTICAL FINGER WAVING 82
SHADOW WAVE 82
REMINDERS AND HINTS ON FINGER WAVING 83

Chapter 12 **HAIRSTYLING 85**
IMPLEMENTS AND MATERIALS USED IN HAIRSTYLING 87
REMOVING TANGLES FROM HAIR 88
MAKING A PART 88
FINDING THE NATURAL PART 89
PIN CURLS 89
Pin Curl Comb-Out 90
Curl and Stem Direction 91

CLOCKWISE AND COUNTERCLOCKWISE CURLS 91
SHAPING FOR PIN CURL PLACEMENTS 92
PIN CURL FOUNDATIONS OR BASES 93
PIN CURL TECHNIQUES 95
Anchoring Pin Curls 98
EFFECTS OF PIN CURLS 99
Vertical Waves 99
Horizontal Waves 99
Interlocking Movement 99
Diagonal Waves 100
Waved Bangs 100
French Twist 100
RIDGE CURLS 101
SKIP WAVE 101
CASCADE OR STAND-UP CURL 102
Effect of Stand-Up Curls 102
SEMI-STAND-UP CURLS 103
ROLLER CURLS 103
BARREL CURLS 105
VOLUME AND INDENTATION IN ROLLER TECHNIQUE
(With Cylinder Rollers) 106
CYLINDER CIRCULAR ROLLER ACTION 107
TAPERED ROLLERS 110
HAIR PARTINGS 111
BACK COMBING AND BACK BRUSHING TECHNIQUES 112
COMB-OUT 113
ARTISTRY IN HAIRSTYLING 115
Facial Types 115
Special Considerations 118
Profile 120
NOSE SHAPES 121
EYES 122
Styling for Women Who Wear Glasses 123
HEAD SHAPES 125
BRAIDING 126
DEFINITIONS PERTAINING TO HAIRSTYLING 128

Chapter 13 **THE ART AND STYLING OF ARTIFICIAL HAIR 131**
WHY WIGS WORN 132
TYPES OF WIGS 132
Human Hair Wigs 132
TAKING WIG MEASUREMENTS 135
ORDERING THE WIG 135
FITTING THE WIG 136
CLEANING WIGS 137
Conditioning the Wig 139
SHAPING WIGS 139

SETTING AND STYLING WIGS 141
PUTTING ON AND TAKING OFF A WIG 142
WIG COLORING 142
Color Rinses 142
Semi-Permanent Tints 143
Permanent Tints 143
HAIRPIECES AND EXTENSIONS 144
Safety Precautions 145
DEFINITIONS PERTAINING TO WIGS 146

Chapter 14 **PERMANENT WAVING 149**
HISTORY OF PERMANENT WAVING 150
COLOR WAVING 151
NEUTRAL AND ACID BALANCED SOLUTIONS 151
PERMANENT WAVING 151
Pysical Action 151
Chemical Action 152
SCALP AND HAIR ANALYSIS 152
PRE-PERMANENT SHAPING AND SHAMPOOING 155
Shampooing for a Permanent Wave 155
Shaping Suggestions for a Permanent Wave 156
Shaping Percautions 156
CURLING RODS 156
Types of Rods 157
CHEMICALS 157
Waving Lotions 157
Neutralizers 158
SECTIONING AND BLOCKING 158
Suggested Hair Blockings and Rod Sizes 159
PATTERNS FOR SECTIONING AND BLOCKING 159
WINDING OR WRAPPING THE HAIR 162
Strand Relation to the Head 162
End Papers 162
Other End Paper Wraps 164
Piggyback Wrap 164
TEST CURLS 165
Pre-Permanent Test Curl Method 166
Test Curl-Wave Development Method 166
Safety Precautions 166
APPLICATION OF WAVING LOTION 167
Applying the Waving Lotion 167
Processing Time 168
Wave Pattern Formation 168
Over-Processing 169
Under-Processing 169
NEUTRALIZATION 169
Preparation 170

Method of Neutralization 170
Removing Neutralizer 170
COLD WAVING (ALKALINE) 171
Important Reminders 173
Cleanup 173
BODY (PERMANENT) WAVING 173
Processing and Neutralizing 173
Advantages 173
HEAT PERMANENT WAVING 174
Neutral and Acid-Balanced Lotions 174
Objectives of Heat Application 174
Neutralizers 176
PERMANENT WAVING FOR MEN 176
Release Statement 177
Permanent Wave Record 177
REMINDERS AND HINTS ON PERMANENT WAVING 178
SPECIAL PROBLEMS 179
Reconditioning Treatments 179
Special Permanent Wave Fillers 179
Aftercare 179
Waving Tinted or Lightened Hair 179
Hair Tinted With Metallic Dye 179
Curl Reduction 180
Permanent Wavign hair With Partial Permanent 180

Chapter 15 **HAIR COLORING** **181**
COLOR THEORY 182
Primary Colors 182
Secondary Colors 183
Tertiary Colors 183
Complementary Colors 183
Concentration 183
CLASSIFICATIONS OF HAIR COLORING 183
Temporary Hair Coloring 184
Semi-Permanent Hair Coloring 184
Permanent Hair Coloring 185
ANILINE DERIVATIVE TINTS 187
Allergy 187
Patch Test 187
PREPARATION FOR HAIR COLORING 188
Consultation 188
Basic Rules for Color Selection 190
Strand Test 190
Keeping Hair Color Records 191
Release Statement 192
TEMPORARY COLORS 192
Materials and Implements 193

Methods of Application 193
Cleanup 193
Alternate Methods 193
SEMI-PERMANENT COLOR 193
Advantages 194
Types 194
Implements and Materials 194
Cleanup 195
PERMANENT HAIR COLORS 196
Single Process Tints 196
Single Process Tint Procedure for Virgin Hair (Tinting to a Lighter Shade) 196
Materials and Implements 196
Preliminary Steps 198
Cleanup 199
Tinting to a Darker Shade 199
Tinting Long Hair 199
Single Process Tint Retouch 199
HIGHLIGHTING SHAMPOO COLORS 199
PRE-LIGHTEN OR PRE-SOFTEN 200
SAFETY PRECAUTIONS 200
HAIR LIGHTENING 201
Action of Hair Lighteners 201
Effects of Lighteners 201
Problems in Hair Lightening 203
TYPES OF LIGHTENERS 203
HYDROGEN PEROXIDE 204
LIGHTENING VIRGIN HAIR 204
Preliminary Test Results 204
Materials and Implements 205
Procedure 205
LIGHTENER RETOUCH 206
Retouch Procedure 206
Precautions 207
Spot Lightening 208
TONERS 208
Pre-Lightening for Toners 208
Toner Application 208
Toner Retouch 210
SPECIAL EFFECTS HIGHLIGHTING 210
Methods for Highlighting 210
SPECIAL PROBLEMS IN HAIR COLORING 212
Damaged Hair 212
Reconditioning Procedure 212
Fillers 213
Tint Removal 214
Removing Coating Dyes 215

TINT BACK TO NATURAL COLOR 215
Procedure 215
DEFINITIONS PERTAINING TO HAIR COLORING 216

Chapter 16 **CHEMICAL HAIR RELAXING AND SOFT CURL PERMANENT 219**
CHEMICAL HAIR RELAXING PRODUCTS 220
Chemical Hair Relaxers 220
Neutralizer 220
Protective Base for Sodium Hydroxide 220
No-Base Relaxers 220
BASIC STEPS 221
Processing 221
Neutralizing 221
Conditioning 221
Recommended Relaxer Strength 221
ANALYSIS OF CLIENT'S HAIR 221
Client's Hair History 221
Scalp Examination 222
CHEMICAL HAIR RELAXING PROCESS (with Sodium Hydroxide) 223
Equipment, Implements and Materials 223
Preparation 223
Procedure 224
Applying Conditioner-Filler 224
Applying the Relaxer 225
Strand Testing 226
Rinsing Out Relaxer 226
Shampooing/Neutralizing 226
APPLYING CONDITIONER 227
SODIUM HYDROXIDE RETOUCH 227
CHEMICAL HAIR RELAXING PROCESS (with Ammonium Thioglycolate) 227
Thio Retouch 228
Other Relaxers 228
CHEMICAL BLOWOUT 228
Equipment, Implements and Materials 228
SAFETY PRECAUTIONS FOR CHEMICAL BLOWOUT 229
SOFT CURL PERMANENT 230
Implements and Materials 231
Procedure 231
Aftercare 233
SAFETY PRECAUTIONS 234

Chapter 17 **THERMAL HAIR STRAIGHTENING 235**
HAIR PRESSING 235
HAIR CHARACTERISTICS 236

SCALP CHARACTERISTICS 237
HAIR AND SCALP EXAMINATION 237
RECORD CARD 237
CONDITIONING TREATMENTS 237
PRESSING OIL OR CREAM 238
EFFECTS OF HAIR STRAIGHTENING 238
HAIR SECTIONING 238
PRESSING COMBS 238
Heating the Comb 239
Cleaning the Comb 239
SOFT PRESS METHOD FOR NORMAL, CURLY HAIR 239
Implements and Materials 239
Preparation 239
Procedure 240
Touch-ups 241
Safety Precautions 241
Release Statement 241
Reminders and Hints on Soft Pressing 242
SPECIAL PROBLEMS 242
Pressing Fine Hair 242
Pressing Short, Fine Hair 242
Pressing Coarse Hair 242
Pressing Tinted, Lightened or Gray Hair 242

Chapter 18 **THERMAL WAVING, CURLING AND BLOW-DRY STYLING 243**
THERMAL WAVING AND CURLING 244
Thermal Irons 244
USING NON-ELECTRIC THERMAL IRONS 245
Temperature of Thermal Irons 245
Testing Thermal Irons 245
Care of Non-Electric Thermal Irons 245
Rolling the Thermal Irons 246
THERMAL WAVING WITH NON-ELECTRIC THERMAL (MARCEL) IRONS 247
Procedure for Left-Going Wave 247
Right-Going Wave 248
Joining or Matching the Waves 249
THERMAL CURLING WITH ELECTRIC THERMAL IRONS 249
Using Electric Thermal Irons 249
Care of Electric Thermal Irons 249
THERMAL IRONS CURLING METHODS 251
Preparation 251
Other Types of Curls 254
VOLUME THERMAL IRON CURLS 255
Volume Base Curls 255
Full Base Curls 255
Half Base Curls 255

Off Base Curls 255
Hints on Thermal Curl Styling 256
ARRANGING THE HAIR IN A SUITABLE HAIRSTYLE 256
SAFETY MEASURES 257
BLOW DRY STYLING 258
Equipment, Implements and Materials 258
The Blow Dryer 258
Combs and Brushes 259
Cosmetics Used in Blow Dry Styling 259
Hints for Blow-Dry Styling 260
Brushes and Combs 260
Blow Dryer 261
Shaping Hair with Styling Comb 263
SAFETY PRECAUTIONS 264

Chapter 19 **MANICURING** **265**
EQUIPMENT, IMPLEMENTS, COSMETICS AND MATERIALS 266
Equipment 266
Implements 266
Cosmetics 269
Materials 270
Shape of Nails 270
PREPARATION OF THE MANICURE TABLE 271
Procedure 272
GIVING A PLAIN MANICURE 272
Procedure 272
Completion 274
Final Cleanup 275
SAFETY RULES IN MANICURING 276
Shaping of Nails 276
HAND MASSAGE 277
Procedure 277
TYPES OF MANICURE 278
Nail Wrapping 279
Removing a Nail Wrap 281
Liquid Nail Wrap 281
Other Nail Problems 281
ARTIFICIAL NAILS 281
Sculptured Nails 281
Implements and Materials 282
Removing Sculptured Nails 283
Repairs and Fill-ins for Sculptured Nails 283
SAFETY PRECAUTIONS 284
Press-on Artificial Nails 284
Implements and Materials 284
Removing Polish 285
Removing Press-on Nails 285

Reminders and Hints on Artificial Nails 285
Dipped Nails 285
Manicure with Hand and Arm Massage 286
PEDICURING 287
Equipment, Implements and Materials 287
Preparation 287
Procedure 288
Foot Massage Procedure 289
Completion 289
Leg Massage 290

Chapter 20 **THE NAIL AND ITS DISORDERS** **291**
NAIL STRUCTURE 292
STRUCTURES ADJOINING THE NAIL 292
Nail Bed 292
Matrix 292
Lunula 292
Parts Surrounding the Nail 293
NAIL GROWTH 293
NAIL MALFORMATION 293
NAIL DISORDERS 294
Nail Irregularities 294
Nail Diseases 296

Chapter 21 **THEORY OF MASSAGE** **299**
HOW MANIPULATIVE MOVEMENTS ARE ACCOMPLISHED 300
Basic Manipulations Used in Massage 300
Joint Movements 303
MOTOR NERVE POINTS OF THE FACE AND NECK 303
Physiological Effects of Massage 304

Chapter 22 **FACIALS** **305**
BASIC FACIAL 306
Preparation 306
Equipment, Implements and Materials 306
Procedure 307
Reminders and Hints in Facial Massage 309
MASSAGE MANIPULATIONS 310
Facial Manipulations 310
Chest, Back and Neck Manipulations 312
SPECIAL PROBLEMS 313
Facial for Dry Skin 313
Facial for Oily Skin and Blackheads 314
Treatment for Whiteheads 315
Facial for Acne 315
Equipment, Implements and Materials 315
Diet for Acne 316

PACKS AND MASKS 316
Pack Facials 316
Equipment, Implements and Materials 316
Egg Pack 316
Hot Oil Mask Facial 317
Equipment, Implements and Materials 317

Chapter 23 **FACIAL MAKEUP 319**
MAKEUP APPLICATION 319
Draping 320
Implements and Materials 320
Makeup Kit 321
Contouring Cosmetics 321
Lip Color 321
Eye Makeup 321
Procedure for a Professional Makeup Application 322
MAKEUP TECHNIQUES FOR THE BLACK WOMAN 326
Foundation 326
Powder 326
Cheek Color 326
Eye Color 326
Lip Color 326
CORRECTIVE MAKEUP AND FACIAL CONTOURING 328
MAKEUP FOR FACIAL TYPES 328
CORRECTING FACIAL FLAWS 333
Corrective Makeup for Eyes 334
Corrective Makeup for Lips 335
Eyebrow Arching 335
Incorrect Shaping 335
Correct Shaping 336
Implements, Supplies and Materials 336
ARITIFICIAL (FALSE) EYELASHES 337
Equipment, Implements and Materials for Applying
Artificial Lashes 338
Procedure for Applying Strip Eyelases 338
Removing Artificial Eyelashes 339
Applying Individual Eyelashes (Eye Tabbing) 339
Sparse Eyelashes 341
Removing Individual Lashes 342
Hints for Removing False Eyelashes 342
SAFETY PRECAUTIONS 342
LASH AND BROW TINT 343
Materials and Implements 343
Preparation 343
Procedure 343

Chapter 24	**SUPERFLUOUS HAIR REMOVAL**	**345**
	ELECTROLYSIS	346
	Electrology Definitions	346
	METHODS OF PERMANENT HAIR REMOVAL	347
	SHORTWAVE METHOD	347
	Equipment, Implements and Materials	347
	Preparation of Client	347
	Preparing the Machine	348
	Analysis	348
	Inserting the Needle into the Follicle	349
	After-treatment Procedure	349
	Regrowth	350
	REMINDERS AND HINTS ON ELECTROLOGY	350
	ELECTRONICALLY-CHARGED TWEEZER	350
	TEMPORARY METHODS	351
Chapter 25	**CELLS**	**355**
	CELL GROWTH AND REPRODUCTION	356
	Metabolism	357
	TISSUES	357
	Organs	357
	SYSTEMS	357
Chapter 26	**THE SKIN AND ITS DISORDERS**	**359**
	THE SKIN	360
	HISTOLOGY OF THE SKIN	361
	How the Skin is Nourished	362
	NERVES OF THE SKIN	363
	Sensory Nerves of the Skin	363
	SKIN ELASTICITY	363
	SKIN COLOR	364
	GLANDS OF THE SKIN	364
	FUNCTIONS OF THE SKIN	365
	DISORDERS OF THE SKIN	365
	Definitions Pertaining to Skin Disorders	366
	LESIONS OF THE SKIN	366
	Definitions Pertaining to Primary Lesions	366
	Definitions Pertaining to Secondary Lesions	367
	Definitions Pertaining to Disease	367
	DISORDERS OF THE SEBACEOUS (OIL) GLANDS	368
	DEFINITIONS PERTAINING TO DISORDERS OF THE SUDORIFEROUS (SWEAT) GLANDS	370
	DEFINITIONS PERTAINING TO PIGMENTATIONS OF THE SKIN	371
	DEFINITIONS PERTAINING TO HYPERTROPHIES	371

Chapter 27 THE HAIR AND DISORDERS OF THE SCALP AND HAIR **373**
HAIR 373
Structures Associated with Hair Root 374
Structures Connected to Hair Follicles 376
Hair Structure 376
HAIR DISTRIBUTION 377
HAIR GROWTH 377
Hair Replacement 378
LIFE AND DENSITY OF HAIR 379
COLOR OF HAIR 379
Graying of Hair 379
HAIR DEFINITIONS AND TECHNICAL TERMS 379
Definitions of Directional Hair Growth 380
HAIR ANALYSIS 380
Condition 380
Texture 381
Porosity 381
Elasticity 381
SCALP DISORDERS 382
Dandruff 382
Alopecia 382
Contagious Disorders 383
Staphylococci Infections 384
HAIR DISORDERS 385
Non-Contagious Disorders 385

Chapter 28 ANATOMY **387**
THE SKELETAL SYSTEM 388
Bones of the Skull 389
Bones of the Cranium Affected by Massage 389
Bones of the Face Affected by Massage 389
THE MUSCULAR SYSTEM 390
Origin, Insertion and Belly of Muscles 390
Stimulation of Muscles 390
THE NERVOUS SYSTEM 391
Division of the Nervous System 392
Nerve Cells and Nerves 392
THE BRAIN AND SPINAL CORD 393
FATIGUE AND ITS CORRECTION 393
THE CIRCULATORY SYSTEM 394
The Heart 394
Blood Vessels 395
THE BLOOD AND ITS FUNCTIONS 395
Primary Functions of the Blood 395
Circulation of the Blood 396
THE LYMPH-VASCULAR SYSTEM 396
THE ENDOCRINE SYSTEM 396

THE EXCRETORY SYSTERM 396
THE RESPIRATORY SYSTEM 397
THE DIGESTIVE SYSTEM 397
Digestion and Skin and Hair 398

Chapter 29 **ELECTICITY AND LIGHT THERAPY 399**
ELECTRICITY 399
ELECTRICAL MEASUREMENTS AND SAFETY DEVICES 400
GALVANIC CURRENT 401
Phoresis 402
FARADIC CURRENT 402
SINUSOIDAL CURRENT 403
HIGH-FREQUENCY CURRENT 403
Methods of Application 404
ELECTRICAL EQUIPMENT 405
SAFETY PRECAUTIONS 407
LIGHT THERAPY 408
How Light Rays are Produced 409
Ultra violet Rays 409
Safety 411
Infrared Rays 411
Visible Lights 411

Chapter 30 **CHEMISTRY 413**
MATTER 414
Atoms 415
Molecules 415
Chemical Activity 415
Forms of Matter 415
ELEMENTS AND COMPOUNDS 416
Properties of Common Elements, Compounds and Mixtures 417
Changes in Matter 418
Oxidation and Reduction 418
Acidity and Alkalinity 419
CHEMISTRY OF WATER 419
Soft Water 419
SHAMPOOING 420
Shampoo Molecules 420
Types of Shampoos 421
CONDITIONERS 422
Instant Conditioners 423
Conditioners Combined with Styling Lotions 423
Protein Penetrating Conditioners 423
Neutralizing Conditioners (pH Balancers) 423
Moisturizing Conditioners 423
Other Conditioners 423

PERMANENT WAVING 424
Composition of Hair 424
Peptide Bonds 424
Cross-Bonds 424
CHANGES IN HAIR CORTEX DURING PERMANENT WAVING 425
Thio Solution in Permanent Waving 425
Neutralizer 425
Acid and Neutral Permanent Waving 426
Protein Fillers 426
Wet Waving and Curling 426
CHEMICAL HAIR RELAXING (STRAIGHTENING) 427
HAIR COLORING 428
Temporary Hair Color 428
ACTION OF HAIR TINTS 428
Temporary Color 429
Semi-Permanent Color 429
Permanent Hair Tints 429
Vegetable Tints (Henna) 430
Metallic Dyes 431
Compound Dyes 431
Color Strippers 431
HAIR LIGHTENING 431
Lightening Products 432
TONERS 432
COLOR FILLERS 432
CHEMISTRY AS APPLIED TO COSMETICS 432
Physical and Chemical Classifications of Cosmetcs 433
PRIMARY COSMETIC INGREDIENTS 435
COSMETICS FOR CLEANSING 436
Depilatories 436
Kinds of Soaps 436
COSMETICS FOR SKIN AND FACE 437
COSMETICS FOR MAKEUP 439
Cheek Color (Rouge) 439
Eye Makeup 440
Miscellaneous Cosmetics 440
SCALP LOTIONS AND OINTMENT 441
Hair Dressings 441
Hair Sprays 441

Chapter 31 **SALON SURVIVAL 443**
WHAT YOU SHOULD KNOW ABOUT OPENING A SALON 444
Location 444
Visibility 444

Competition 444
Study the Area 444
Study the Lease 444
Parking Facilities 445
Written Agreements 455
PLANNING THE PHYSICAL LAYOUT 455
Reception Area 446
REGULATIONS, BUSINESS LAWS AND INSURANCE. 446
ADVERTISING 446
BUSINESS OPERATION AND PERSONNEL MANAGEMENT . . .447
Allocation of Money. 448
BOOKING APPOINTMENTS 448
GOOD BUSINESS ADMINISTRATION 449
Daily Records. 449
Service Records 450
Appointment Record 450
BUSINESS LAW FOR THE SALON 450
Individual Ownership. 450
Partnership. 450
Corporation 451
Before Buying or Selling an Established Salon 451
Agreement to Buy a Salon 451
Protection in Making a Lease 451
Protection Against Fire, Theft and Lawsuits. 451
IMPORTANT TERMS TO KNOW. 452
TELEPHONE USE IN THE SALON 453
Effective Telephone Techniques 456
Booking Appointments by Phone 456
How to Adjust Complaints by Phone 457
Answering Price Objections 458
REMINDERS FOR PROPER TELEPHONE USAGE 459
SELLING IN THE BEAUTY SALON 459
Selling Principles 460
Personality in Selling 461
SALES PSYCHOLOGY 461
Sales Techniques 462
Selling Beauty Services and Accessories 463
Selling Supplies 464
FIRST AID 464
Artificial Respiration 466
Breathing Obstruction (Abdominal Thrust) 468
Glossary 469
Index 488

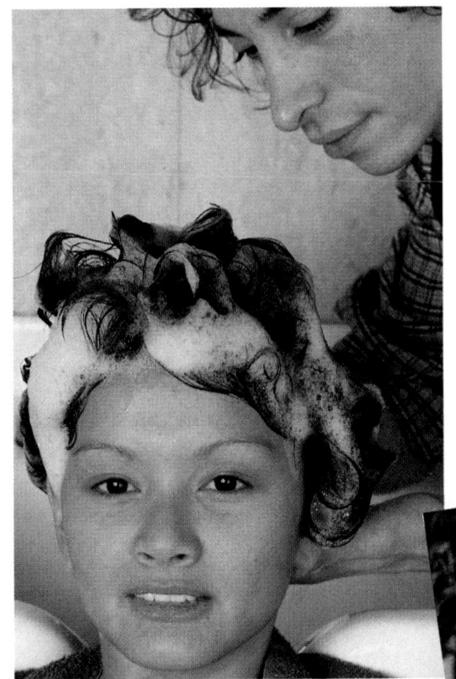

Shampoo Technician

Manicurist

Cosmetology Career Options

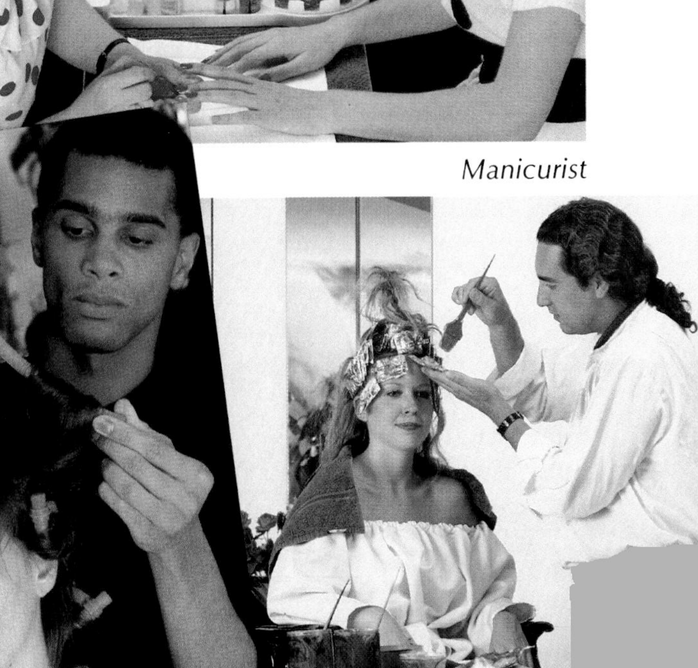

Hair Colorist

Hairstylist

Chemical Specialist

Esthetician

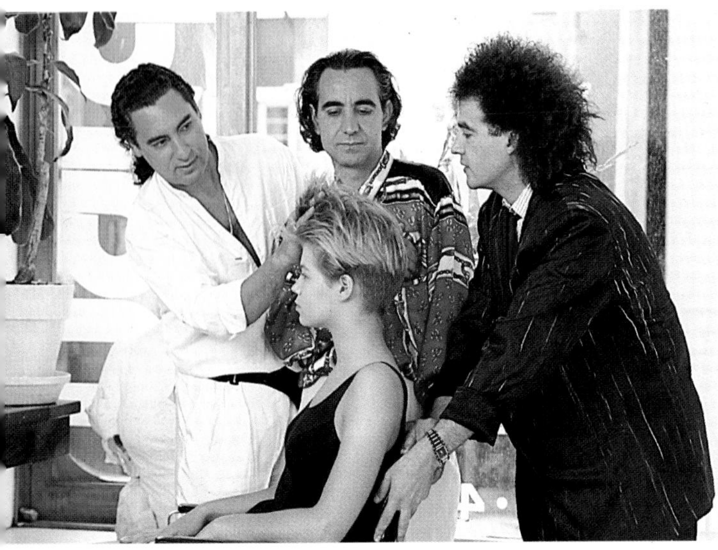

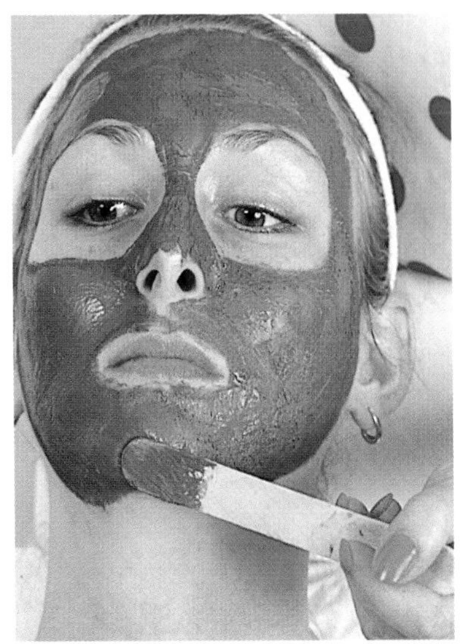

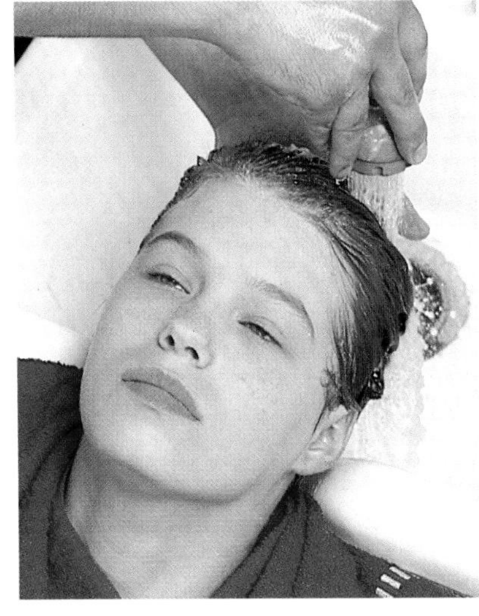

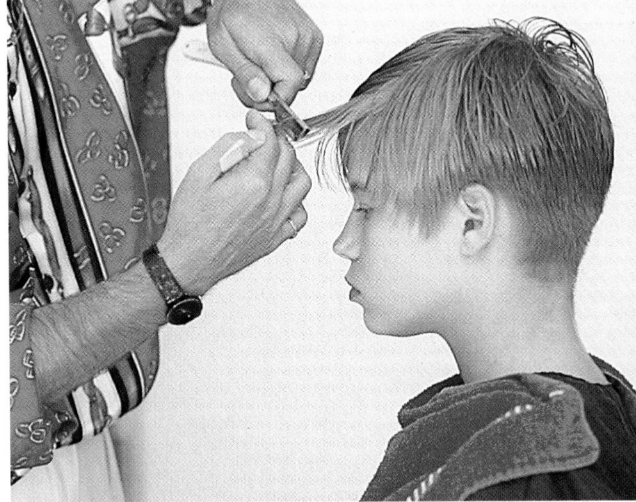

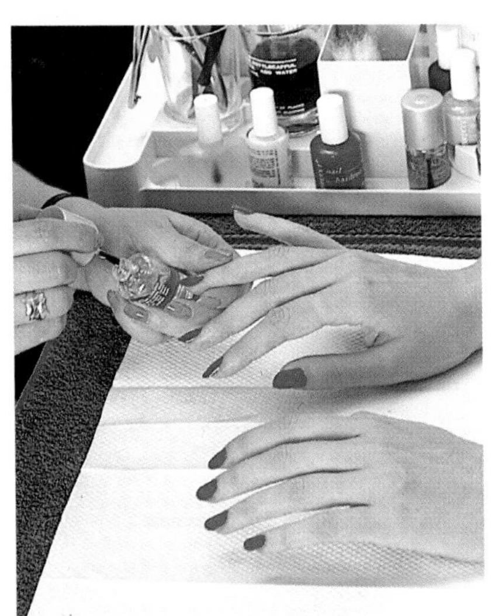

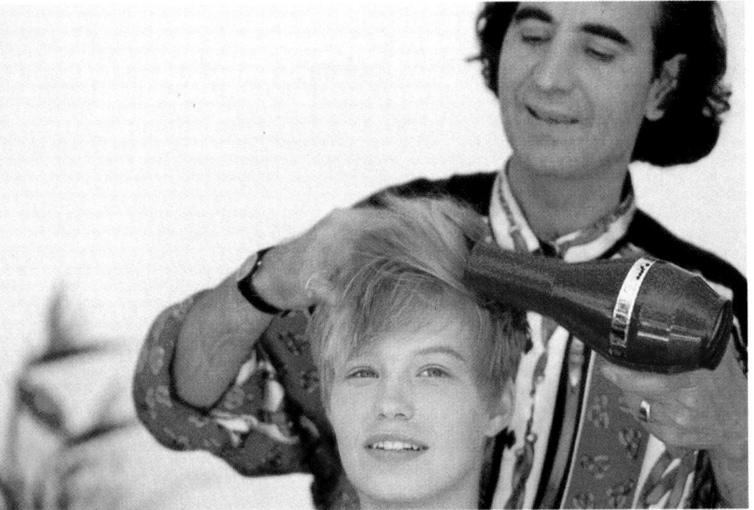

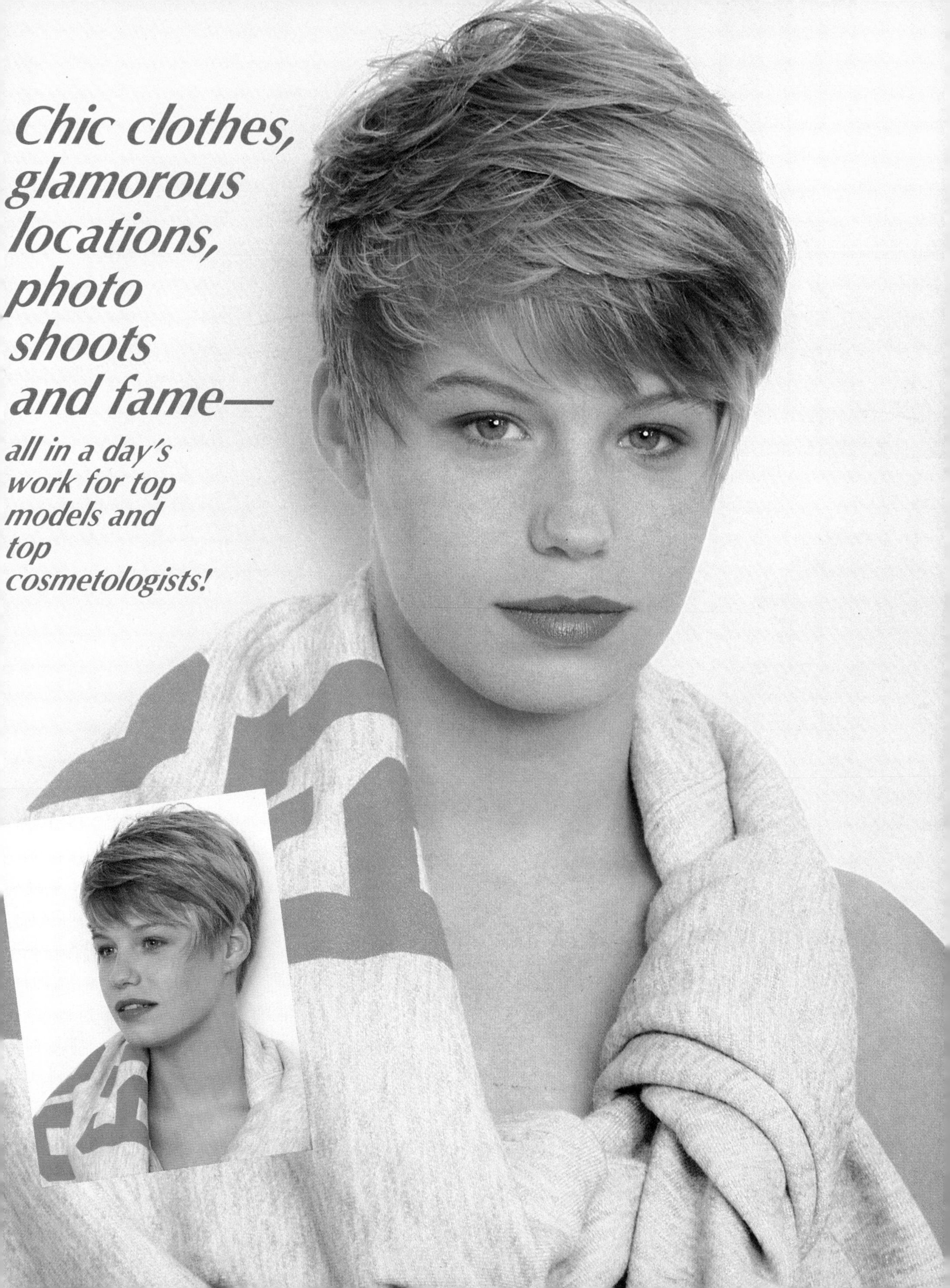
Chic clothes, glamorous locations, photo shoots and fame—
all in a day's work for top models and top cosmetologists!

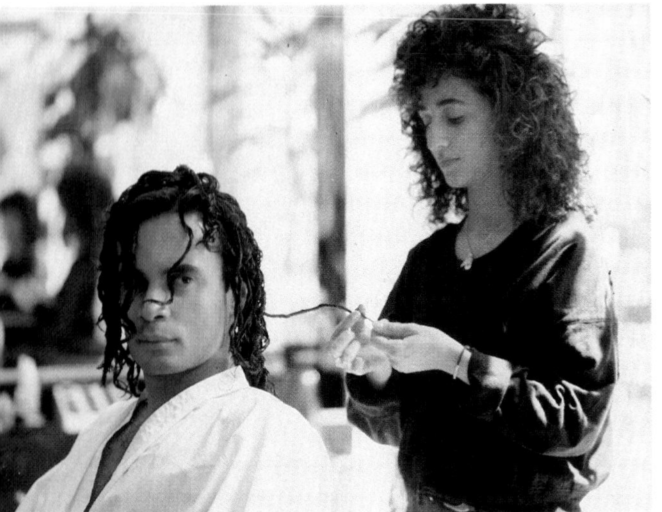
Men's Styling

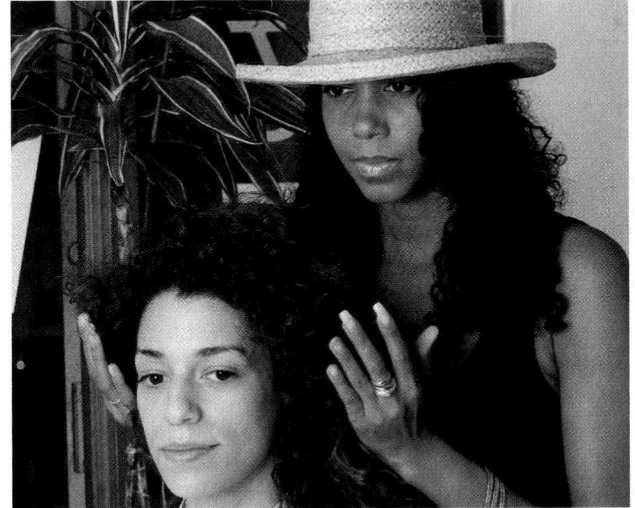
Image Building

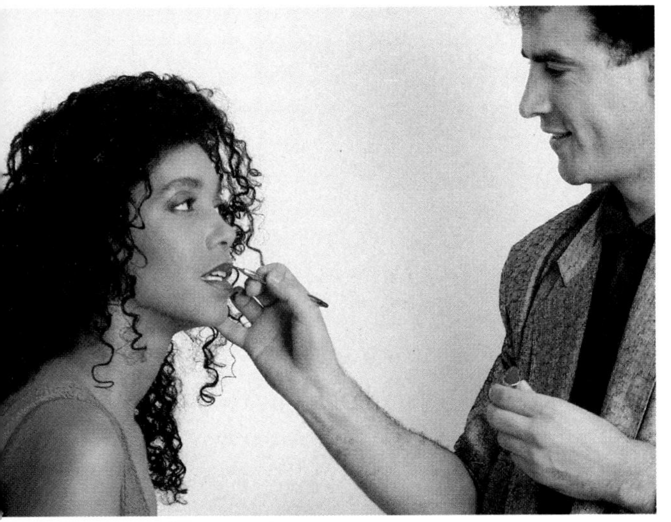
Makeup Artistry

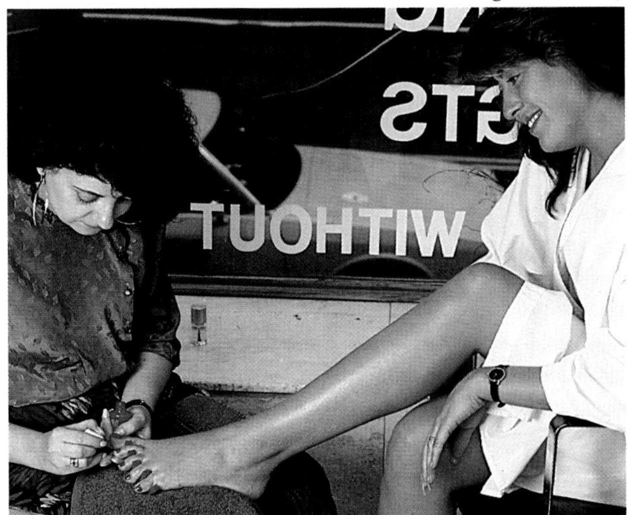
Pedicuring

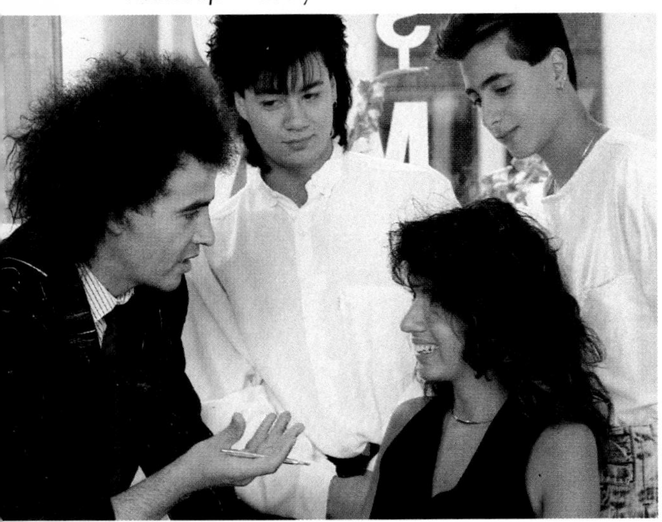
Consultation

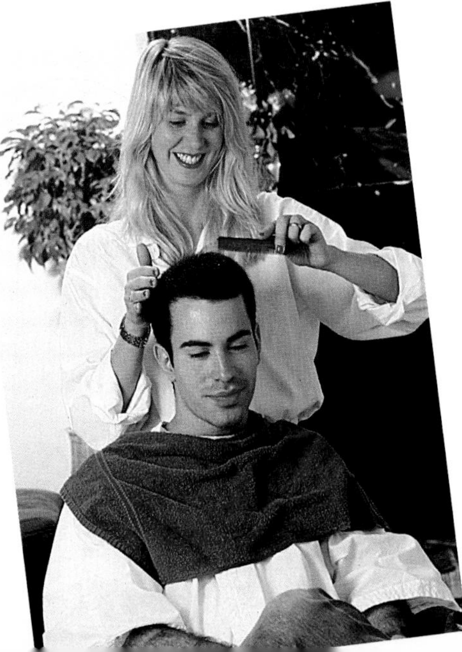
Haircutting

Chapter 1

HYGIENE AND GOOD GROOMING

LEARNING OBJECTIVES

The student successfully mastering this chapter will be able to:

1. *Name the rules of hygiene and good grooming.*
2. *Discuss how healthy thoughts contribute to a healthy body.*
3. *List the requirements for good personal hygiene.*
4. *Give the details of good grooming.*
5. *Define the relationship of cleanliness to good health and success as a cosmetologist.*

Good health is required for the successful practice of cosmetology. Without it, you cannot work efficiently or enjoy the pleasures of life. With it, constructive work and happiness are possible.

In keeping with the profession, cosmetologists should be examples of good health, so that they will increase their value to themselves, to their employers and to the community.

Hygiene is a science that deals with healthful living. It includes both personal and public hygiene.

Personal hygiene concerns the intelligent care taken by the individual to preserve health by following the rules of healthful living, such as:

1. Cleanliness
2. Oral hygiene
3. Good posture
4. Sufficient exercise
5. Relaxation
6. Adequate sleep
7. Balanced diet
8. Wholesome thoughts

Public hygiene or **sanitation** refers to the steps taken by the government to promote public health. The government takes the responsibility of protecting the health, safety and welfare of its citizens by seeing that they are provided with:

1. Pure air
2. Pure food
3. Pure water
4. Adequate sewerage
5. Control of disease
6. Adequate medical facilities

Beauty problems also can become **health problems.** A clear complexion, fine-textured skin, sparkling eyes and luxuriant hair may project a healthy condition. A dull, sallow complexion may be indicative of:

1. Sluggish circulation
2. Lack of fresh air
3. Irregular elimination
4. Improper diet
5. Poor health

HYGIENIC RULES

To improve your health and appearance, you must follow hygienic rules of living.

Eating well-balanced meals at regular intervals and drinking a sufficient amount of water will keep the digestive system functioning properly and produce better elimination. One of the basic causes of poor health is a faulty diet. Avoid such poor eating habits as:

1. Not eating enough of the right kinds of food, which can lead to loss of weight, lower resistance or nutritional diseases
2. Overeating, which taxes the digestive system and organs of elimination

Exercise and recreation in the form of running, walking, dancing, sports and gym activities develop endurance and keep the body fit. A few of the benefits resulting from regularly exercising are:

1. Improvement in the body's absorption of food
2. Improvement in blood circulation
3. Larger supply of life-giving oxygen to the body, due to the increased action of the heart and lungs

Moderate amounts of sunshine add vigor and help to supply the body with essential vitamin D.

Fatigue caused by work, exercise, mental effort or worry should always be followed by a period of rest or relaxation. Overexertion and lack of rest tend to drain the body of its vitality. Therefore, an adequate amount of sleep, not less than seven hours, is necessary. This allows the body to recover from the fatigue of the day's activities and replenish itself with renewed energy.

HEALTHY THOUGHTS

The mind and body operate as a unit. A healthy body and mind contribute to a good life. A healthy body is one in which all organs perform their functions normally. Healthy thoughts can be cultivated by self-control. Worry and fear should be replaced by the health-giving qualities of cheerfulness, courage and hope. Outside interests and recreation relieve the strain of boredom and hard work.

Thoughts and emotions influence bodily activities. A thought can cause the face to turn red and increase the heart action. It can either stimulate or depress the functions of the body. Strong emotions, such as worry and fear, have a harmful effect on the heart, arteries and glands. Depression weakens the functions of the organs, thereby lowering the resistance of the body to disease.

A Well-Groomed Female Cosmetologist

A well-groomed cosmetologist is one of the best advertisements for an effectively run salon.

To keep your appearance at its best you must give daily attention to all the important details that make for a clean, neat and charming personality.

Daily Bath and Deodorant Keep the body cleansed and odor-free by taking a daily shower or bath and using an underarm deodorant.

Oral Hygiene Clean and brush the teeth regularly. Use mouthwash to sweeten the breath.

Hairstyle Keep the hair clean and lustrous. Wear an attractive and practical hairstyle at all times.

Clothes Wear a uniform that is spotlessly clean, neat and properly fitted. Wear fresh underclothes.

Facial Makeup Use the correct cosmetics to match your skin tone. Keep your makeup fresh, your eyebrows and lips well-shaped.

Hands and Nails Keep you hands clean and smooth and always have your nails well manicured.

Jewelry Avoid gaudy jewelry. Jewelry should be practical for the workplace and reflect professionalism.

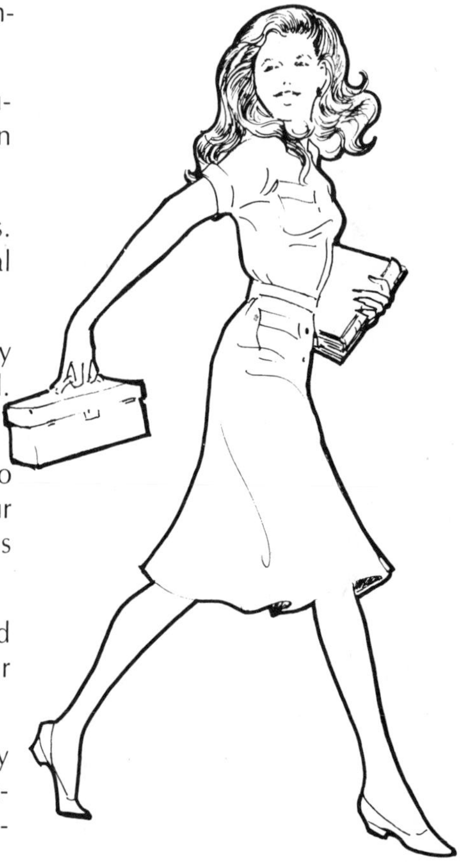

Shoes and Hosiery Wear low-heeled shoes that are well fitted and sensibly styled. Keep your shoes shined and in good condition. Wear clean hose. Watch out for hosiery runs and wrinkles.

Many beauty salon owners consider appearance, visual poise and personality to be as important as technical knowledge and manual skills.

A Well-Groomed Male Cosmetologist

Proper grooming is also important for male cosmetologists. Give careful attention to cleanliness of your uniform, skin, hair, hands and teeth. Keep your beard and mustache neatly trimmed. Keep your breath sweet with mouthwash. Keep your body odor-free by taking a shower or bath daily and using an underarm deodorant.

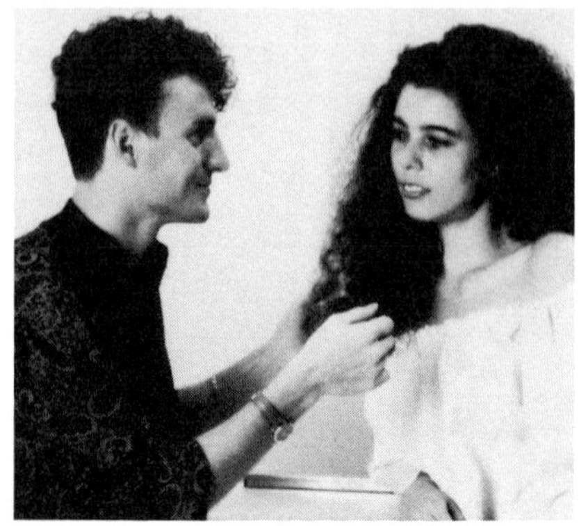

MAINTAIN GOOD HEALTH

To maintain good health, observe the following rules:

1. Get as much clean and fresh air as you can.
2. Drink a sufficient amount of water each day.
3. Follow a balanced diet. Do not overeat.
4. Develop regular elimination habits.
5. Stand, sit and walk with good posture.
6. Engage in recreation and outdoor exercise and get adequate sleep.
7. Have regular physical examinations.

SUMMARY

The cosmetologist must observe cleanliness in the following ways:

1. Keep the body clean by taking a daily bath or shower.
2. Avoid body odor by using a deodorant.
3. Keep teeth and gums in good condition. Brush teeth at least twice daily.
4. Have a dental examination every six months.
5. Avoid bad breath by rinsing your mouth with a good mouthwash.
6. Never wear shoes without clean hose or socks.
7. Keep shoes clean and in good condition.
8. Wear clean underclothes and a clean uniform each day.
9. Keep hair well groomed.
10. Keep hands and fingernails in good condition.
11. Wash hands before and after serving each client.
12. Avoid the common use of towels, drinking cups, cosmetics, hairbrushes and combs.

REVIEW QUESTIONS

Hygiene and Good Grooming

1. *List eight basic requirements for good personal hygiene.*
2. *Which three mental qualities help to promote good health?*
3. *What are the requirements for good personal hygiene?*
4. *Give the details of good grooming.*
5. *What is the relationship of cleanliness to good health and success as a cosmetologist?*

Chapter 2

VISUAL POISE

LEARNING OBJECTIVES

The student successfully mastering this chapter will be able to:

1. *Recognize the benefits of good posture.*
2. *Describe the basic standing procedure.*
3. *Describe the correct sitting procedure.*

Most of your time as a professional cosmetologist will be spent on your feet. Correct posture, therefore, is very important because it helps to prevent fatigue, will improve your personal appearance and permit you to move with ease and grace.

GOOD POSTURE

Good posture is an important part of personal care. Its continued practice assists in the prevention of many physical problems. In addition, it is a self-disciplinary factor that contributes to the development of other good habits, which are elements that determine a gracious and pleasing personality. When present, they indicate a poised, well-ordered individual.

Many salon owners consider appearance, visual poise and personality to be as important as technical knowledge and manual skills.

Stand Correctly **Regular exercise** keeps the muscles of the body in good condition and assists in forming the habit of good posture. Practice will train the muscles to hold the body correctly. Good posture is a matter of habit. Avoid slouching, humped shoulders and spinal curvature while working. To walk and stand correctly, distribute the body weight so that you achieve proper body balance.

For the basic standing position:

1. Turn the left foot out at a 45° (0.875 radius) angle.
2. Point the right foot straight ahead on a straight line.
3. Bend the right knee slightly over the line of the left knee.
4. Flex the left knee slightly.

Centerline The centerline of the body extends from the center of the head, through the neck, shoulder, hip, knee and arch of the foot.

Body Weight Body weight is balanced along the body's centerline and supported by the weight-bearing arches of the feet.

Good Posture Head up, Chin level with floor
Chest up
Shoulders relaxed
Lower abdomen flat

FIVE DEFECTIVE BODY POSTURES

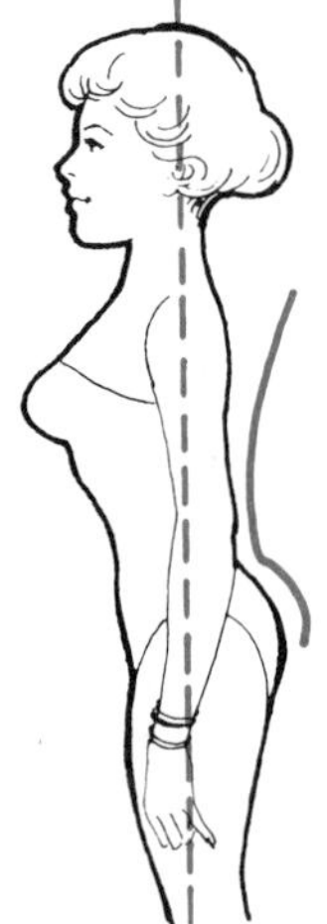

Stiff-rigid—poor posture

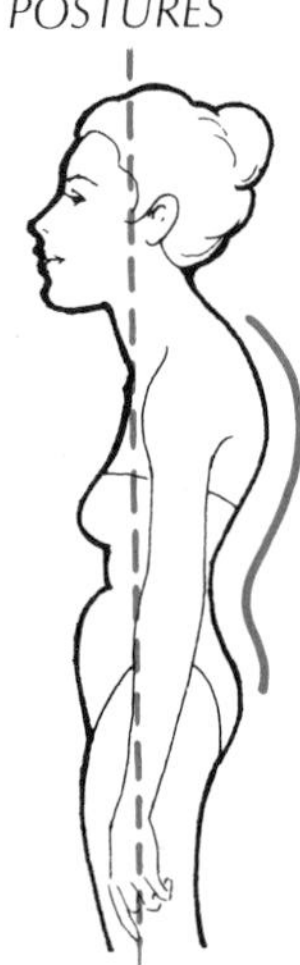

Slumped-humped—poor posture

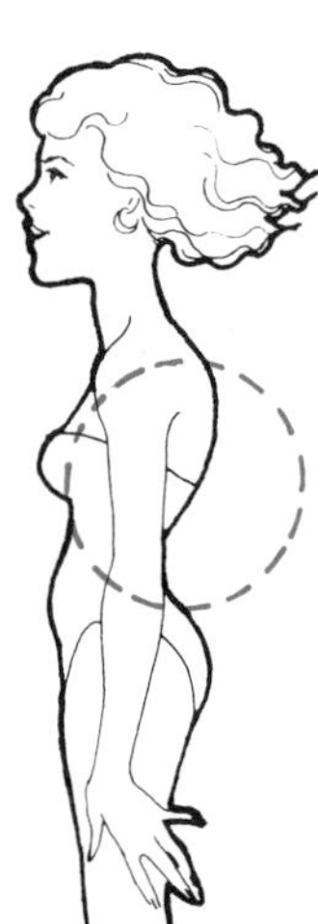

*Sway-back or lordosis (**LOR**-do-sis)*

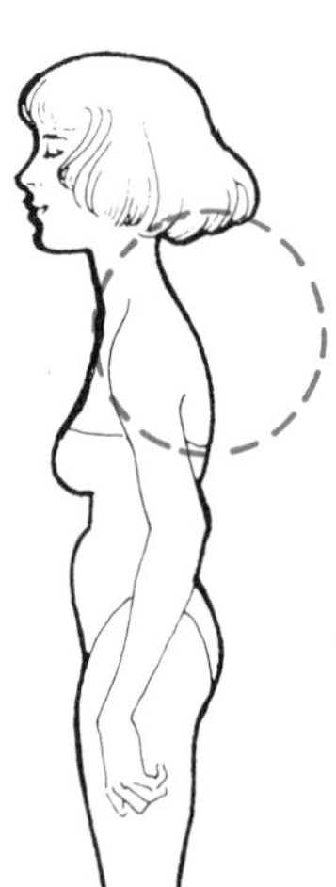

*Drooped shoulders—kyphosis (ki-**FO**-sis)*

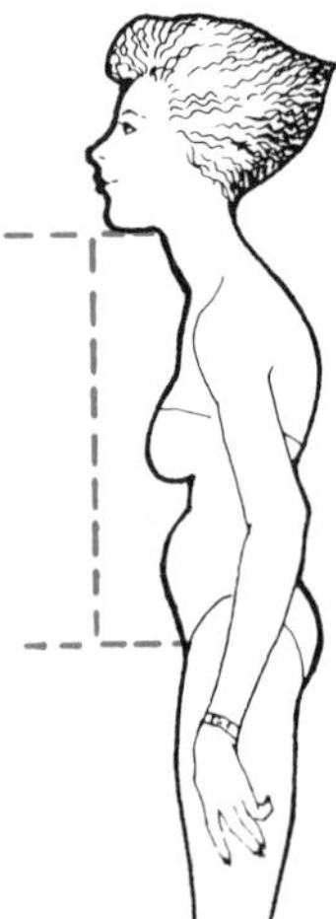

*Sway-back and drooped shoulders—scoliosis (**SKO**-le-o-sis)*

POSTURE WHEN GIVING A SHAMPOO

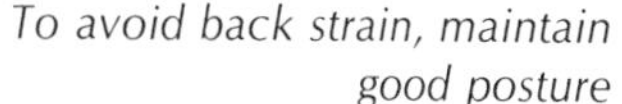
To avoid back strain, maintain good posture

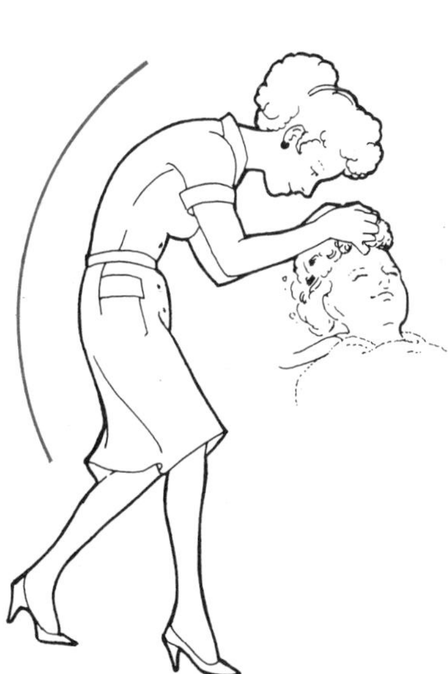
Poor posture

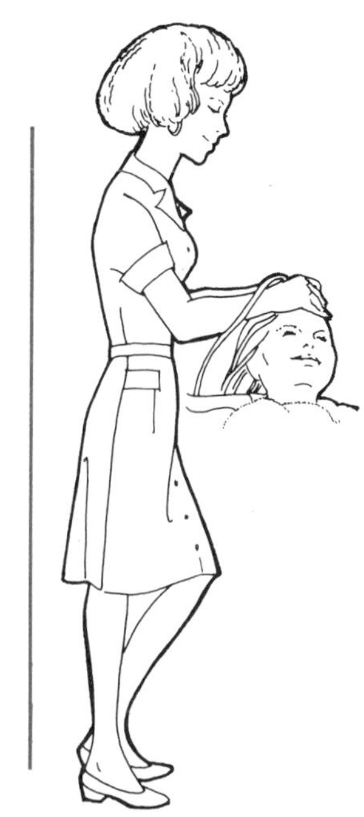
Good posture

COMFORT FOR CLIENT AND COSMETOLOGIST

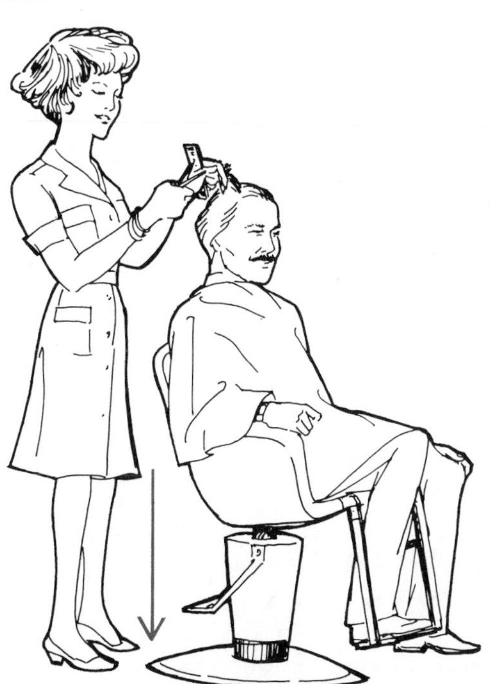
Short cosmetologist, tall client—lower the chair.

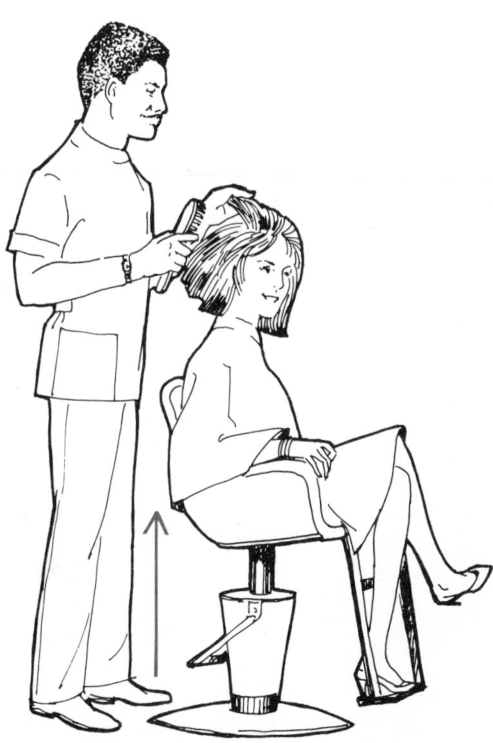
Short client, tall cosmetologist—raise the chair.

CORRECT BODY USE

Correct Sitting Technique

Never fall into a chair. Always glide gracefully into a sitting position. When sliding to the back of the chair, place both hands on the front edge of the chair, at the sides of the hips. Raise the body slightly and slide back. Do not wiggle back.

Rules for a Good Sitting Position

1. Keep the feet close together.
2. Keep the knees together.
3. Place the feet out slightly farther than the knees.
5. Keep the soles of your shoes on the floor.

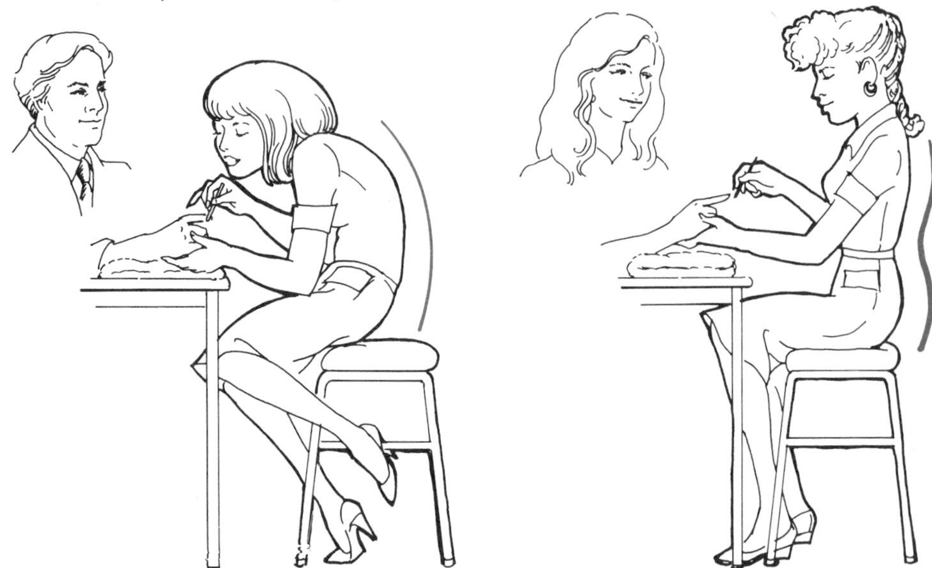

Poor sitting posture *Good sitting posture*

When giving a manicure, assume a correct sitting position to avoid fatigue and back strain. Sit with the lower back against the chair, leaning slightly forward. If a stool is used, sit on the entire stool. Keep the chest up. Rest body weight on the full length of the thighs.

To avoid back strain while reading, writing or studying, whether in school, at work or at home, sit toward the back of the chair. Do not sit in a slouching position at any time.

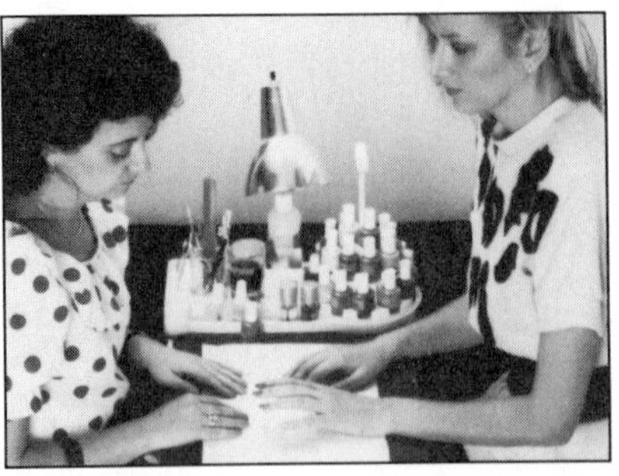

Correct Stooping Technique

To pick up an article from the floor.

1. Place the feet close together.
2. Keep the back perpendicular to the floor as the knees bend.
3. Lift with the muscles of the legs and buttocks, not with the back.

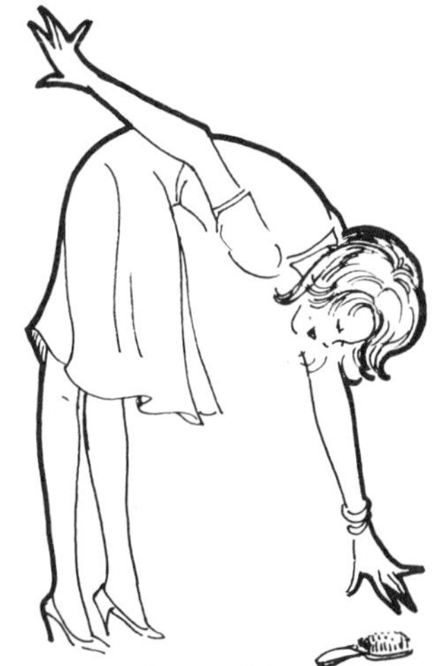

Incorrect stooping position

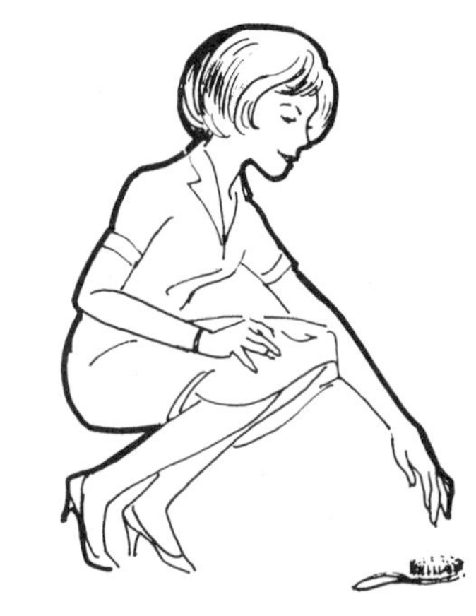

Correct stooping position

Correct Lifting Technique

When you lift something heavy, be sure to use the weight lifter's method or you might cause a rupture or a slipped disk. Lift with your back straight, pushing with the heavy thigh muscles, never the back muscles.

Caution

Have some idea of the weight of the object you are lifting. You can hurt your back just as severely by lifting a light object your muscles expect to be heavy as you can by lifting a heavy object incorrectly.

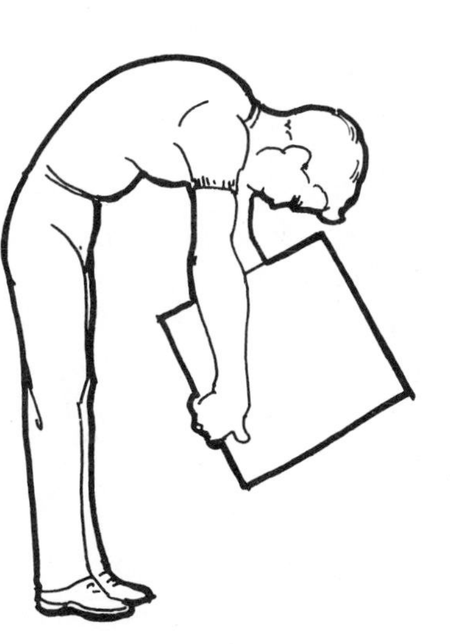

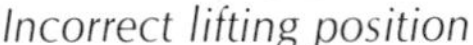

Incorrect lifting position

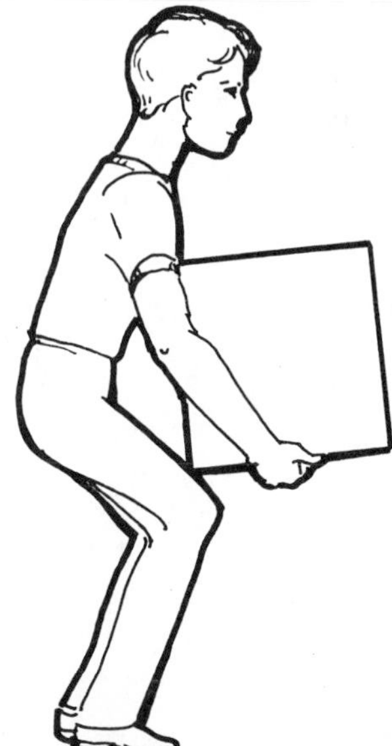

Correct lifting position

Foot Care

High heels are often responsible for poor posture, malformed feet and aching backs. The weight of the body is thrown forward, putting a strain on the feet and back.

Low, broad heels give the body support and balance which help to maintain good posture. Low-heeled shoes are more comfortable and tend to offset fatigue resulting from prolonged standing.

The cosmetologist should give the feet the following daily care:

1. After bathing, apply cream or oil and massage each foot for five minutes.
2. Remove cream and apply an antiseptic foot lotion.
3. Keep the toenails filed smooth.
4. Corns, bunions or ingrown nails should receive care from a podiatrist.

Wearing well-fitted, low-heeled shoes and giving the feet a few minutes of daily care are also steps to good posture and success.

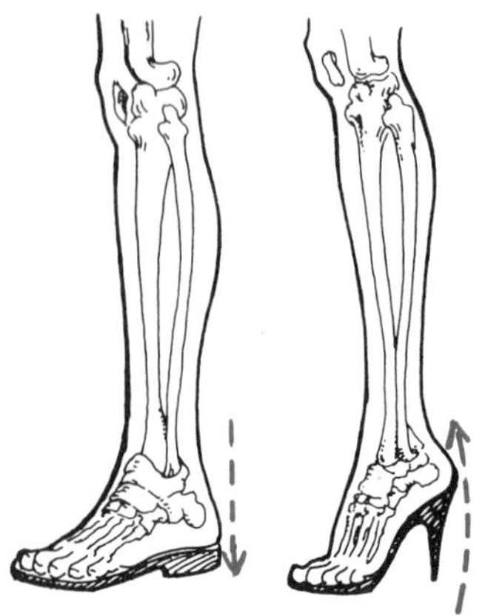

For comfort and to help maintain good posture, wear well-fitted, low-heeled shoes.

Normal and Weak Arches

A normal foot is narrow in the middle and wide at the heel and toes. Good arches are characteristic of the normal footprint.

A weak foot is caused by a weak arch. Its footprint is wider in the middle than a normal footprint.

Fallen arches, or flat feet, are a common ailment. A flat foot leaves a footprint that is almost the same throughout its entire length.

Weak and flat feet can be strengthened by massage and exercise or can be helped by wearing arch supports and proper shoes. These remedial measures should be taken only after consultation with a foot specialist.

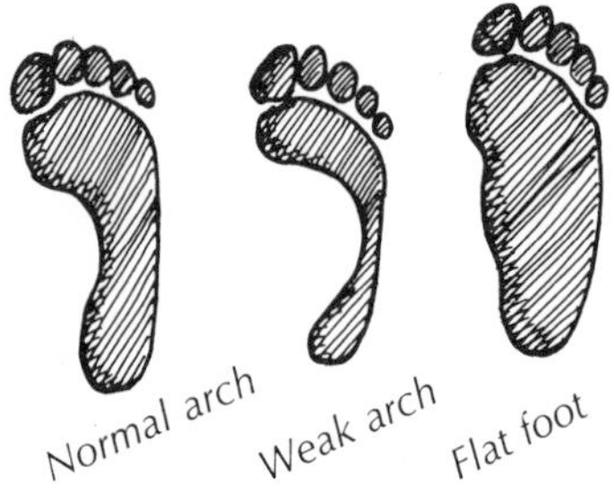

REVIEW QUESTIONS

Visual Poise

1. *What are three benefits of correct posture?*
2. *How does regular exercise assist in forming the habit of good posture?*
3. *In a basic stance or standing position, place the left foot at a .... degree angle and point the right foot straight ahead.*
4. *For a good standing posture, keep the head ....; chin level with ....; chest ....; shoulders relaxed and lower abdomen ....*
5. *For a good sitting posture, keep the feet and knees close ....*
6. *For a comfortable sitting posture, keep the soles of the feet on the ....*
7. *When giving a manicure, sit with the lower back against the ....*
8. *Why is correct sitting position important when giving a manicure?*
9. *How should one sit to avoid back strain?*
10. *Why should the cosmetologist wear low, broad-heeled shoes?*
11. *Why should the cosmetologist give his or her feet daily care?*
12. *The cosmetologist who stands for long periods of time should wear well-fitted, ... shoes.*

Chapter 3

PERSONALITY DEVELOPMENT

LEARNING OBJECTIVES

The student successfully mastering this chapter will be able to:

1. *List the reasons for cultivating a pleasing personality.*
2. *Identify the qualities needed for a pleasing personality.*
3. *Determine the relationship of personality and success for a cosmetologist.*

Your **personality** is the key to a successful career in cosmetology. Personality is the outward reflection of your inner feelings, habits, attitudes and values. It is the total effect you have on other people.

Only you can form the pattern of the "ideal individual" you hope to be. Only you can develop a personality that will help open the door to a life filled with pleasant and useful experiences.

A pleasant personality and a good character are as vital to a successful career in cosmetology as are expert technical ability and an attractive appearance.

Without a pleasing personality, a cosmetologist's fine workmanship or attractive appearance will be overlooked. A person is not born with a personality; it is acquired according to the way individuals meet their everyday problems. By developing the ability to handle both the good and the bad experiences of life, you will develop a better personality.

DESIRABLE QUALITIES TO CULTIVATE

Attitude has a great deal to do with personality. It influences your likes and dislikes and your response to people, events and things. People who meet difficult situations with calmness and who are cheerful, pleasant and easy to get along with have a healthy attitude toward life.

Behavior. Control your temper. Once you have spoken, you cannot recall a single word. One person with emotional controls off balance can throw others into a state of confusion. Everything you say or do (good or bad) starts a chain of reactions that can have continuing and lasting effect. When you become master of your own behavior, you can cultivate those characteristics that are desirable and discard those that are unwanted.

Thoughts. How and what you think are parts of your personality, so do everything you can to improve the quality of your thoughts. If you want people to listen when you speak, know what you are talking about and be able to say it well. Increase your word power by reading good newspapers, magazines and books. Learn new words each day by looking up in the dictionary the unfamiliar ones you encounter in conversation and reading.

A **pleasant voice** is needed; words alone are not enough. A properly pitched tone of voice must be used if speech is to be pleasing. A **monotone** voice is dull and uninteresting.

Everyone strives for **emotional stability**. Those who achieve it realize how much it contributes to their appreciation of life. If you want to be admired, develop the ability to live life to its fullest. Emotional stability will help you in this task. Learn to suppress the signs that betray emotions, such as facial expressions, or gestures of anger, impatience, envy or greed.

Be gracious. Learn to display pleasant emotions. A smile of greeting, a word of welcome, the willingness to assume the responsibilities of friendship, fitting into new environments, meeting new people with charm and grace, all express the quality of graciousness.

Good manners reflect your thoughtfulness of others. Good manners should be easy to develop. They include all the little things, such as saying "Thank you," "Please," treating others with respect, exercising care of other people's property, tolerating and understanding other people's efforts and being considerate of those with whom you work. Courtesy is one of the keys to a successful career.

Be well groomed. The first impression you have of a person is how he or she looks. This is true of the impression the other person has of you. Make sure you are clean and attractively styled. Your clothing should be immaculately clean, your hands smooth and your nails properly manicured. Your grooming goes hand-in-hand with good posture, whether standing, walking or sitting.

Have a sense of humor. Cultivate your sense of humor. Take yourself less seriously. When you can laugh at yourself, you will have gained the ability to properly evaluate your position in society.

Remember, your personality is the key to success. Be sure to develop yours to the utmost.

Voice and Conversation

A pleasant voice, interesting conversation and the use of good English contribute to success; they will serve you well as a professional cosmetologist because clients will enjoy being with you and will seek your services.

Success is not attained within the salon alone. Success depends on personal contacts, membership in associations and active participation in many social and cosmetology functions. Some of these must include association meetings, trade shows, conventions, workshops and social gatherings with the people who create, develop and direct cosmetology activities.

Your voice should project your most attractive characteristics. These are:

1. **Sincerity**—honesty of mind or intention
2. **Intelligence**—the act of understanding
3. **Friendliness**—friendly behavior
4. **Vitality**—vigor and liveliness
5. **Flexibility**—pliable, not rigid, in voice tones
6. **Expressiveness**—the expression of one's individuality

The **tone of voice** can be used to express the emotions of anger, joy, hate, love, jealousy, friendliness and envy. Your voice should be clear and understandable. If the spoken words cannot be understood, a good voice tone is useless.

To be successful, a pleasing voice is needed:

1. To greet the clients
2. For conversation
3. To sell yourself
4. To sell services and products
5. To build business
6. To talk on the telephone

Conversation involves the use of voice, words, intelligence, tact and personality.

The correct use of words is vital to the art of conversation. The most serious violations of good speech are the use of slang, vulgarisms and poor grammar.

Topics of conversation should be as noncontroversial as possible. Friendly relations are easily achieved through pleasant conversations. Such relationships build a better business.

Topics to Discuss in Conversation

1. Client's cosmetic and hair care needs
2. Client's own activities
3. Fashions
4. Literature
5. Art
6. Music
7. Education
8. Travel
9. Civic affairs
10. Vacations

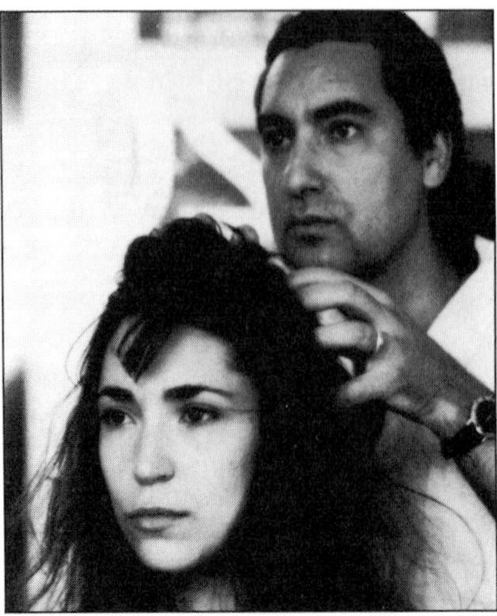

Try to understand the client's state of mind and personality type. Your conversation should be directed toward the client's interests. Fit your conversation to the client's mood.

The ability to carry on pleasant and relevant conversations with clients is an asset to all cosmetologists.

How to Acquire Conversational Charisma

The following steps can help you achieve the charisma that contributes to success in the beauty profession:

1. Guide the conversation.
2. Do not be argumentative.
3. Be a good listener.
4. Do not monopolize the conversation.
5. Do not pry into personal affairs.
6. Talk about ideas rather than people.
7. Use simple language that can be understood.
8. Never gossip. Gossip is small talk used by uninteresting people.
9. Be pleasant.
10. Use proper English.

Never Discuss the Following Topics

1. Your own personal problems
2. Religion
3. Other client's bad behavior
4. Your love affairs
5. Your financial status
6. Poor workmanship of fellow workers
7. Your health problems
8. Information given to you in confidence

Unpopular persons annoy or irritate others. To become popular, develop a desirable personality by adhering to the following rules:

1. Don't be bossy.
2. Don't be sarcastic.
3. Don't ridicule people.
4. Don't lose your temper.

5. Don't be rude to others.
6. Don't start an argument.
7. Don't talk continually.
8. Don't spread gossip.
9. Don't use profanity, slang or poor grammar.
10. Don't monopolize the conversation.

YOUR PERSONALITY CHART

An **attractive personality** is one of your greatest assets in life. It is the charm revealed in your speech, appearance, behavior and manners. It is the total effect you have on other people. How you behave in school, business or social life can either add or take away from your personality.

Try to make your answers to the following questions project a true picture of your inner and outer self. First evaluate yourself. If your rating is low, consult your teacher or friends to find out what can be done to enrich and improve it. Analyze your personality every three months to find out what progress you are making.

Personality Quiz

Check the proper boxes in this personality quiz to find out if you have the personality qualities listed below.

1. **Female.** Do you give careful attention to personal grooming such as your clothes, hair, makeup, hosiery and shoes?
   ☐ Always ☐ Sometimes ☐ Never
   Male. Do you give careful attention to personal grooming, such as your clothes, socks, shoes, hair, shave, mustache and hair in nose?
   ☐ Always ☐ Sometimes ☐ Never
2. Do you check your posture when sitting, standing and walking?
   ☐ Always ☐ Sometimes ☐ Never
3. Do you change undergarments daily and avoid bad breath and body odor at all times?
   ☐ Always ☐ Sometimes ☐ Never
4. Are you loyal to others?
   ☐ Always ☐ Sometimes ☐ Never
5. Are you friendly and courteous to others?
   ☐ Always ☐ Sometimes ☐ Never
6. Are you truthful in dealing with others?
   ☐ Always ☐ Sometimes ☐ Never
7. Can you get along and work well with others?
   ☐ Always ☐ Sometimes ☐ Never
8. Can you accept responsibility?
   ☐ Always ☐ Sometimes ☐ Never
9. Do you have confidence in your knowledge and ability?
   ☐ Always ☐ Sometimes ☐ Never
10. Do you have a good tone of voice and choice of words?
   ☐ Always ☐ Sometimes ☐ Never

Rating Your Personality

Give yourself 10 points for **Always;** 5 points for **Sometimes;** and zero (0) for **Never.** Compare your final rating with the following standards:

Excellent personality 85-100%
Good personality 75-85%
Fair personality.. 60-75%
Poor personality... 59% or less

Note

About two-thirds of all job dismissals are due to bad manners, poor personality and inability to get along with people. It is to your advantage, therefore, to do all you can to improve your personality.

REVIEW QUESTIONS

Personality Development

1. *What are the reasons for a cosmetologist to cultivate a pleasing personality?*
2. *What are the nine desirable qualities to cultivate for a pleasing personality?*
3. *What is the relationship between personality and success for a cosmetologist?*

Chapter 4

PROFESSIONAL ETHICS

LEARNING OBJECTIVES

The student successfully mastering this chapter will be able to:

1. *List the rules of the cosmetologist's code of ethical conduct.*
2. *Maintain a professional attitude toward clients.*

Cosmetology refers to the art and science of beautifying and improving the skin, nails and hair. Cosmetology offers a professional career to those students who receive a thorough technical training, develop the proper image and service-oriented personality and observe professional ethics.

ETHICS

Ethics relate to the proper conduct and business dealings of cosmetologists with their employers, clients and co-workers. Simply stated, a cosmetologist's code of ethical conduct is based on the Golden Rule, namely, "Do unto others as you would have them do unto you."

Ethical conduct helps to build confidence and increase your clientele. The individual cosmetologist should live up to the following rules of ethics:

1. Give courteous and friendly service to all clients.
2. Treat all clients honestly and fairly; do not show favoritism.
3. Be fair, courteous and show respect for the feelings and rights of others.

4. Keep your word and fulfill your obligations.
5. Cherish a good reputation. Set an example of good conduct and behavior.
6. Be loyal to your employer, manager and associates.
7. Practice only the highest standards of sanitation at all times.
8. Obey all provisions of the state cosmetology laws.
9. Believe in the cosmetology profession. Practice it faithfully and sincerely.
10. As a student:
    a) Be loyal to, and cooperate with, school personnel and fellow students.
    b) Comply with school and clinic rules and regulations.

Questionable practices, extravagant claims and unfulfilled promises violate the rules of ethical conduct. They cast an unfavorable light on cosmetology in general and upon the individual student, cosmetologist and beauty salon in particular.

A PROFESSIONAL ATTITUDE TOWARD CLIENTS

Greet a client by name, with a pleasing tone of welcome in your voice. See that personal belongings are cared for. Be sure your client is comfortable. Notice your client's mood. Often the client will prefer quiet and relaxation. Confine your own conversation to cosmetic needs. If the client wishes to talk, be a good listener. Never repeat a tidbit of gossip — you risk your client's confidence in you. **Never gossip about anyone.**

Off-color stories are distasteful to most people and have no place in a salon.

Good habits and practices acquired during your school training lay the foundation for a successful career in cosmetology. To become successful, you should:

1. Be ethical by following the rules of proper personal behavior.
2. Make a good impression on others.
3. Cultivate confidence and a pleasing personality.
4. Pay attention to the minor details that will make clients like you.
5. Be cordial when greeting clients in person or over the telephone.
6. Cultivate a pleasing voice.
7. Listen attentively when others speak.
8. Address clients by their names — Miss or Mrs. Smith. Never use "Honey," "Dearie," and so forth.
9. Handle all clients with tact. Develop an even temperament.
10. Set a good example for what you are selling. An attractive personal appearance is your best advertisement.
11. Train yourself to be capable and efficient in your work.

TO BE SUCCESSFULL...
BE PUNCTUAL. Get to work on time and you won't miss any clients.

TARDINESS never pays.

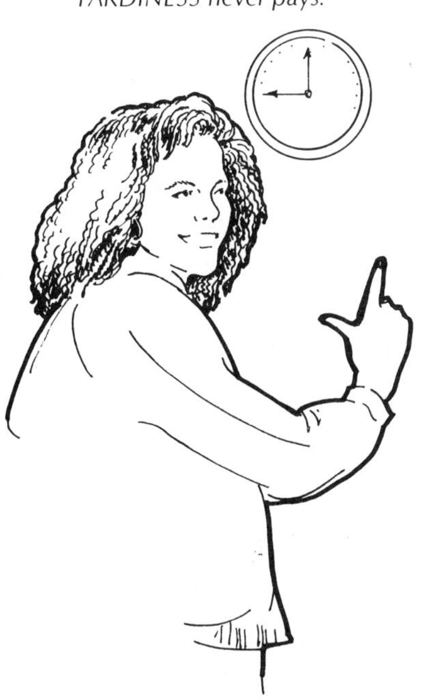

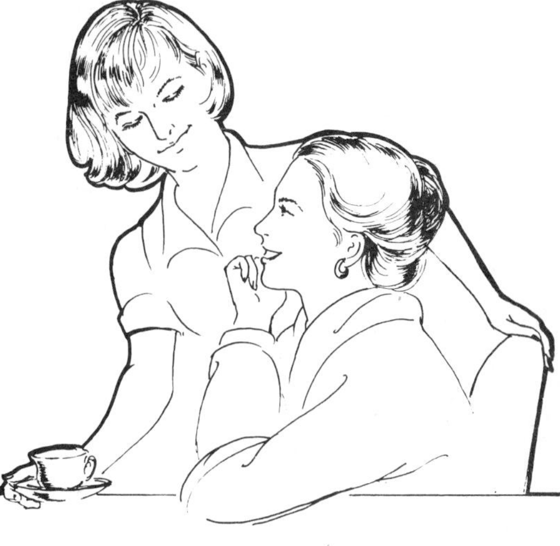

BE COURTEOUS. Treat people with the same kindness you would want to be treated with and everyone will like you.

DISCOURTESY is inexcusable.

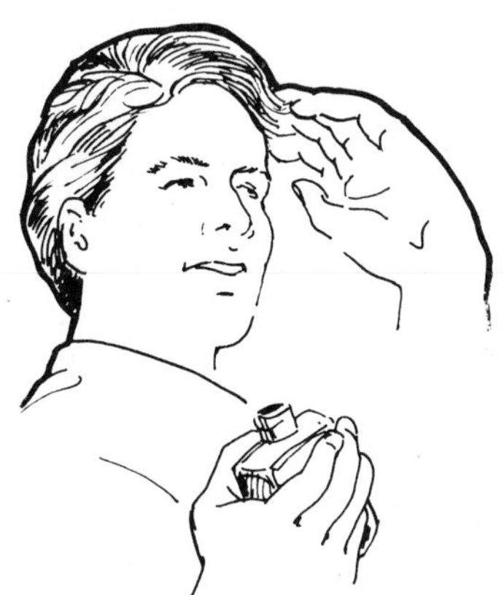

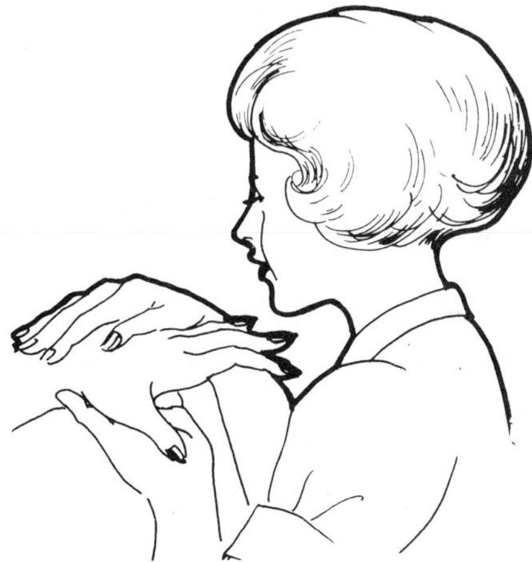

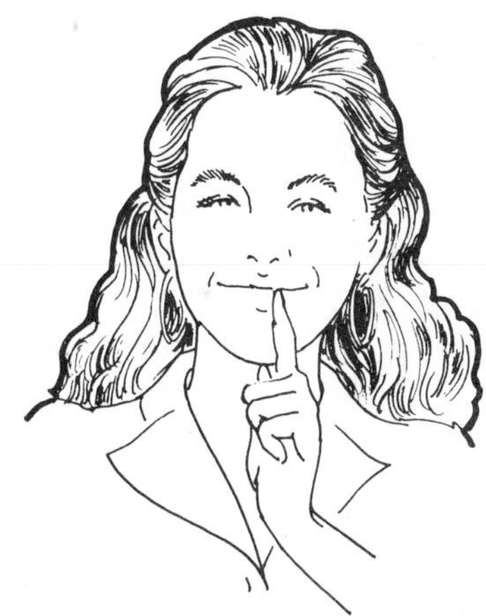

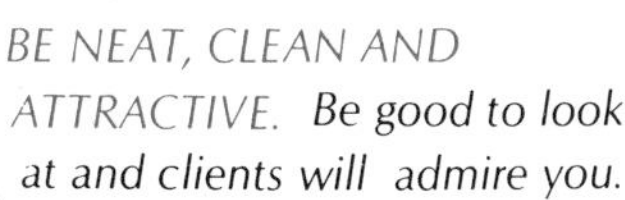

BE NEAT, CLEAN AND ATTRACTIVE. Be good to look at and clients will admire you.

CARELESSNESS of hygiene is offensive.

BE GENTILE. You will be remembered for this valued characteristic.

HARSH, rough treatment chases clients away.

MIND YOUR OWN BUSINESS. Clients will trust you. GAB and they won't like you.

TO BE SUCCESSFUL you must learn to do the little things that will make people like you and want to come back to see you again and again.

12. Be punctual in arriving at work and keeping appointments.
13. Plan each day's schedule. Avoid long waiting periods.
14. Learn to talk intelligently about your work.
15. Develop business and sales abilities along with common sense. Use tact when suggesting additional services to clients.
16. Avoid criticizing, condemning or complaining.
17. Be prompt and judicious in adjusting a client's complaints.

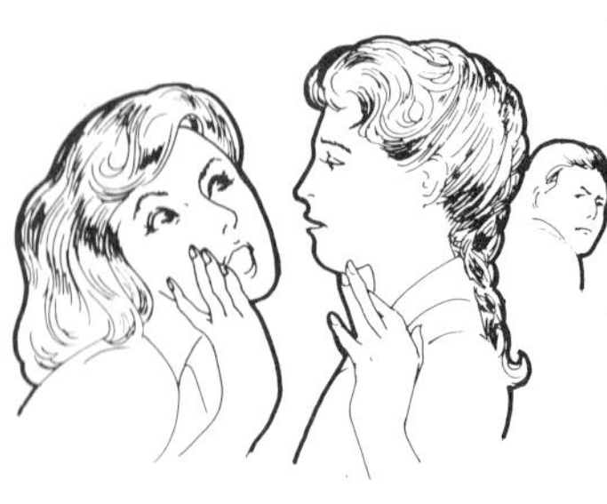

Nobody likes a person who gossips.

To be successful the cosmetologist should avoid:

1. Bad breath and body odor.
2. Chewing gum and smoking in the presence of clients.
3. Speaking in a loud or harsh voice.
4. Criticizing the services of fellow workers.
5. Discussing personal problems with clients.
6. Lounging on the arms of chairs, on tabletops or in the reception room.
7. Poor posture when working; dragging the feet when walking.
8. Playing the television or radio loudly in the presence of clients.
9. Spreading gossip or using profane or sarcastic language.
10. Making statements that are untrue or unduly critical; this lowers the dignity of cosmetology as a profession.
11. Know the rules and regulations that govern the practice of cosmetology in your state.

The successful cosmetologist extends **courtesy** to state board members and inspectors. These people are acting in the line of duty and they contribute to the higher standards of cosmetology.

The successful cosmetologist must know the laws, rules and regulations that govern cosmetology and must comply with them. By such compliance, the cosmetologist is contributing to the health, welfare and safety of the community.

REVIEW QUESTIONS

Professional Ethics

1. *Define the cosmetologist's code of ethical conduct.*
2. *Explain why it is important to maintain a professional attitude toward clients.*
3. *Why should the cosmetologist never repeat gossip to clients?*
4. *Why is it desirable that the cosmetologist always be gentle in the performance of services?*
5. *Why is it important to avoid statements that are untrue or unduly critical?*

Chapter 5

BACTERIOLOGY

LEARNING OBJECTIVES

The student successfully mastering this chapter will be able to:

1. *Gain an understanding of bacteriology.*
2. *Identify the various types and classifications of bacteria.*
3. *Explain how bacteria grow and reproduce.*
4. *Recognize the relationship of bacteria to the spread of disease.*

Bacteriology (*bak-teer-i-**OL**-o-jee*), **sterilization**, (*ster-i-li-**ZAY**-shon*) and **sanitation** (*san-i-**TAY**-shon*) are subjects of practical importance to cosmetologists because they have a direct bearing on their own welfare as well as that of their clients'. To protect individual and public health, cosmetologists should know when, why and how to use good sterilization and sanitation practices.

In order to understand the importance of sanitation and sterilization, a basic understanding of how **bacteria** (*bak-**TEER**-i-ah*) affect our daily lives is necessary.

BACTERIOLOGY

Bacteriology is the science that deals with the study of **micro-organisms** (*mi-**KROH**-or-ga-niz-ems*) called bacteria.

Cosmetologists should understand how the spread of disease can be prevented and they must become familiar with the precautions necessary to protect their health as well as that of their clients'. Knowledge of the relationship between bacteria and disease will help students understand the need for school and salon cleanliness and sanitation.

State boards of cosmetology and health departments require the use of sanitary measures while serving the public. Contagious disease, skin infections and blood poisoning are caused either by the conveyance of infectious bacteria from one individual to another or by unsanitary implements (such as combs, brushes, hairpins, clips, rollers and the like) used first on an infected person and then on others. Dirty hands and fingernails are other sources of infectious bacteria.

Bacteria

Bacteria are minute, one-celled vegetable micro-organisms found nearly everywhere. They are especially numerous in dust, dirt, refuse and diseased tissues. Bacteria are also known as **germs** (*jurms*) or **microbes** (***MI***-*krohbs*).

Bacteria can exist almost anywhere and are found on the skin, in water, air, decayed matter, secretions of body openings, on clothing and under the nails.

Bacteria can be seen only with the aid of a microscope. Fifteen hundred rod-shaped bacteria will barely reach across a pinhead.

Types of Bacteria

There are hundreds of different kinds of bacteria. However, all bacteria are classified into two types, depending on whether they are beneficial or harmful.

1. **Non-pathogenic** (*non-path-o-**JEN**-ik*) **organisms** (*beneficial or harmless types*) constitute the majority of all bacteria. They perform many useful functions such as decomposing refuse and improving the fertility of the soil. To this group belong the **saprophytes** (*sap-**RO**-fyts*), which live on dead matter and do not produce disease.
2. **Pathogenic** (*path-o-**JEN**-ik*) **organisms** (*microbes or germs*) are harmful and, although in the minority, produce disease when they invade plant or animal tissues. To this group belong the **parasites** (***PAR**-a-syts*), which require living matter for their growth.

It is because of pathogenic bacteria that cleanliness and sanitary conditions are necessary in a beauty school or salon.

Pronunciations of Terms Relating to Pathogenic Bacteria

Singular		**Plural**	
coccus	(***KOK**-us*)	cocci	(***KOK**-si*)
bacillus	(*ba-**SIL**-us*)	bacilli	(*ba-**SIL**-i*)
spirillum	(*spi-**RIL**-um*)	spirilla	(*spi-**RIL**-a*)
staphylococcus	(*STAF-i-lo-**KOK**-us*)	staphylococci	(*STAF-i-lo-**KOK**-si*)
streptococcus	(***STREP**-to-KOK-us*)	streptococci	(***STREP**-to-KOK-si*)
diplococcus	(***DIP**-lo-KOK-us*)	diplococci	(***DIP**-lo-KOK-si*)

treponema pallida (*trep-o-**NE**-mah **PAL**-i-dah*)

syphilis (***SIF**-i-lis*)

Three general types types of bacteria

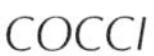

COCCI — BACILLI — SPIRILLA

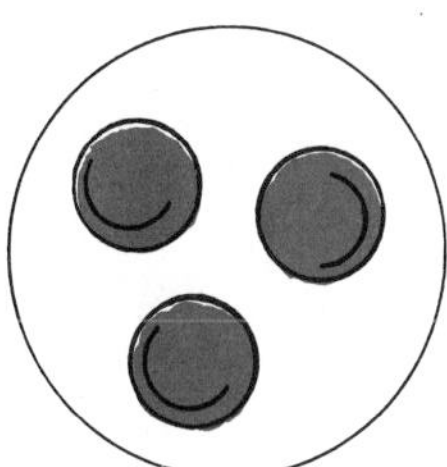

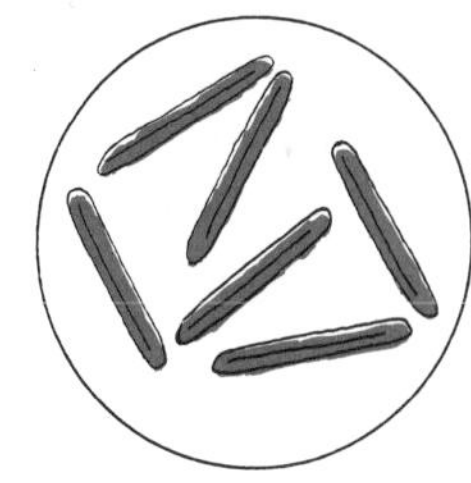

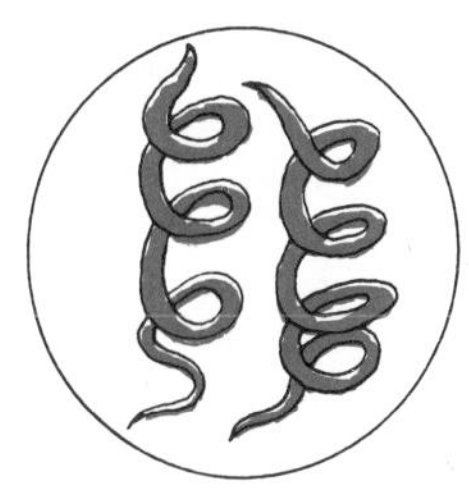

Groupings of bacteria

DIPLOCOCCI — STREPTOCOCCI — STAPHYLOCOCCI

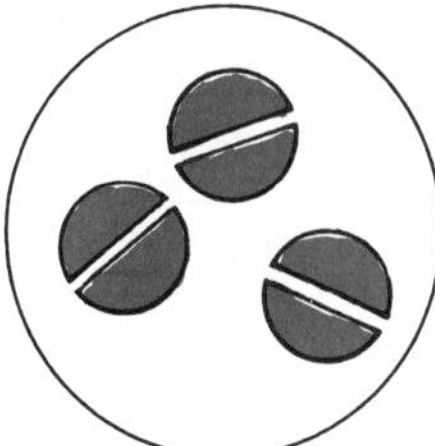

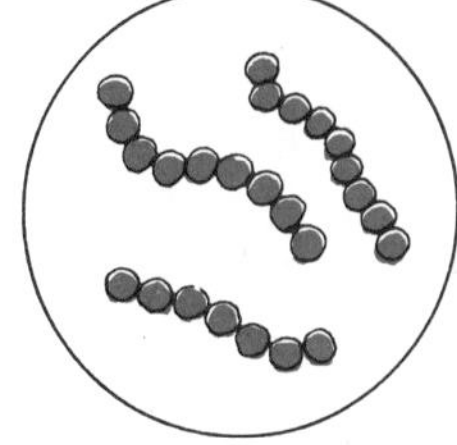

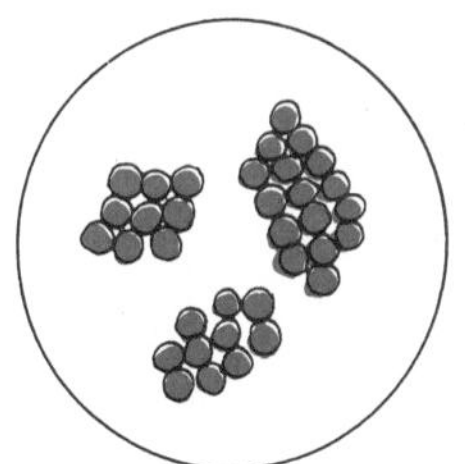

Six disease-producing bacteria

TYPHOID BACILLUS SHOWING FLAGELLA — TUBERCLE BACILLUS (Tuberculosis) — DIPHTHERIA BACILLUS

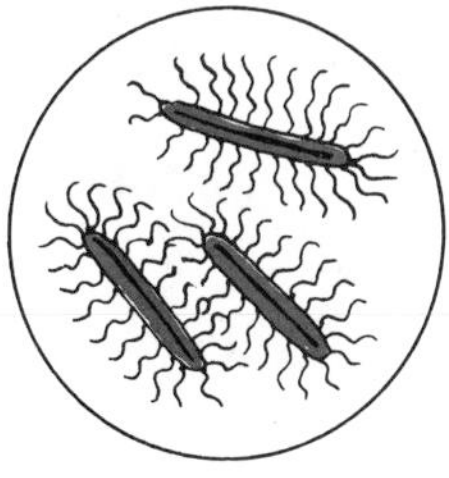

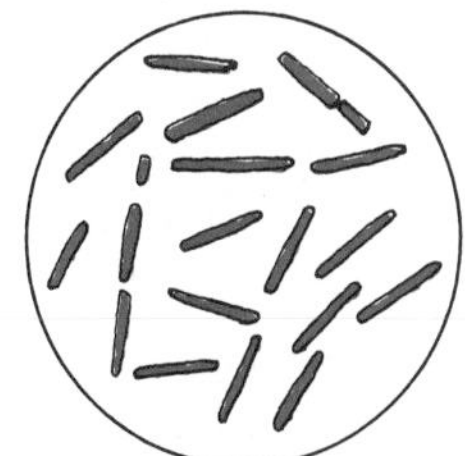

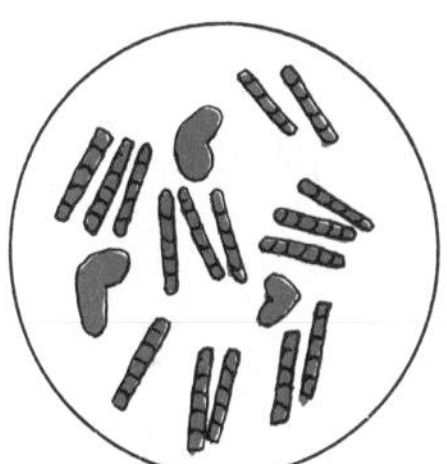

INFLUENZA BACILLUS — CHOLERA (Microspira) — TETANUS BACILLUS WITH SPORES

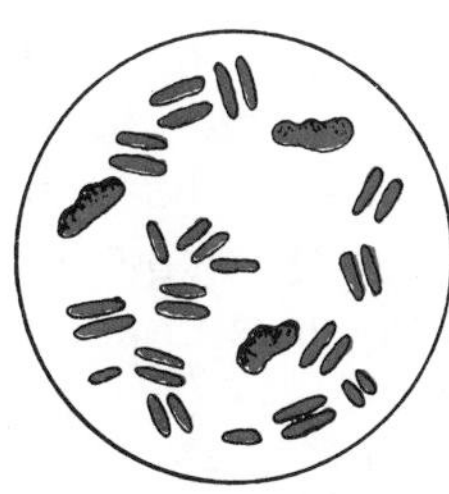

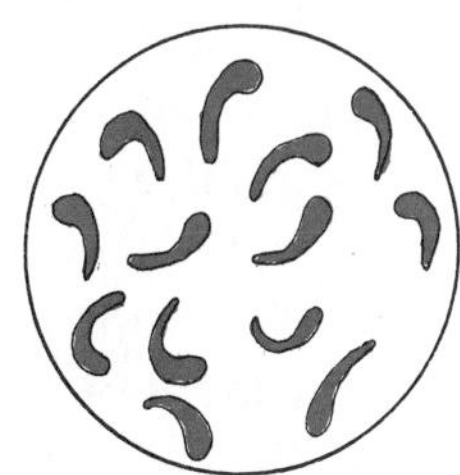

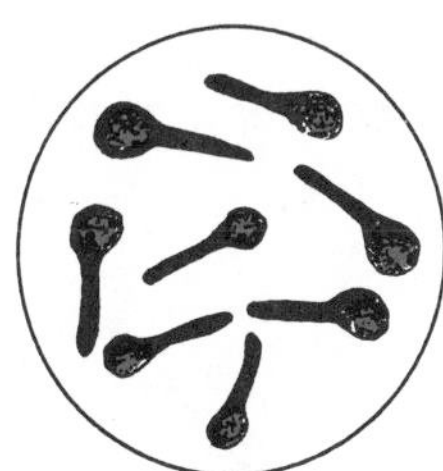

To Avoid the Spread of Disease

KEEP YOURSELF CLEAN. KEEP YOUR SURROUNDINGS CLEAN. KEEP EVERYTHING YOU COME IN CONTACT WITH CLEAN. SEE THAT EVERYTHING YOU USE IS CLEAN.

Classifications of Pathogenic Bacteria

Bacteria have distinct shapes which aid in their identification. Pathogenic bacteria are classified as follows:

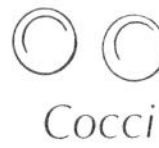
Cocci

1. **Cocci** are round-shaped organisms that appear singly or in the following groups:
   a) **Staphylococci** are pus-forming organisms that grow in bunches or clusters. They cause abscesses, pustules and boils.
   b) **Streptococci** are pus-forming organisms that grow in chains. They cause diseases, such as blood poisoning.
   c) **Diplococci** grow in pairs. They cause pneumonia.

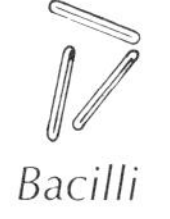
Bacilli

2. **Bacilli** are rod-shaped organisms that are either short, thin or thick in structure. They are the most common and produce diseases such as tetanus (lockjaw), influenza, typhoid fever, tuberculosis and diphtheria. Many bacilli are **spore** producers.

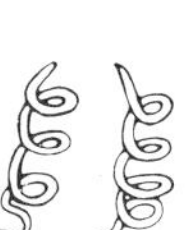
Spirilla

3. **Spirilla** are curved or corkscrew-shaped organisms. They are further subdivided into several groups, of chief importance being the **Treponema pallida**, which cause **syphilis**.

Bacterial Growth and Reproduction

Bacteria generally consist of an outer cell wall and internal protoplasm. They manufacture their own food from the surrounding environment, give off waste products and grow and reproduce.

Bacteria can exhibit two distinct phases in their life cycle: the **active** or **vegetative** stage and the **inactive** or **spore-forming** stage.

Active or Vegetative Stage

During the active stage, bacteria grow and reproduce. These microorganisms multiply best in warm, dark, damp or dirty places where sufficient food is present.

When conditions are favorable, bacteria reproduce very fast. As food is absorbed, the bacterial cell grows in size. When the limit of growth is reached, the bacterial cell divides crosswise into halves forming two cells. From one bacterium as many as 16 million germs can develop in half a day.

When conditions are unfavorable, bacteria die or become inactive.

Inactive or Spore-Forming Stage

Certain bacteria, such as the anthrax and tetanus bacilli, form **spherical spores** with tough outer coverings during their inactive stage in order to withstand periods of famine, dryness and unsuitable temperatures. In this stage, spores can be blown about and are not harmed by disinfectants, heat or cold.

When favorable conditions are restored, the spores change into the active or vegetative form, then grow and reproduce.

Movement of Bacteria

The ability to move about is limited to the bacilli and spirilla; the cocci rarely show active motility (self-movement). To move about, bacteria use hairlike projections, known as **flagella** (*fla-**JEL**-a*) or **cilia** (***SIL**-i-a*), which extend from the sides or the end. A whiplike motion of these hairs propels bacteria around in liquid.

Bacterial Infections

Pathogenic bacteria become a threat to health when they enter the body. An infection occurs if the body is unable to cope with the bacteria and their harmful toxins. A local infection is indicated by a boil or pimple that contains pus. A general infection results when the bloodstream carries the bacteria and their toxins to all parts of the body, as in blood poisoning or syphilis.

The presence of pus is a sign of infection. Staphylococci are the most common pus-forming bacteria. Found in pus are bacteria, waste matter, decayed tissue, body cells and blood cells, both living and dead.

A disease becomes **contagious** (*kon-**TAY**-jus*) when it spreads from one person to another by contact. The term **communicable** also refers to a disease that is transmitted by contact. Some common contagious disorders that would prevent a cosmetologist from working are tuberculosis, common cold, ringworm, scabies, head lice and viral infections.

The chief sources of contagion are unclean hands, unclean implements, open sores, pus, mouth and nose discharges and the common use of drinking cups and towels. Uncovered coughing, sneezing and spitting in public also spreads germs.

There can be no infection without the presence of pathogenic bacteria.

Pathogenic bacteria can enter the body by way of:

1. A break in the skin, such as a cut, pimple or scratch
2. The mouth (breathing or swallowing air, water or food)
3. The nose (air)
4. The eyes or ears (dirt)

The body fights infection by means of:

1. The unbroken skin, which is the body's first line of defense
2. Body secretions, such as perspiration and digestive juices
3. White blood cells within the blood that destroy bacteria
4. Antitoxins that counteract the poisons produced by bacteria

Infections can be prevented and controlled through personal hygiene and public sanitation.

Other Infectious Agents

Filterable viruses (*fil-**TER**-a-bil VI-rus-es*) are living organisms so small that they can pass through the pores of a porcelain filter. They cause the common cold and other **respiratory** (***RES**-pi-ra-tour-ee*) and **gastro-intestinal** (*GAS-troh-in-**TES**-ti-nal*) infections.

Parasites are organisms that survive on other living organisms without giving anything in return.

Plant parasites or **fungi** (***FUN**-ji*), such as molds, mildews and yeasts, can produce contagious diseases, such as ringworm and **favus** (***FA**-vus*).

Animal parasites are responsible for contagious diseases. For example, the itch mite causes scabies and the louse causes **pediculosis** (*pe-DIK-u-**LOH**-sis*).

Contagious diseases caused by parasites should never be treated in the school of salon. Clients should be referred to their physicians.

IMMUNITY

Immunity (*i-**MYOO**-ni-tee*) is the ability of the body to resist infection by destroying bacteria once they have gained entrance. Immunity against disease can be natural or acquired and is a sign of good health. **Natural immunity** means natural resistance to disease, which is partly inherited and partly developed by hygienic living. **Acquired immunity** is achieved after the body has overcome certain diseases by itself or when it has received inoculations against these diseases.

A human disease carrier is a person who is immune to a disease yet serves as a host to germs that can infect others.

Typhoid (***TI**-foid*) **fever** and **diphtheria** (*dif-THEER-i-a*) can be transmitted in this manner.

Bacteria can be destroyed by disinfectants and by intense heat achieved by boiling, steaming, baking or burning, as well as by ultra-violet rays. (This subject is covered in chapter 6, **Sterilization and Sanitation**.)

REVIEW QUESTIONS

Bacteriology

1. *Define bacteriology and explain why it is important to cosmetologists.*
2. *What are the various types and classifications of bacteria?*
3. *How does bacteria grow and reproduce?*
4. *What is the relationship of bacteria to the spread of disease?*

Chapter 6

STERILIZATION AND SANITATION

LEARNING OBJECTIVES

The student successfully mastering this chapter will be able to:

1. *Define the following terms relating to sterilization and sanitation: antiseptic, disinfectant (bactericide or germicide), fumigant and sanitize.*
2. *List the two main methods of sterilization and sanitation and give an example of each.*
3. *Explain the use of sodium hypochlorite compounds, quats, formalin and alcohol as sanitation agents.*
4. *List safety precautions for the use of chemical sanitation agents.*
5. *List at least eight sanitation rules pertinent to the salon.*
6. *Explain how public sanitation is a matter of importance to the cosmetology student.*

STERILIZATION AND SANITATION

Sterilization is the process of cleansing an object by destroying or retarding the growth of bacteria, both beneficial and harmful.

Health departments and state boards of cosmetology recognize that it is impossible to completely sterilize all implements and equipment in the beauty school or salon. Therefore, it is generally recognized that implements and equipment are sanitized, not sterilized. Implements requiring sterilization will be covered later.

Throughout the entire text the term **sanitize** will be used to indicate all forms of sanitation.

Sanitation is of practical importance to the cosmetologist because it deals with methods used to prevent the growth of germs, particularly those responsible for infections and contagious diseases.

Definitions Pertaining to Sanitation

Antiseptic (*an-ti-**SEP**-tik*)—A chemical agent that can kill or retard the growth of bacteria.

Asepsis (*ay-**SEP**-seez*)—Freedom from disease germs.

Bactericide (*bak-**TEER**-i-sid*)—A chemical agent having the power to destroy bacteria (germs or microbes).

Disinfect (*dis-in-**FEKT***)—To destroy bacteria on any object.

Disinfectant (*dis-in-FEK-tant*)—A chemical agent having the power to destroy bacteria (germs or microbes).

Fumigant (***FYOO**-mi-gant*)—Vapor used to keep clean objects sanitary.

Germicide (***JUR**-mi-sid*)—A chemical agent having the power to destroy germs (bacteria or microbes).

Sanitize (***SAN**-i-tiz*)—To render objects clean and sanitary.

Sepsis (***SEP**-sis*)—Poisoning due to pathogenic bacteria.

Sterile (***STER**-il*)—Free from all germs.

Sterilize (***STER**-i-liz*)—To make free from all bacteria (harmful or beneficial) by the act of sterilizing.

Methods of Sterilization and Sanitation

Chemicals are the most effective sanitizing agents used in salons for checking the growth of bacteria. The chemical agents used for sanitizing purposes are antiseptics and disinfectants.

1. An **antiseptic** is a substance that can either kill bacteria or retard their growth without killing them. As a general rule, antiseptics are safe for use on the skin.
2. A **disinfectant** destroys most bacteria and is used to sanitize implements.

Several chemicals can be classified as both antiseptic and disinfectant. A **strong solution** may be used as a disinfectant and a **weak solution** as an antiseptic. Examples: alcohol or **quats** (*kwats*).

Requirements of a Good Disinfectant

1. Easy to prepare
2. Quick acting
3. Almost odorless
4. Noncorrosive
5. Economical
6. Nonirritating to skin

There are many prepared and ready-to-use chemical disinfectant agents on the market. If these are used, select the ones that have been approved by your board of health or state board of cosmetology. Chemicals commonly used in the beauty salon are:

1. **Sodium hypochlorite** (*SOH-di-um HY-po-chlor-it*)—To sanitize implements.
2. **Quaternary ammonium compounds** (quats) (*KWAH-ter-nah-re ah-MO-ne-um KOM-pounds*—[*kwats*]—To sanitize implements.
3. **Formaldehyde** (*for-MAL-de-hid*)—To sanitize implements.
4. **Alcohol**—To sanitize sharp-cutting instruments and electrodes.
5. **Prepared commercial products** that clean floors, sinks and toilet bowls.

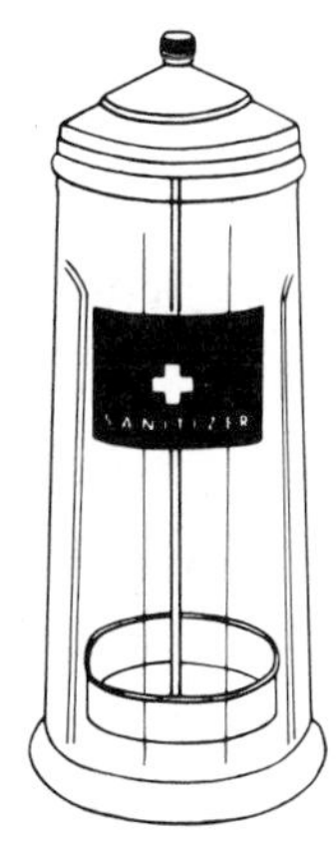

Wet sanitizer

A **wet sanitizer** is any receptacle large enough to hold a disinfectant solution in which the objects to be sanitized are completely immersed. A cover is provided to prevent contamination of the solution. Wet sanitizers can be obtained in various sizes and shapes.

Before immersing objects in a wet sanitizer containing a disinfectant solution, be sure to:

1. Remove hair from combs and brushes.
2. Wash them thoroughly with hot water and soap.
3. Rinse them thoroughly.

This procedure prevents contamination of the solution. In addition, soap and hot water remove most of the bacteria.

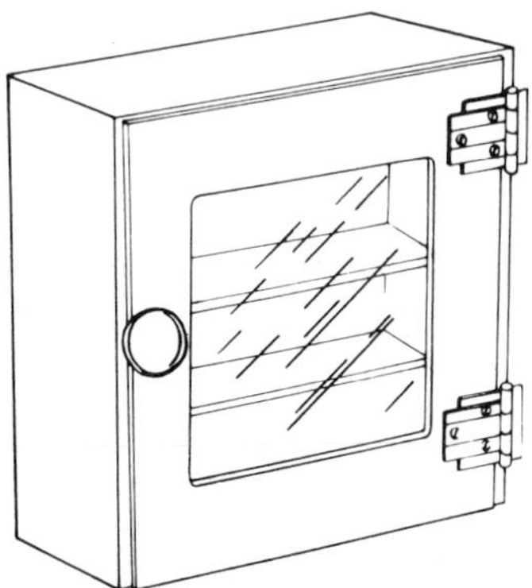
Dry or cabinet sanitizer

After the implements are removed from the disinfectant solution, they must be rinsed in clean water, wiped dry with a clean towel and stored in a dry cabinet sanitizer or ultraviolet ray sanitizer until needed.

A **dry** or **cabinet sanitizer** is an airtight cabinet containing an active fumigant. The sanitized implements are kept clean by being placed in the cabinet until needed.

How to prepare a fumigant. Place 1 tablespoon (15 ml) of borax and 1 tablespoon (15 ml) of formalin on a small tray on the bottom of the cabinet. This will create formaldehyde vapors. Replace chemicals regularly as they lose their strength, which depends on how often the cabinet door is opened and closed.

Formalin and other effective fumigants are also available in tablet form. Follow the manufacturer's directions.

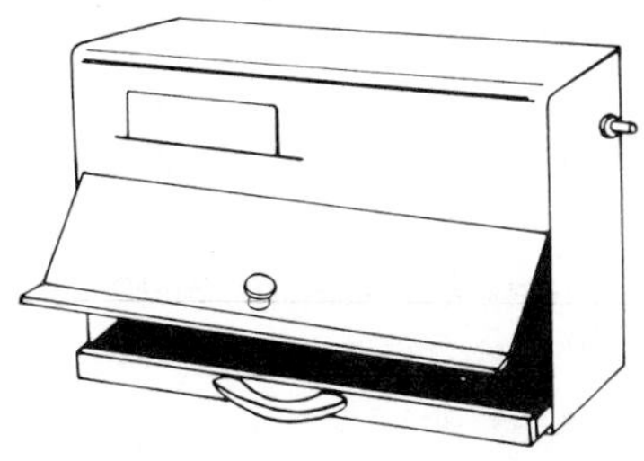
Ultraviolet ray sanitizer

Ultraviolet ray electrical sanitizers are effective for keeping combs, brushes and implements clean until ready for use.

CHEMICAL SANITIZING AGENTS

Sodium Hypochlorite

Sodium hypochlorite (common household bleach) compounds are frequently used to provide the sanitizing ability of chlorine. One of the key advantages of chlorine is its ability to destroy viruses. A 10% solution with an immersion time of 10 minutes is recommended. Many prepared disinfectants contain sodium hypochlorite. Follow the manufacturer's directions for mixing and for immersion time.

Quaternary Ammonium Compounds

Quaternary ammonium compounds (quats) are a broad range of surface-active chemical agents that are important in the salon. Quats are formulated into products that you will be using as disinfectants, cleansers, sterilizers and fungicides for sanitation purposes that we will discuss in this chapter. Quats can also be formulated into shampoos, conditioning products, and various skin care products that will be covered in later chapters.

The advantages of quats as sanitation agents are that they are odorless, colorless, nontoxic, stable and offer a short disinfection time. Immersion time can be as long as 20 minutes, depending on the strength of the solution.

Caution

Before using any sanitizing agent, read and follow the manufacturer's directions. Find out if the product can be used in naturally soft or hard water, or water that has been softened. Inquire whether it contains a rust **inhibitor** (in-hib-i-tor). Should the product lack a rust inhibitor, the addition of 1/2% **sodium nitrite** (so-de-um ni-trit) to the solution prevents the rusting of metallic implements.

Formalin

Formalin is an effective sanitizing agent which can be used as a disinfectant. As purchased, formalin is approximately 37% to 40% of formaldehyde gas in water. Formalin should be used with great care, because inhalation can damage mucous membranes and contact with the skin can cause irritation. Due to its potential harm, formalin is most commonly added to prepared sanitizing agents and is used in various strengths, as follows:

25% solution (equivalent to 10% formaldehyde gas)—used to sanitize implements. Immerse implements in the solution for at least 10 minutes. (Preparation: 2 parts formalin, 5 parts water, 1 part glycerine.)

10% solution (equivalent to 4% formaldehyde gas)—used to sanitize combs and brushes. Immerse them for at least 20 minutes. (Preparation: 1 part formalin, 9 parts water.)

Sanitizing with Chemical Disinfectants

1. Wash the implements thoroughly with soap and hot water.
2. Use a plain, hot water rinse to remove all traces of soap.
3. Immerse the implements in a wet sanitizer (containing approved disinfectant) for the required time.
4. Remove the implements from the wet sanitizer, rinse in water and wipe dry with a clean towel.
5. Store the sanitized implements in individually wrapped cellophane envelopes in a cabinet sanitizer or in an ultraviolet ray cabinet until ready to be used.

Sanitizing with Alcohol

To sanitize **electrodes** and **implements,** use 70% alcohol or 99% isopropyl alcohol.

70% alcohol refers to ethyl or grain alcohol.

99% isopropyl alcohol has the same sanitizing strength as 70% ethyl alcohol.

Implements having a fine cutting edge are best sanitized by rubbing the surface with a cotton pad dampened with 70% alcohol. This application prevents the cutting edges from becoming dull. Time should be 10 minutes and the alcohol should evaporate naturally for contact-effective sanitation.

Electrodes (*i-lek-trohds*) can be safely sanitized by gently rubbing the exposed surface with a cotton pad dampened with 70% alcohol for five minutes. Then place the articles into a dry sanitizer or ultra violet ray sanitizer until ready for use.

Sanitizing Floors, Sinks and Toilet Bowls

To sanitize floors, sinks and toilet bowls in the salon use a commercial product, such as Lysol or pine needle oil. **Deodorants** also are useful to offset offensive smells and impart a refreshing odor.

Whichever disinfectant is used, make sure that it is properly diluted as suggested by the manufacturer.

IT IS ALWAYS A PLEASURE FOR CLIENTS TO RECEIVE SERVICES IN A BEAUTY SALON THAT IS SPOTLESS. GET INTO THE HABIT NOW. KEEP EVERYTHING CLEAN AND IN ORDER.

Proportions For Making Percentage Solutions

100% Active Liquid Concentrate	*Strength*
5 drops of liquid to 1 oz. (30 ml) water or 1 teaspoon (5 ml) of liquid to 12 oz. (.36 l) water or	1%
10 drops of liquid to 1 oz. (30 ml) water or 2 teaspoons (10 ml) of liquid to 12 oz. (.36 l) water	2%
4 teaspoons (20 ml) of liquid to 12 oz. (.36 l) water	4%
5 teaspoons (25 ml) of liquid to 12 oz. (.36 l) water	5%
10 teaspoons (50 ml) of liquid to 12 oz. (.36 l) water	10%

* Consult your state board of cosmetology or health department for a list of approved disinfectants to be used in beauty salons.

Table of Equivalents

Ordinary measured glass	8 oz. (0.237 l)
1 pint	16 oz. (0.475 l)
1 quart	32 oz. (0.95 l)
1/2 gallon	64 oz. (1.9 l)

SAFETY PRECAUTIONS

The use of chemical sanitizing agents involves certain dangers, unless safety measures are taken to prevent mistakes and accidents. Follow these safety rules:

1. Purchase chemicals in small quantities and store them in a cool, dry place; otherwise, they could deteriorate when exposed to air, light and heat.
2. Carefully weigh and measure chemicals.
3. Keep all containers labeled, covered and under lock and key.
4. Do not smell chemicals or solutions because some of them have pungent odors and can irritate the membranes of your nose.
5. Avoid spilling when diluting chemicals.
6. Keep a complete first aid kit on hand.

SANITIZING RULES

Chemical solutions in sanitizers should be changed regularly.

Manicuring implements must be kept in a disinfectant solution (70% alcohol) during a manicure.

All articles must be clean and free from hair before being sanitized.

Combs and **brushes** must be sanitized after each client has been serviced.

Shampoo bowls must be sanitized before and after each use.

All manicuring implements must be sanitized after use.

Sanitize electrical appliances by rubbing their surface with a cotton pad dampened with 70% alcohol.

All cups, finger bowls or **similar objects** must be sanitized prior to being used for another client.

Note The immersing of implements in a chemical solution should conform to state board of cosmetology regulations issued by your state.

PUBLIC SANITATION

Public sanitation is the application of measures to promote public health and to prevent the spread of infectious diseases.

The importance of sanitation cannot be overemphasized. Professional services bring the cosmetologist in direct contact with the client's skin, scalp, hair and nails. By using the best sanitary practices, you can insure the protection of the client's health and your own.

Disinfectants Commonly Used in Beauty Salons

NAME	FORM	STRENGTH	HOW TO USE
Quaternary Ammonium Compounds (Quats)	Liquid or Tablet	1:1000 solution	Immerse implements in solution for 20 minutes.
Formalin	Liquid	25% solution	Immerse implements in solution for 10 minutes.
Formalin	Liquid	10% solution	Immerse implements in solution for 20 minutes.
Ethyl or Grain alcohol	Liquid	70% solution	Sanitize sharp cutting implements & electrodes.
Cresol (lysol)	Liquid	10% soap solution	Cleanse floors, sinks and toilets.

Antiseptics Commonly Used in Beauty Salons

NAME	FORM	STRENGTH	HOW TO USE
Boric acid	White crystals	2–5% solution	Cleanse the eyes.
Tincture of iodine	Liquid	2% solution	Cleanse cuts and wounds.
Hydrogen peroxide	Liquid	3–5% solution	Cleanse skin and minor cuts.
Ethyl or grain alcohol	Liquid	60% solution	Cleanse hands, skin and minute cuts. Not to be used if irritation is present.
Formalin	Liquid	5% solution	Cleanse shampoo bowl, cabinet and so on.
Chloramine-T (chlorazene; chlorozol)	White crystals	1/2% solution	Cleanse skin and hands, and for general use.
Sodium hypochlorite (javelle water; zonite)	White crystals	1/2% solution	Rinse the hands.

Other approved disinfectants and antiseptics are being used in beauty salons. Consult your state board of cosmetology or your health department.

Various governmental agencies protect community health by providing for a wholesome food and water supply and the quick disposal of refuse. These steps are only a few of the ways in which public health is safeguarded.

Drinking water should be odorless, colorless and free from any foreign matter. Crystal-clear water might be unsanitary because of the presence of pathogenic bacteria, which cannot be seen with the naked eye.

The **air within a beauty salon** should not be dry, stagnant, or have a stale, musty odor. Room temperature should be about 70° Fahrenheit (21° Celsius).

The salon can be ventilated by an exhaust fan or an air-conditioning unit. Air-conditioning has the advantage of permitting changes in the quality and quantity of air brought into the salon. Temperature and moisture content of the air can be regulated by air-conditioning.

A **person with an infectious disease** is a source of contagion to others. Hence, cosmetologists with colds or other contagious diseases must not be permitted to serve clients. Likewise, clients obviously suffering from an infectious disease must not be accommodated in a salon. In this way, the best interests of other clients are served.

The **public** has learned the importance of sanitation and is now demanding that every possible sanitary measure be used in the salon for the promotion of public health.

The **state board of cosmetology** and **board of health** in each state or locality have formulated sanitary regulations governing salons. Every cosmetologist must be familiar with these regulations and obey them.

SUMMARY

Adherence to the following sanitary rules will result in cleaner, better service to the public:

1. Every salon must be well lighted, heated, ventilated, and kept in a clean and sanitary condition.
2. Walls, curtains and floor coverings in a salon must be washed and kept clean.
3. All salons must be supplied with hot and cold running water. Drinking facilities (individual paper cups and/or fountain) should be provided.
4. All plumbing fixtures must be properly installed and work effectively.
5. The premises must be kept free from rodents, vermin, flies and all insects.
6. The salon is not to be used for eating, sleeping or living quarters.
7. All hair, cotton or other waste material must be removed from the floor without delay, deposited in a closed container, and removed from the premises frequently.

8. Rest rooms must be kept in a sanitary condition and have a soap dispenser and individual paper towels.
9. Each cosmetologist must wear a clean uniform while working on clients.
10. The cosmetologist **must cleanse** the hands thoroughly **before** and **after** serving a client and **after leaving the rest room.**
11. A freshly laundered towel must be used for each client. Clean towels must be stored in a sanitized, closed cabinet. Soiled towels and linens must be placed immediately after use in containers provided for this purpose. Keep dirty towels away from clean towels.
12. Headrest coverings and neck strips **must be changed for each client.**
13. **Do not permit** the shampoo cape to come in contact with the client's skin.
14. The common use of powder puffs, lip color, cheek color, solid soap, sponges, combs, brushes or styptic pencils is **prohibited.**
15. Keep lotions, ointments, creams and powders in clean, closed containers. Use clean spatulas to remove creams or ointments from jars. Use sterile cotton to apply lotions and powders. Recover cosmetic containers after each use.
16. For manicuring, provide a sanitary container or finger bowl with an individual paper cup for each client.
17. Discard emery boards after use on a client.
18. Soiled combs, brushes, towels or other used material must be removed from tops of workstations immediately after use.
19. Clippies, hairpins or bobby pins must not be placed in the mouth.
20. Combs or implements must not be carried in pockets of the uniform.
21. Clippies, curlers, bobby pins or hairpins must be sanitized after each use.
22. All implements and articles used must first be sanitized and then placed in a dustproof or airtight container or in a cabinet sanitizer.
23. Objects dropped on the floor are not to be used until they are sanitized.
24. Dogs, cats, birds or other pets should not be permitted in a beauty school or salon.

Reminders

1. The **responsibility for sanitation** rests with **each student** in the school and **each cosmetologist** in the salon. The manager must provide the necessities for school and salon sanitation.
2. You **must** obey the rules issued by the health department and the state board of cosmetology regarding acceptable methods of sanitation.

REVIEW QUESTIONS

Sanitation

1. *Define the following terms: antiseptic, disinfectant, fumigant and sanitize.*
2. *What are the two main methods of sanitation? Give an example of each method.*
3. *How are sodium hypochlorite compounds, quats, formalin and alcohol used as sanitation agents?*
4. *What are the safety precautions for the use of chemical sanitation agents?*
5. *What are at least eight sanitation rules that apply to the salon?*
6. *Why is public sanitation a matter of importance to the cosmetology student?*

Chapter 7

DRAPING

LEARNING OBJECTIVES

The student successfully mastering this chapter will be able to:

1. *List the steps in the preparation for draping.*
2. *Demonstrate draping for wet services.*
3. *Demonstrate draping for dry services.*
4. *Demonstrate draping for thermal services.*

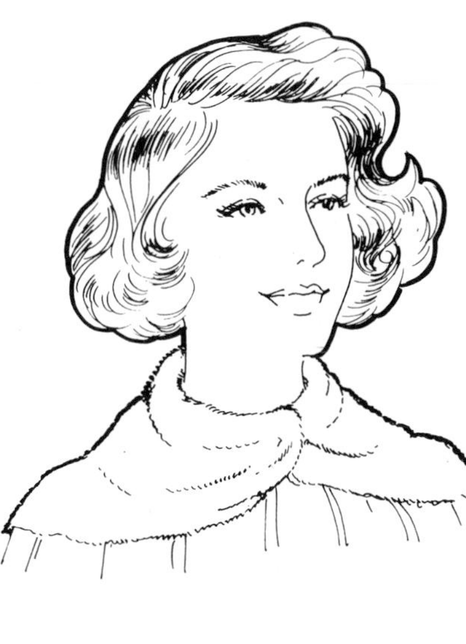

The protection of the client must be the first consideration at all times. Whenever cosmetology services are being performed, the cosmetologist's primary responsibilities are:

1. To provide for the client's comfort.
2. To protect the client's clothing from damage by any of the chemicals or cosmetic solutions being used.
3. To protect the client from injury.
4. To provide competent, professional services to the client.

Draping correctly for the various services offered is an important part of the cosmetologist's job. Properly draping the client is the "first line of defense" for the protection of the skin and clothing from stains and damage. In addition the client feels more confident, relaxed and comfortable knowing that the cosmetologist is concerned with personal safety.

Note

There are many ways to drape a client for various salon services. Only some of the methods are discussed and illustrated here. Your instructor may use different techniques, which are equally acceptable. Basically, however, every method of draping is designed to accomplish the same objective, which is the protection of your clients and their clothing.

PREPARATION FOR DRAPING

Before draping a client for any kind of hair service, the following steps should be followed:

1. Seat the client comfortably.
2. Select and arrange the required materials and supplies.
3. Wash and sanitize the hands.
4. Ask the client to remove all neck and hand jewelry, earrings and glasses, and put them safely away. Have the client remove contact lenses before a permanent wave, hair relaxing, color or lightening service.
5. Turn the collar to the inside, making sure that it is straight and will not wrinkle (fig. 1).

Fig. 1

DRAPING FOR WET HAIR SERVICES

A neck towel is used for sanitation as well as protection. Special care must be exercised to make certain that the cape does not come into direct contact with the client's skin, because the cape is used on many clients and could be a carrier of disease or infection. For any wet hair service, make sure that the towel protects the client from accidental wetting.

Procedure

If the towel is short, it can be folded on the bias, which will add length and give a higher "collar" for more protection.

1. Place the cape loosely across the front of the client (fig. 2).
2. Drape the towel across the crown area of the client's head (fig. 2).
3. Slide the towel down around the neck, leaving 1/3 of the width of the towel draped over the shoulders and 2/3 of the width of the upright around the neck (fig. 3).

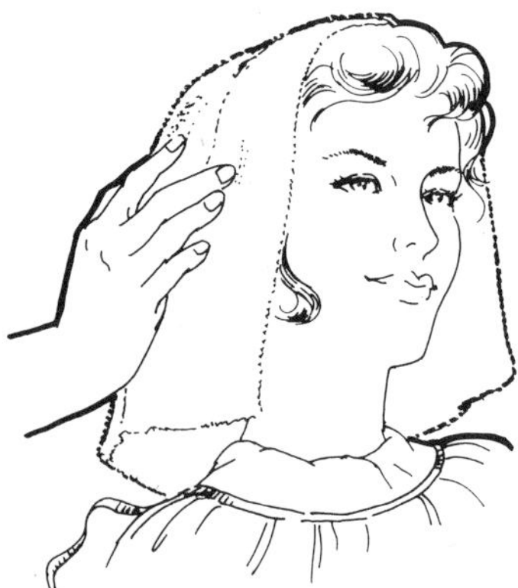

Fig. 2 Place cape loosely in front of client. Sliding towel down around client's neck.

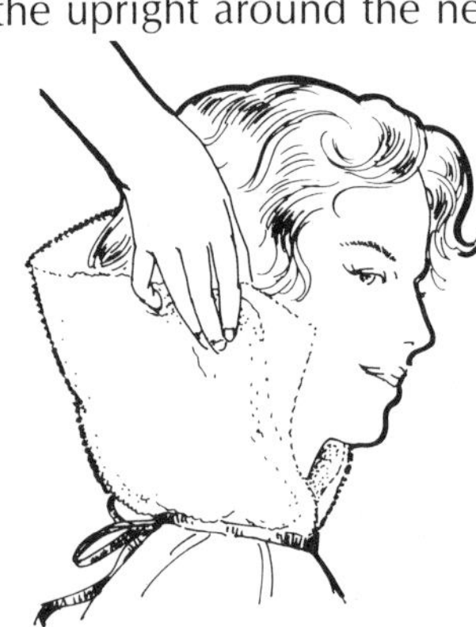

Fig. 3 Adjust and tie cape over towel.

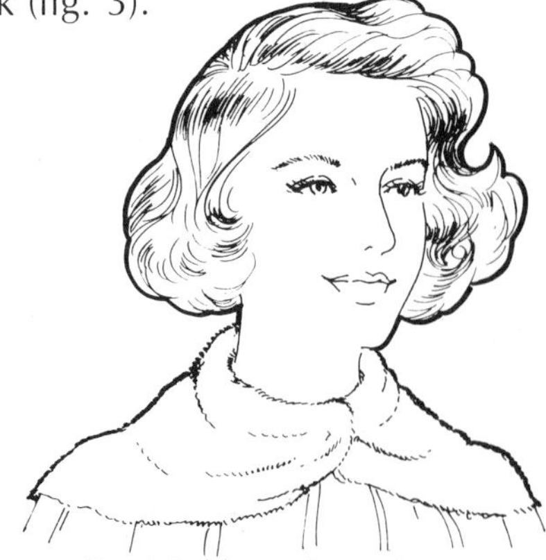

Fig. 4 Fold towel over in cape effect.

4. Adjust the cape over the towel and fasten the cape band around the neck.
5. Fold the upright portion of the towel down and over to create a cape effect (fig. 4).

The client and clothing are now completely protected against any dripping liquid.

Additional draping for chemical services: A second towel may be used over the cape for additional protection before applying chemicals to the hair. Drape over the shoulders and fasten in the front with a large clip or clamp. Your instructor might also advise that the client's clothing be replaced with a protective smock.

DRAPING FOR DRY HAIR SERVICES

Draping for dry hair services differs somewhat from the techniques previously outlined. The cape is used in much the same manner, and great care must be exercised to be certain that the cape does not touch the client's skin. However, in draping for dry services, less emphasis is placed on the use of towels; neck strips are more commonly used for sanitary as well as protective purposes.

Procedure

1. Place the neck strip around the neck of the client (fig. 5).
2. Fold the ends of the neck strip and tuck them in (fig. 5).
3. Adjust the cape carefully around the neck with the ends of the neck band overlapping at the back of the neck.
4. Be certain that the neck band of the cape rests in the center of the neck strip around the entire neck (fig. 6).
5. Fasten the cape so that it fits snugly around the neck (fig. 6).
6. Fold the uncovered portion of the neck strip down over the cape neck band, make sure the cape does not touch the skin (fig. 7).

The client is now protected against hair clippings and water drippings.

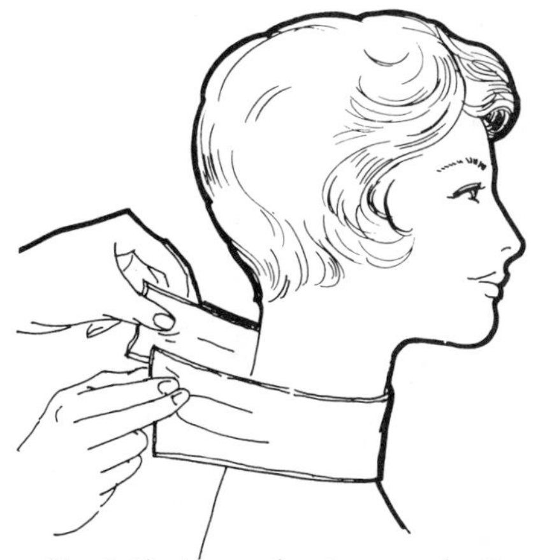

Fig. 5 Placing neck strip around neck; folding ends over and tucking in.

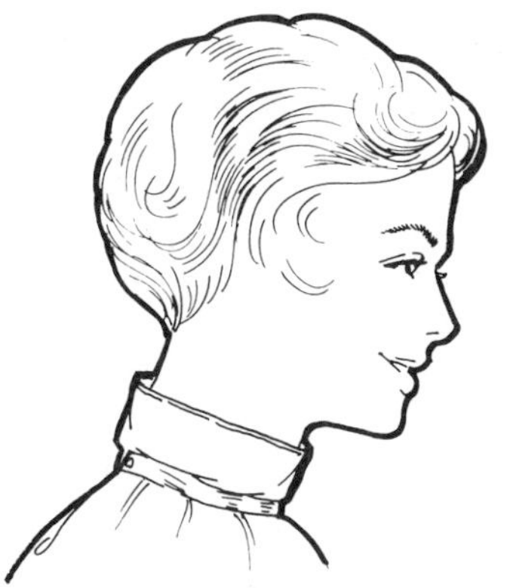

Fig. 6 Tie, pin attached cape over neck strip.

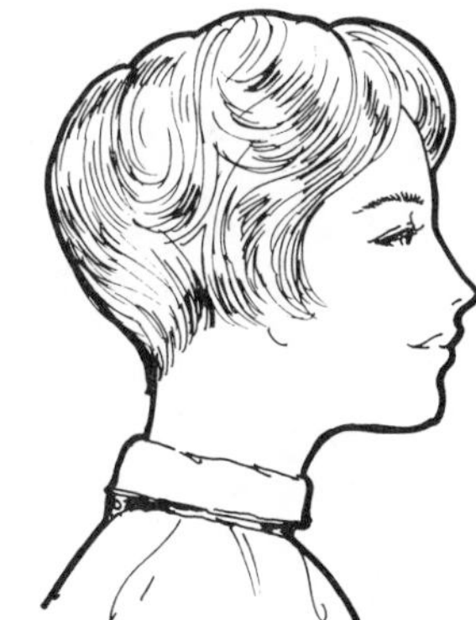

Fig. 7 Fold neck strip down over cape neck band. Cape should not touch the client's skin.

DRAPING FOR THERMAL SERVICES

When draping for thermal curling or waving, a plastic cape will create a fire hazard. It is advisable to use a cotton or linen cape for these services.

DRAPING FOR A COMB-OUT

Draping for a comb-out is the same as draping for dry hair shaping. The only differences are that the cape used for a comb-out is usually shorter and is fastened in front to avoid interference with the back and nape comb-out (fig. 8).

Comb-out capes do not have to be waterproof and can be made of soft colorful material. This type of cape is more attractive to the client. However, this cape should be laundered more frequently to maintain its freshness and cleanliness.

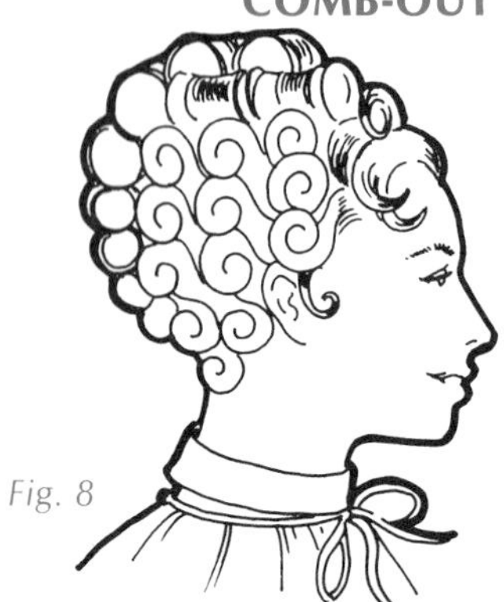

Fig. 8

DRAPING FOR FACIALS

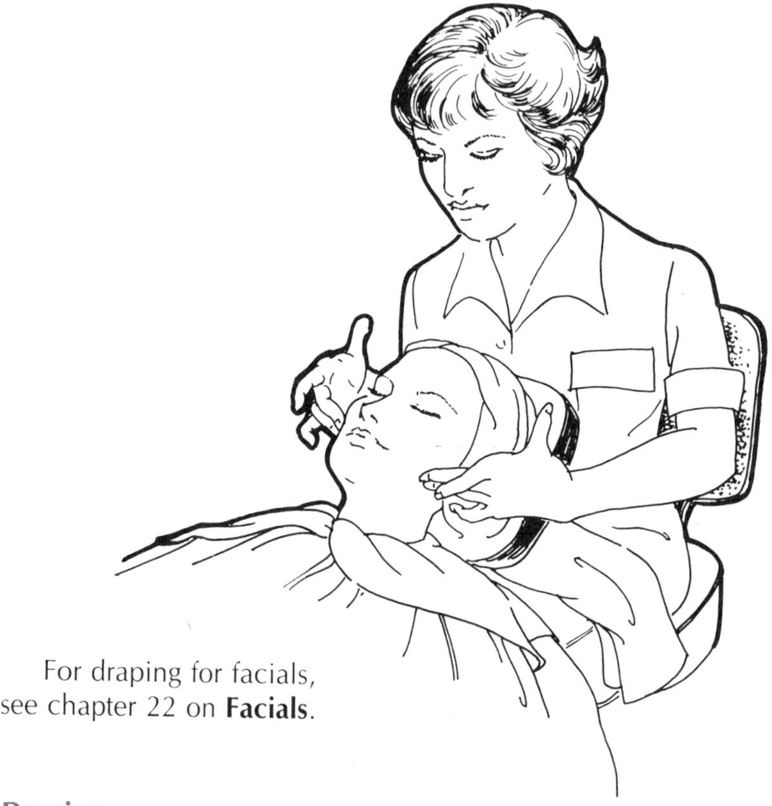

For draping for facials, see chapter 22 on **Facials**.

REVIEW QUESTIONS

Draping

1. *What are the differences for draping for a comb-out?*
2. *What are the steps for preparing the client for draping?*
3. *How is draping accomplished for wet services?*
4. *How is draping accomplished for dry services?*
5. *How is draping accomplished for thermal services?*

Chapter 8

SHAMPOOING AND RINSING

LEARNING OBJECTIVES

The student successfully mastering this chapter will be able to:

1. *List the reasons for good hygienic care of the hair and scalp.*
2. *State why a cosmetologist should have a sound background in professional methods of shampooing.*
3. *Identify various types of shampoos.*
4. *Demonstrate the procedure for shampoo manipulations.*
5. *Show the accepted methods of cleansing the hair and scalp.*
6. *Explain when and how to use various types of shampoos.*
7. *Explain the effect of hair rinses on the hair.*
8. *Identify various types of rinses.*
9. *Explain when and how to use the various types of rinses.*

SHAMPOOS

Shampooing is usually the first service that you will be asked to perform in a salon. A shampoo is the basis of all hairdressing services and every operator should be able to give a shampoo. A shampoo can be considered a valuable selling aid. A customer who is pleased with a shampoo is more likely to accept the recommendation of the cosmetologist for additional services. Therefore, the operator who gives a professional shampoo becomes a valuable employee.

Shampoos are primarily given to clean the hair and scalp and add luster to the hair. A scalp massage helps to increase the blood circulation, stimulates the scalp and relaxes the client. If the customer is pleased with the results, there is a good possibility of a return visit.

The hair and scalp must be cleansed to remove the oil, perspiration, scales and dirt. If this accumulation remains on the scalp, it becomes a breeding place for disease-producing bacteria and can lead to scalp disorders.

Today's shampoos are specially formulated to cleanse the hair and scalp while not leaving either harshly affected. Strong soaps and detergents are fast disappearing from the market. All shampoos should cleanse the hair of excess oils, debris and dirt. They should be able to be used in both hard and soft water. Shampoos for cleansing normal hair should have a pH range of 4.5 to 5.5.

Water

Chemically, water is composed of hydrogen and oxygen. Depending on the kinds and quantities of other minerals present, water can be classified as either **hard** or **soft**. You must know the type of water that is available to be able to select the correct shampoo.

Soft water is best for use in salons. It has been chemically softened and allows the shampoo to lather freely.

Hard water contains minerals such as calcium and magnesium, which do not allow soap shampoos to lather. The mineral will also dry the hair, leaving it feeling harsh. A chemical process can be used to soften hard water.

Selecting the Correct Shampoo

The hairstylist should first discuss the desired service with the customer. Identify possible disorders, noting allergies and hair, skin or scalp problems. The operator must identify the type of problem and its cause. Check if the problem is due to a permanent wave, tint, lightener, rinse or even some medical or physical reason. Do a complete hair evaluation and analysis for each client before selecting the best shampoo.

Hair is not considered normal if it has been:

Lightened	Sun bleached
Toned or tinted	Abused by use of harsh shampoos
Permanently waved	Damaged by improper care
Chemically relaxed	Damaged by exposure to elements

Required Materials and Implements

Remember to gather all necessary materials and implements before beginning to shampoo. A client expects a cosmetologist to be prepared and does not want to be left waiting at the basin.

Draping the Client for a Shampoo

It is important to drape the client correctly, so that full protection is given to both person and clothing. (For the correct method of draping, refer to chapter 7 on **Draping**.)

HAIR BRUSHING TECHNIQUE

Brushing the hair is an important part of the shampoo and conditioning service.

Never brush the hair before:

1. Applying a tint, lightener or toner.
2. Giving a permanent wave or chemical relaxer.
3. Checking the scalp for irritations.

Why It Is Important to Brush the Hair and Scalp

1. To make hair shine
2. To groom hair; to make it neat and tidy
3. To remove knots, tangles and back combing
4. To remove dust, dirt and cosmetics
5. To loosen and remove dandruff and dry skin from the scalp
6. To stimulate the oil glands and the circulation of the blood
7. To spread oil along the hair shaft
8. To soothe nerves
9. To keep the hair and scalp clean and healthy
10. To remove loose hairs

How to Brush the Hair and Scalp

1. Part the hair from the center front to the nape of the neck.
2. Part the hair from ear to ear, across the top of the head.
3. Part the section one inch from the center of the head, right front section.
4. Hold the hair between the finger and thumb.
5. Lay the brush with the bristles away from you and against the scalp.
6. Sweep the bristles the full length of the hair, moving toward the ends of the hair.
7. Make a second parting one inch from the first parting.
8. Continue this procedure until all the hair has been thoroughly brushed.
9. Be gentle but firm in your movement; do not hurt the scalp.

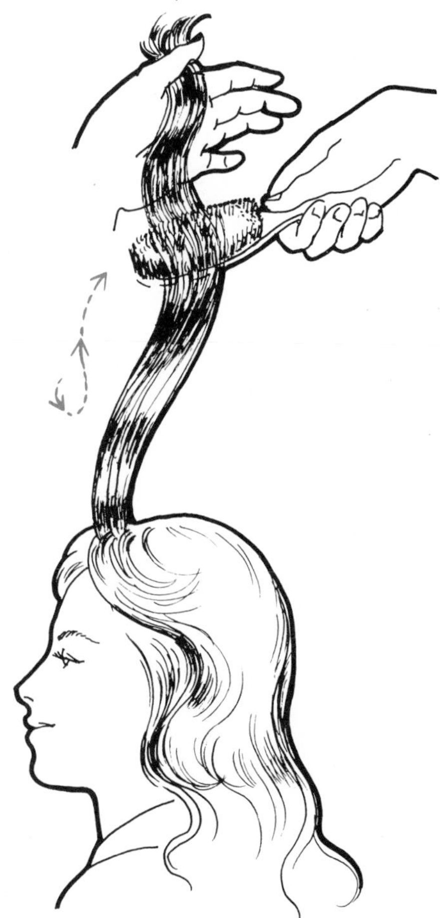

Brushing the hair

SHAMPOO PROCEDURE

Materials

Shampoo	Towels
Brushes	Combs
Shampoo-cape	Neckstrip
Conditioner	

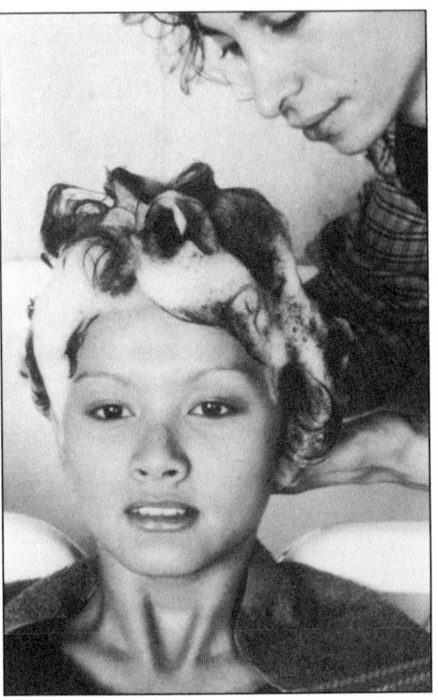

Support the client's head with your right hand and place the cape over the back of the chair.

Plain Shampoo

1. Seat the client comfortably.
2. Select the required materials.
3. Wash and sanitize the hands.
4. Place a neck strip or towel and shampoo cape around the client's neck.
5. Ask the client to remove any jewelry.
6. Examine the condition of the client's hair and scalp.
7. Brush the hair thoroughly.
8. Seat the client at the basin, adjust the chair back and place the cape over the back of the chair.

Note Explain to the customer that you are going to adjust the chair and gently hold the neck and head in your hands.

Procedure

You must be able to use both hands with equal ease and work from either side of the basin.

Turn on the cold water first and gradually add warm water until you obtain the proper temperature to suit your client.

Test the temperature by spraying the water on the inner side of your wrist.

Adjust the temperature of the water, keeping your fingers curved over the nozzle so that you immediately know if the temperature has changed.

Make sure that the pressure of the water is not too strong so the spray doesn't splash the customer.

1. Wet the hair thoroughly with warm water. Lift the hair and work with your free hand to make certain it is saturated right to the scalp. Place your hand so that it protects the client's face, ears and neck from spray when working around the hairline area.

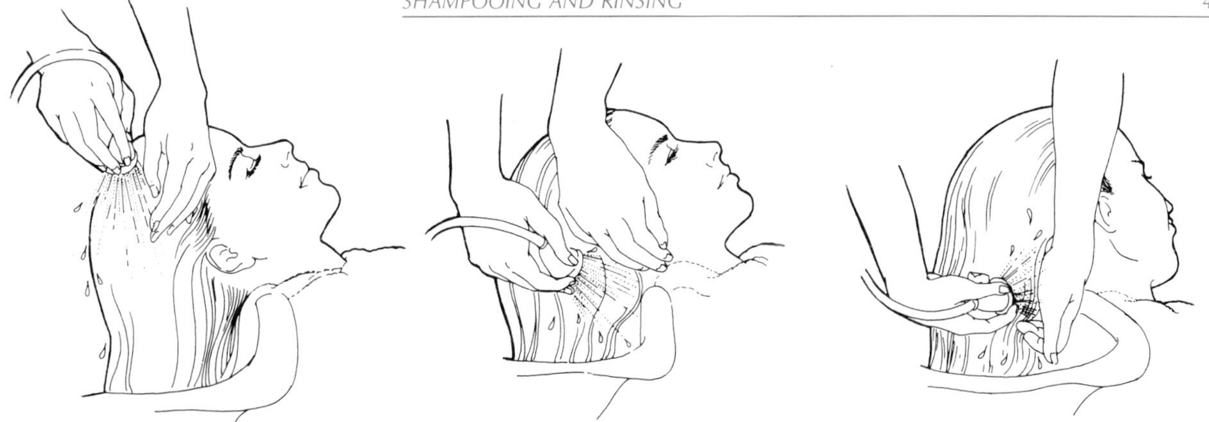

Fig. 1 Protecting the face *Fig. 2 Protecting the ears* *Fig. 3 Protecting the neck*

2. Start the application of shampoo at the front hairline and work down so that the lather flows into the basin. Gently support the client's head with either hand and apply shampoo across the back of the neck. Massage the shampoo into a lather over the entire head.

Reminders In massaging the scalp, do not use firm pressure if the:

Shampoo is to be followed by a lightening treatment

Shampoo is to be followed by a tint treatment

Shampoo precedes a permanent wave

Scalp is tender or sensitive

Customer requests less pressure

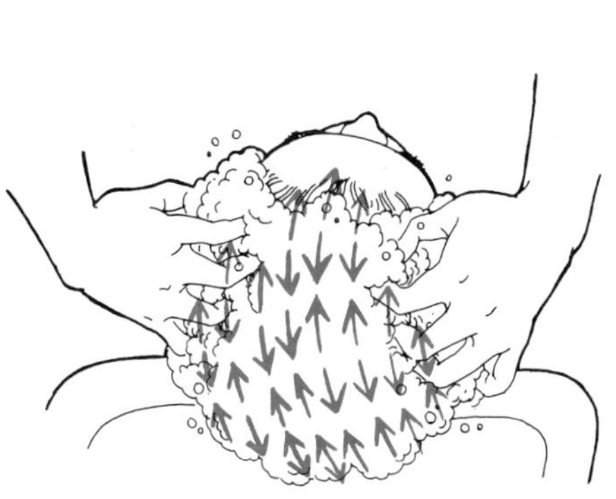

Fig. 4 Manipulate the scalp from hairline at ears to the top of the head

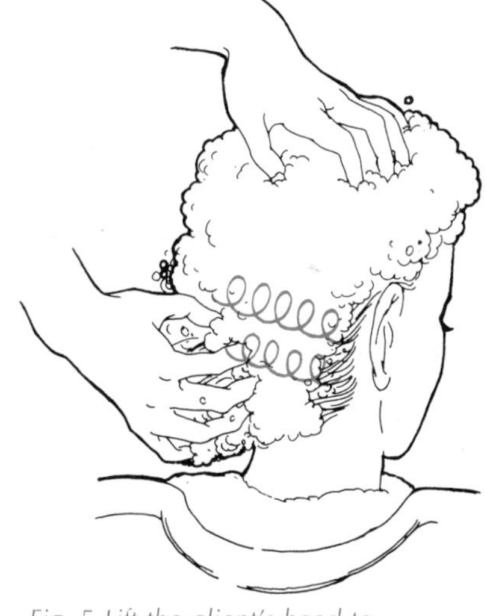

Fig. 5 Lift the client's head to shampoo the nape area.

3. Manipulate the scalp. Starting at the hairline in front of the ears, massage the scalp by using the cushions of the fingers of both hands and work in a back-and-forth movement until the crown is reached.

Continue working to the back of the head, sliding the fingers back 2.5 inches with each movement. Gently lift the client's head, supporting it with the hand. Massage down the back of the head between the ears in the nape area.

Repeat the massage process until the right side of the head is covered. At the left ear, repeat the massage for the left side of the head. Allow the customer to relax against the basin and massage around the hairline with the fingertips in a rotary fashion. Repeat massage movements until the entire scalp has been manipulated.

4. Rinse the hair thoroughly as shown in figs. 1, 2, and 3. Allow the spray of water to flow from the hairline through the crown nape areas into the basin. Lift the hair from the scalp to allow the spray to thoroughly rinse out the shampoo. Cup the spray against the neck area to make sure the water penetrates through to the scalp.

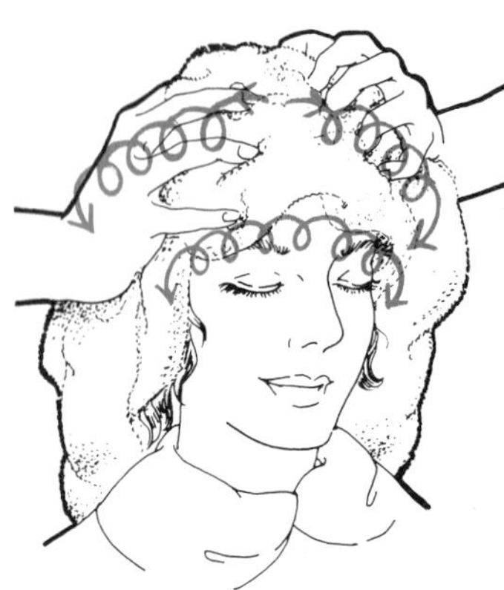

Towel drying the hair

5. If required, reapply shampoo for a second time as outlined in step 2. Less shampoo will be required because this application will lather easily. Follow the same procedure as you did for the first shampoo.

6. Rinse the hair thoroughly.

7. Partially towel dry. Remove excess moisture from the hair at the shampoo bowl and wipe moisture from the face and ears with the ends of the towel. Place the towel over the back of the client's head and drape the head with it. Gently squeeze the towel to remove excess water. Massage the hair gently with towel, using a patting action.

8. Return the client to the styling area and comb out tangles, starting in the nape area and from the ends of the hair.

9. **Remember** to start combing in small sections and **do not** pull the hair.

10. Proceed with styling or the next service.

Cleanup

1. Discard used materials and return unused materials to their correct place.
2. Remove hair from combs and brushes. Wash with hot, soapy water to which disinfectant has been added. Place in a wet sanitizer. Dry the brushes and place them in a dry sanitizer.
3. Place used towels in a covered towel hamper.
4. Wash and sanitize the hands.

Safety Precautions

1. Protect the client's eyes from shampoo.
2. Protect the client's ears by placing sanitized cotton in them if the client is especially sensitive.
3. Test water temperature before applying water to the client's head.
4. Do not scratch the client's scalp with your fingernails.
5. Remove excess moisture from the client's hair before leaving the shampoo basin.
6. Clean and sanitize the shampoo basin after each use.
7. Mop up any water from the floor.

SHAMPOOING LIGHTENED HAIR

Special care must be taken with lightened hair because it can tangle when wet. Use tepid water and a shampoo that is low in alkalinity. Work with your hands underneath the hair to avoid matting. For ease in combing, use conditioners that are specially formulated for lightened hair. Gently towel dry the hair. Do not drag the comb through tangles. The same care should be exercised with tinted, relaxed or damaged hair.

TYPES OF SHAMPOOS

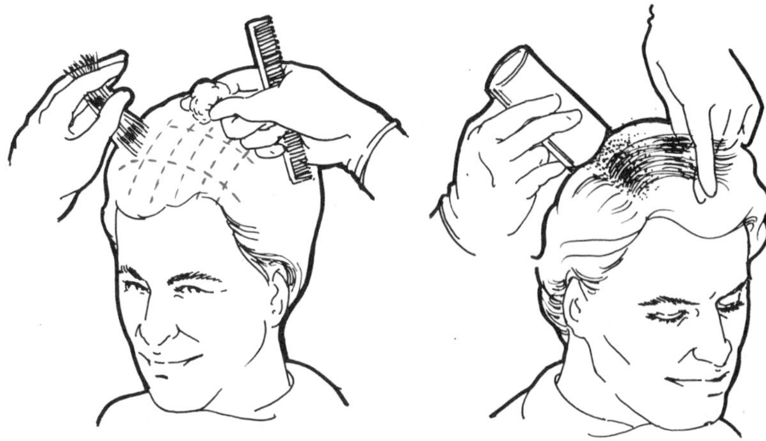

Using a liquid dry shampoo *Using a powder dry shampoo*

Plain Shampoo

Plain or all-purpose shampoos are usually liquid and produce a high lather. Plain shampoo should not be used on tinted, damaged or lightened hair. It will strip or fade the color and can further damage the hair.

Soapless Oil Shampoos

Soapless oil shampoos are made from synthetic detergents in which the oils have been treated with sulfuric acid. They are effective in both hard and soft water. They rinse out easily and do not leave a soap residue on the hair. Nearly all shampoos are of this type.

Liquid Cream Shampoos

Liquid cream shampoos contain oily compounds that make the hair feel silky and soft. Cream shampoos are mostly emulsions.

Cream or Paste Cream Shampoos

Paste cream shampoos are practically the same as the liquid cream except that less water is used.

Acid-Balanced or Nonstrip Shampoos

Shampoos with a pH of between 4.5 and 5.5 are considered to be acid-balanced. Their use will maintain the pH of the hair and skin. They are nonstrip and are recommended for color treated or permanently waved hair.

Antidandruff or Medicated Shampoos

Medicated shampoos are specially formulated to control dandruff flaking without removing the natural moisture from the hair. They must not be used on tinted hair.

Liquid Dry and Powder Shampoos

Liquid dry shampoos are cosmetic products used for cleansing the scalp and hair when the client is prevented by illness from having a regular shampoo. Dry shampoos may be used. They contain an absorbent powder.

Other Types of Shampoos

Protein shampoos are specially formulated from vegetable or animal protein. They add protein to the hair and leave it in manageable condition.

Color shampoos such as henna, give highlights to the hair.

Highlighting shampoos, see chapter 15 on **Hair Coloring**.

HAIR RINSES

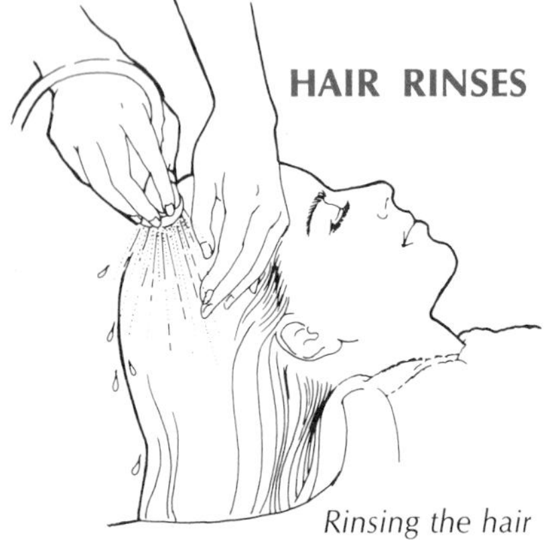

Rinsing the hair

Conditioning rinses temporarily condition the hair by removing alkali and other residues from the hair and scalp. They coat the hair cuticle with a lubricating film, which makes the hair glossy, smooth to touch and easy to detangle and control. Most rinses consist of a few basic ingredients such as acid and protein substances in a creamy liquid form. Oils and waxes help to maintain hair at its normal pH 4.5 to 5.5 to counteract dandruff and give hair a shiny appearance.

Acid rinses are nonstrip. They prevent the stripping of color after a tint or toner and help to close and harden the cuticle that was opened by the alkaline tint or toner.

Instant Conditioning Rinses

Instant conditioning rinses make hair detangling easier. The conditioner coats the hair strand and prevents friction and stress when combing or brushing. They are often called cream rinses.

Color Rinses

Color rinses are used to highlight or add temporary color to the hair. (For additional information see chapter 15 on **Hair Coloring**.)

Medicated Rinses

Medicated rinses help to control dandruff because they have antiseptic ingredients. Follow the manufacturer's instructions.

Stabilizing Rinses

Stabilizing rinses help to restore the hair's acid balance and are used after most chemical services. They are carried into the cortex by a fine penetrating foam.

REVIEW QUESTIONS

Shampooing and Rinses

1. *List five reasons it is important to take good hygienic care of the hair and scalp.*
2. *Why is it important to have knowledge of professional methods of shampooing?*
3. *List seven types of shampoos and when they would be used.*
4. *List the accepted methods of shampooing the hair and scalp.*
5. *Describe the effect of hair rinses on the hair.*
6. *List the various types of rinses described.*
7. *Describe when and how you would use the various types of rinses.*

Chapter 9

SCALP AND HAIR CARE

LEARNING OBJECTIVES

The student successfully mastering this chapter will be able to:

1. *Give reasons for scalp care and its treatments.*
2. *Name the importance of regular scalp manipulation.*
3. *Give the normal and abnormal conditions of the scalp and hair.*
4. *Identify dandruff and its treatment.*
5. *Determine a dry hair and scalp condition and its treatment.*
6. *Determine an oily hair and scalp condition and its treatment.*
7. *Discuss the use of corrective hair treatments.*
8. *Identify alopecia and its possible cause.*
9. *Recognize alopecia areata and its treatment.*

SCALP CARE AND TREATMENTS

The purpose of scalp treatments is to preserve the health of the hair and scalp. Treatments also help prevent dandruff and excessive hair loss.

Cleanliness is a basic requisite for a healthy scalp. The scalp and hair should be kept clean by frequent treatment and shampooing. A clean scalp will resist a variety of disorders.

Scalp manipulations stimulate the circulation of the blood to the scalp, relax and soothe the nerves, stimulate the muscles and the activity of scalp glands, render a tight scalp more flexible and help maintain the growth and health of the hair.

Although shampooing keeps the hair clean, it will not prevent the hair from becoming dry and brittle. The cosmetologist, therefore, should always recommend the proper cosmetic applications to counteract the danger of either a dry and scaly scalp or an excessively oily condition.

Because the scalp and hair are vitally related, many scalp disorders need correction in order to keep the hair healthy. A healthy scalp contributes to the growth of healthy hair. The cosmetologist treats only common and minor conditions.

Do not suggest a scalp treatment:

1. If there are scalp abrasions or if there is a scalp disorder.
2. Immediately prior to the application of a lightener, tint, toner, permanent wave or chemical hair relaxing treatment.

Advise client to consult a physician for serious or contagious scalp ailments. However, conditions caused by neglect, such as tight scalp, overactive or inactive oil glands and tense nerves, can be corrected or alleviated by proper scalp treatments.

Preparing a Client for Scalp Treatment

As in any other salon service, first gather all the necessary equipment according to the kind of scalp treatment you are about to give.

Prepare the client by properly draping, removing all pins and clips from the hair and combing out tangles.

Brush the hair. Brushing should always be an essential part of every scalp treatment. Proper brushing, with a good natural bristle brush will help to stimulate scalp circulation, remove dust and dirt from the hair and give it added luster and sheen. (For instructions on hair brushing, see chapter 8 on **Shampooing and Rinsing**.)

SCALP MANIPULATIONS

Since the same manipulations are given with all scalp treatments, the cosmetologist should learn to give them with a continuous, even motion to stimulate the scalp and/or soothe the client's tension. Scalp massage is most effectively applied as a series of treatments once a week for normal scalp and more frequently for scalp disorders under the direction of a dermatologist.

Anatomy

Knowing the muscles, the location of blood vessels and the nerve points of the scalp and neck will help guide the cosmetologist to those areas in which massage movements are to be directed for the most beneficial results.

Scalp Manipulation Technique

There are several ways in which scalp manipulations may be given. The following routine might be changed to meet your instructor's requirements.

With each massage movement, place the hands under the hair so the length of the fingers, balls of the fingertips and cushions of the palms can stimulate the muscles, nerves and blood vessels of the scalp area.

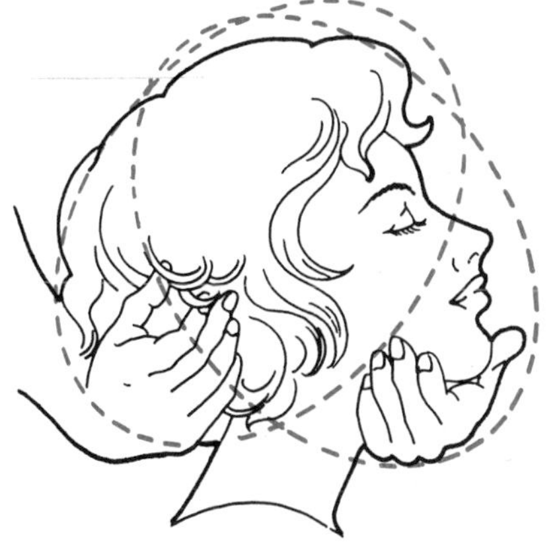

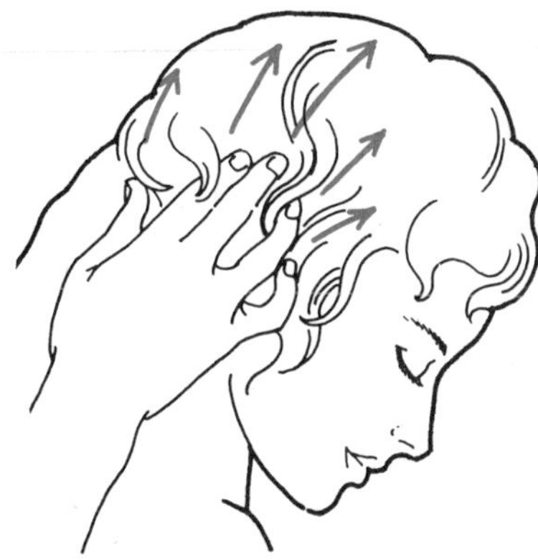

RELAXING MOVEMENT. Cup the client's chin in your left hand; place your right hand at the base of the skull and rotate the head gently. Reverse the position of your hands and repeat.

SLIDING MOVEMENT. Place your fingertips on each side of the client's head; slide your hands firmly upward, spreading the fingertips until they meet at the top of the head. Repeat four times.

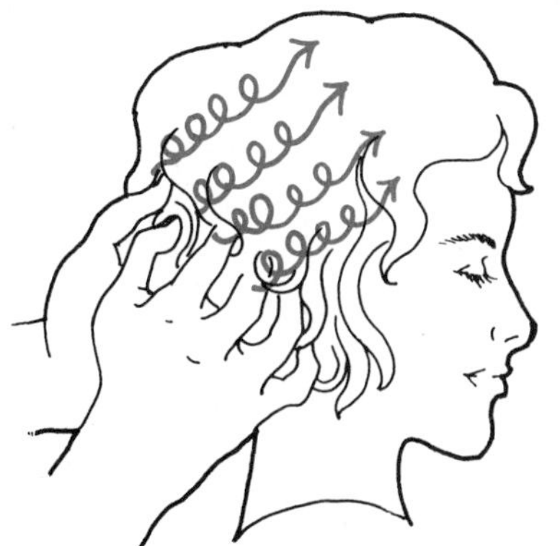

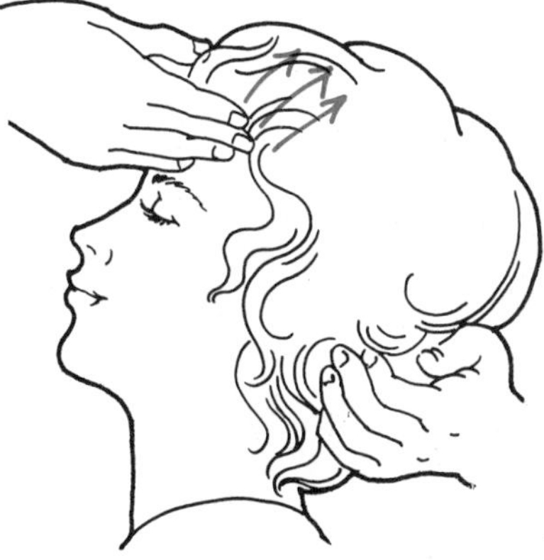

SLIDING AND ROTATING MOVEMENT. Slide your fingertips firmly up the client's scalp, rotate and move the client's scalp. Repeat four times.

FOREHEAD MOVEMENT. Hold the back of the client's head with your left hand. Place stretched thumb and fingers of your right hand on the patron's forehead. Move your hand slowly and firmly upward to 1″ past the hairline. Repeat four times.

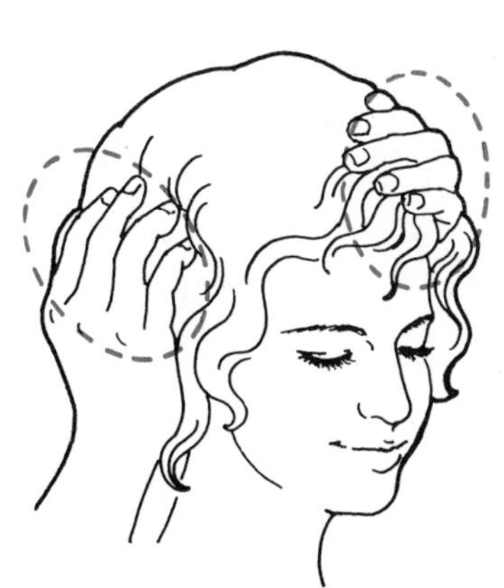

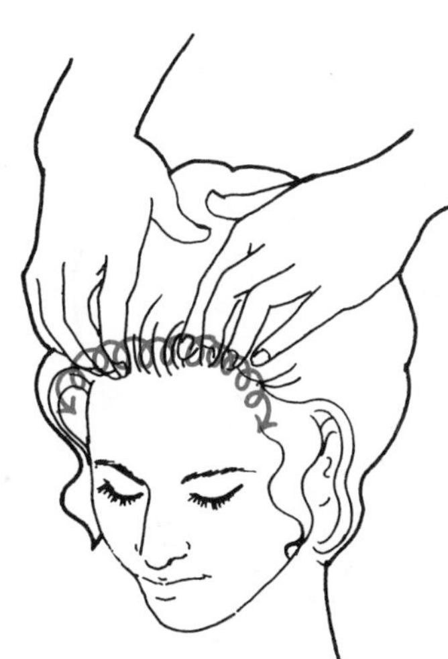

SCALP MOVEMENT. Place the palms of your hands firmly against the client's scalp. Lift the scalp in a rotary movement, first with your hands placed above the ears and then with your hands placed at the front and back of the head.

HAIRLINE MOVEMENT. Place the fingers of both hands at the client's forehead. Massage around forehead by rotating and lifting.

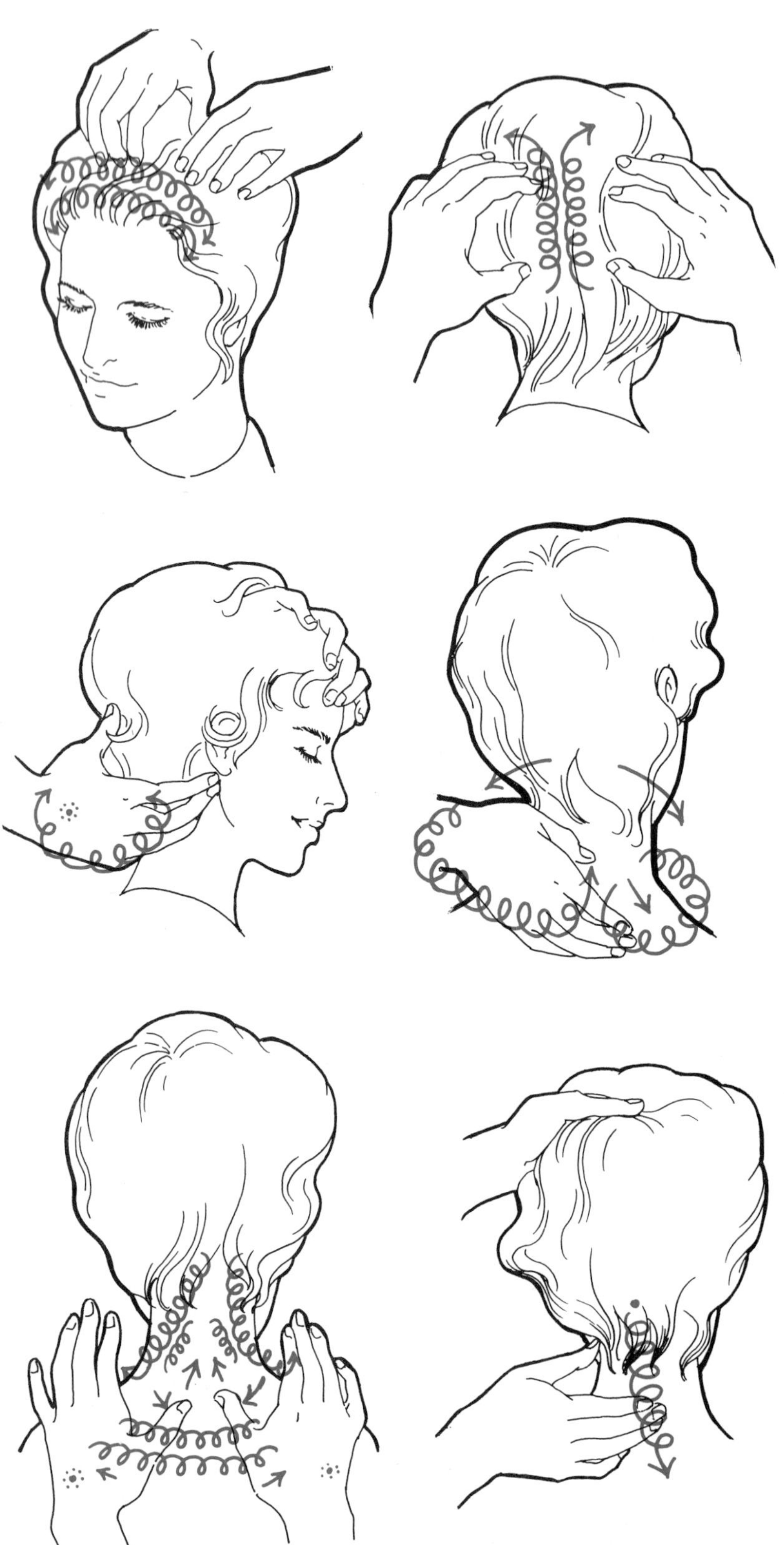

FRONT SCALP MOVEMENT. *Drop back 1″, and repeat the preceding movement over the entire front and top of the scalp.*

BACK SCALP MOVEMENT. *Place the fingers of each hand on the sides of the client's head. Starting below the ears, manipulate the scalp with your thumbs and work up to the crown. Repeat four times. Repeat thumb manipulations working towards the center of the head.*

EAR-TO-EAR MOVEMENT. *Place your left hand on the client's forehead, and massage from the right ear to the left ear along the base of the skull with a rotary movement of the palm of the hand.*

BACK MOVEMENT. *Stand to the left of the client and place your left hand on the head. Using your right hand, rotate from the base of the client's neck, along the shoulder, and back across the shoulder blade to the spine. Slide your hand up the patron's spine to the base of the neck. Repeat on the opposite side.*

SHOULDER MOVEMENT. *Place your palms together at the base of the client's neck. With a rotary movement, catch the muscles in the palms and massage along the shoulder blades to the point of the shoulder and back again. Now massage from the shoulders to the spine and back again.*

SPINE MOVEMENT. *Massage from the base of the client's skull down the spine with a rotary movement. Using firm finger pressure, bring your hand slowly to the base of the client's skull.*

TREATMENT FOR NORMAL HAIR AND SCALP

The purpose of a general scalp treatment is to keep the scalp and hair in a clean and healthy condition. Regular scalp treatments are also beneficial in preventing baldness.

Preparation

1. Assemble all materials and supplies.
2. Help the client with the salon smock.
3. Prepare the client. (Drape properly.)

Procedure

1. Brush the hair for about five minutes.
2. Apply scalp treatment or cream.
3. Apply infrared lamp for about five minutes.
4. Give scalp manipulations for 10 to 20 minutes.
5. Shampoo the hair.
6. Towel dry the hair to remove excess moisture.
7. Apply suitable scalp lotion or styling aid.
8. Style the hair.
9. Clean up your workstation.

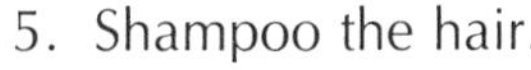

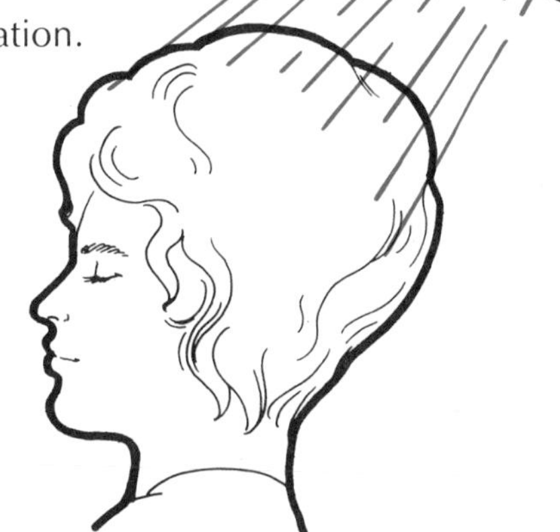

Applying heat with an infrared lamp

DANDRUFF

The principal signs of dandruff are the appearance of white scales on the hair and scalp which might be accompanied by itching of the scalp. Dandruff may be associated with either a dry or oily scalp condition. The more common causes of dandruff are poor circulation of blood to the scalp, improper diet, uncleanliness and infection.

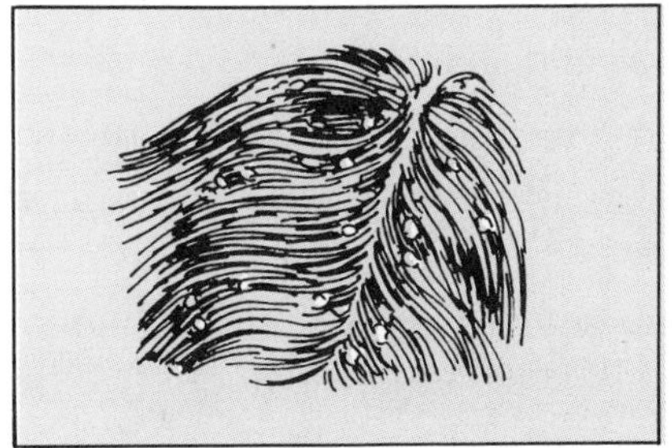

Simple dandruff

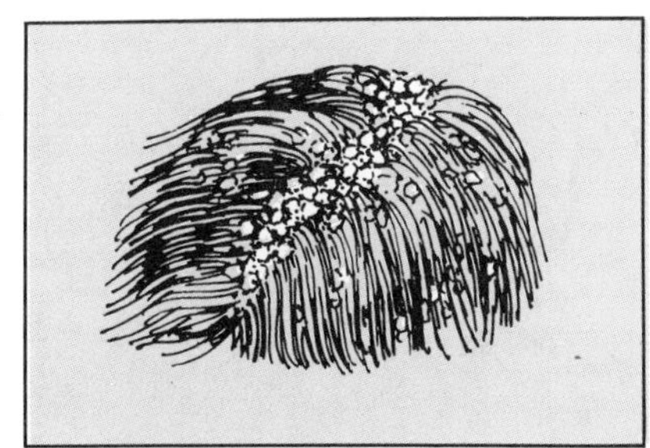

Excessive dandruff

Procedure

1. Prepare the client as for a normal scalp treatment.
2. Brush the client's hair for five minutes.
3. Apply a scalp preparation according to condition (dry or oily).
4. Apply infrared lamp for about five minutes.
5. Give scalp manipulations, using indirect high-frequency current.
6. Shampoo with corrective anti-dandruff lotion.
7. Thoroughly towel dry the hair.
8. Apply a scalp preparation suitable for the condition.
9. Clean up your work station.

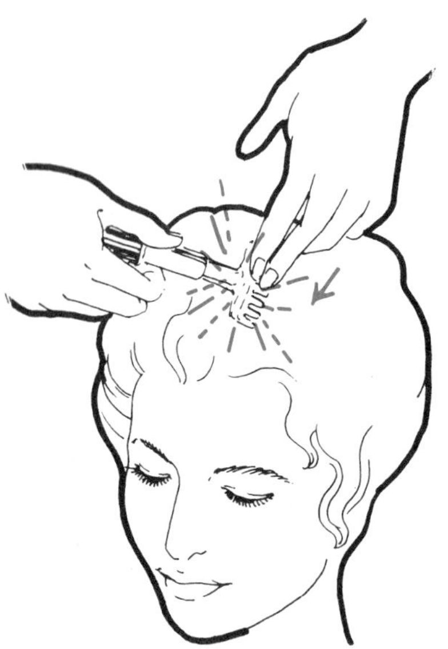

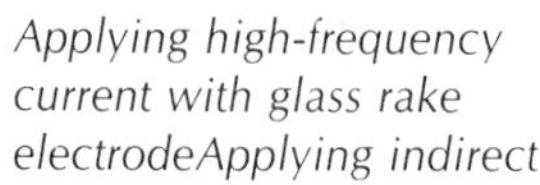

Applying high-frequency current with glass rake electrodeApplying indirect

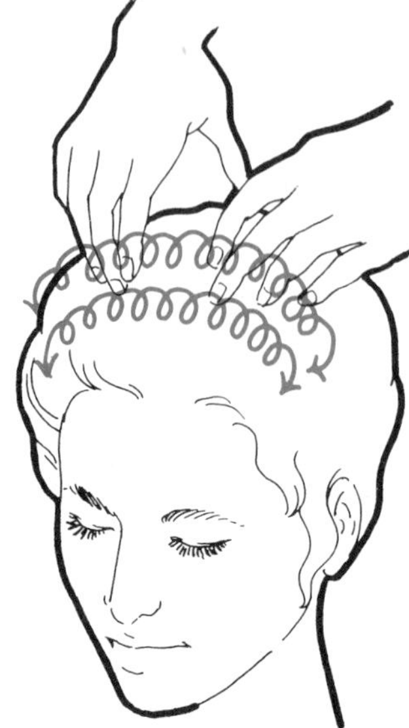

Applying indirect high-frequency current, cosmetologist manipulates the scalp...

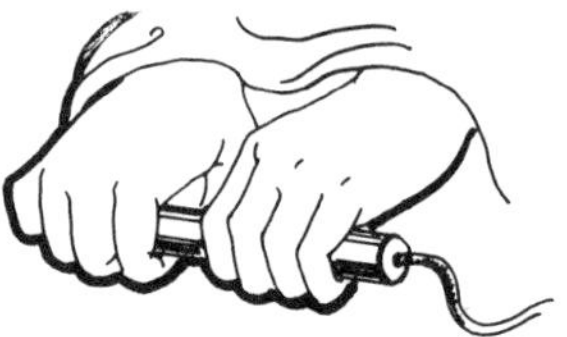

...while the client hold the metal electrode.

DRY HAIR AND SCALP TREATMENT

This treatment should be used when there is a deficiency of natural oil on scalp and hair. Select scalp preparations containing moisturizing and emollient materials. Avoid the use of strong soaps, preparations containing a mineral oil or sulfonated oil base, greasy preparations and lotions with a high alcohol content.

Procedure

1. Prepare the client as for a normal scalp treatment.
2. Brush the client's hair for about five minutes.
3. Apply preparation and gently massage into the scalp as directed by the manufacturer or your instructor.
4. Give a mild shampoo.
5. Towel dry the hair and scalp thoroughly.
6. Apply moisturizing scalp cream sparingly with a rotary, frictional motion.
7. Stimulate the scalp with direct high-frequency current, using the glass rake electrode, for about five minutes.
8. Set, dry and style the hair.
9. Clean up your workstation.

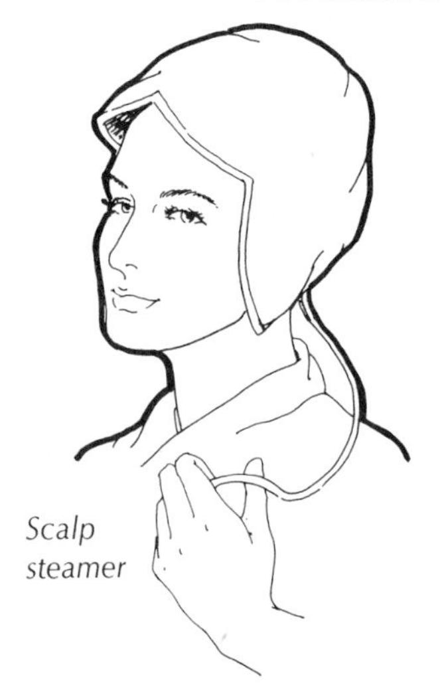

Scalp steamer

OILY HAIR AND SCALP TREATMENT

Excessive oiliness is caused by the overactivity of the sebaceous (oil) glands. Manipulate the scalp and knead it to increase blood circulation to the scalp. Any hardened sebum in the pores of the scalp will be removed with the correct degree of pressing and squeezing. To normalize the function of these glands, excess sebum should be flushed out with each treatment.

Procedure

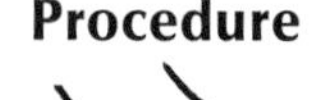

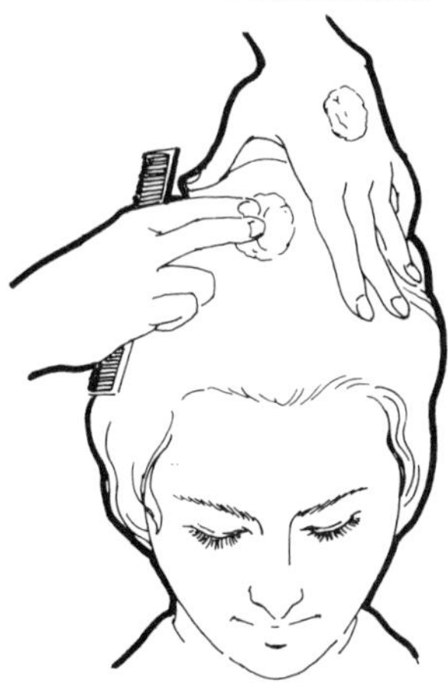

Applying scalp lotion with cotton pledget

1. Prepare the client as for a normal scalp treatment.
2. Brush the client's hair for about five minutes.
3. Apply a medicated scalp lotion to the scalp only with a cotton pledget.
4. Apply infrared lamp for about five minutes.
5. Shampoo with a corrective shampoo for oily scalp.
6. Towel dry the hair.
7. Apply direct high-frequency current for three to five minutes.
8. Apply a scalp tonic containing an astringent base.
9. Set, dry and style the hair.
10. Clean up your workstation.

Caution

Creams or ointments may be applied before using high-frequency current. Hair tonics or lotions with alcoholic content may be applied only ***after*** the application of high-frequency current.

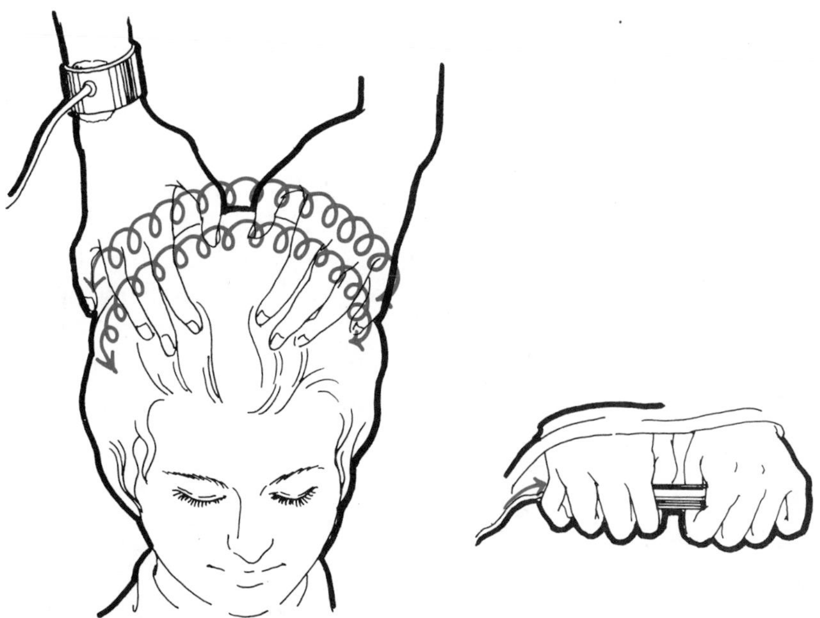

Applying faradic current. Manipulate the scalp while the client holds the electrode.

CORRECTIVE HAIR TREATMENT

A corrective hair treatment deals with the hair shaft, not the scalp. Dry and damaged hair can be greatly improved by conditioners. Hair treatments are especially beneficial and extremely important when given approximately a week or 10 days before, and a week or 10 days after, a permanent wave, tint, lightener, toner or chemical hair relaxing treatment.

Dry hair may be softened quickly with a conditioning preparation applied directly on the hair shaft. The product used for this purpose is usually an emulsion which contains cholesterol and related compounds.

Some conditioners function more effectively when heat is applied to increase penetration into the cortex. The heat applied to the hair opens the cuticle's imbrications and permits significantly more corrective agents to enter the hair. This provides more conditioning and lasting benefits.

Procedure

1. Prepare the client as you would for a normal scalp treatment.
2. Brush the client's hair for about five minutes.
3. Apply a mild shampoo.
4. Towel dry the hair.
5. Apply a conditioner according to the manufacturer's directions.
6. Clean up your workstation.

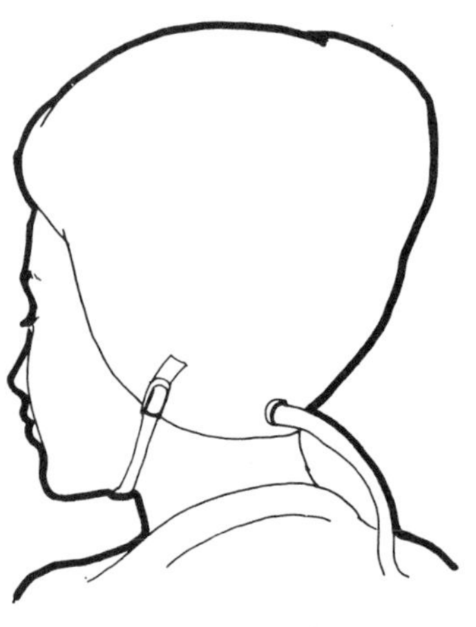

Applying heat

TREATMENT FOR ALOPECIA

Alopecia refers to a condition of premature baldness or excessive hair loss. The chief causes of alopecia are poor circulation, lack of proper stimulation, improper diet, certain infectious skin diseases, such as ringworm, or mild internal disorders. Treatment for alopecia stimulates the blood supply to the scalp and helps revive the papillae.

Procedure

1. Prepare the client as you would for a normal scalp treatment.
2. Brush the client's hair for about five minutes.
3. Apply a medicated scalp ointment as directed by a physician.
4. Apply infrared light for about five minutes.
5. Give scalp manipulations. You may use the faradic or indirect high-frequency current.
6. Use a mild shampoo.
7. Towel dry the hair.

8. Apply direct high-frequency current for about five minutes.
9. Apply medicated scalp lotion.
10. Repeat scalp manipulations; include neck, shoulders and upper back.
11. Clean up your workstation.

TREATMENTS FOR ALOPECIA AREATA

Alopecia areata (*al-o-**PE**-she a-**RE**-a-ta*) is a disorder causing baldness in spots. This condition may be treated under the direction of a physician.

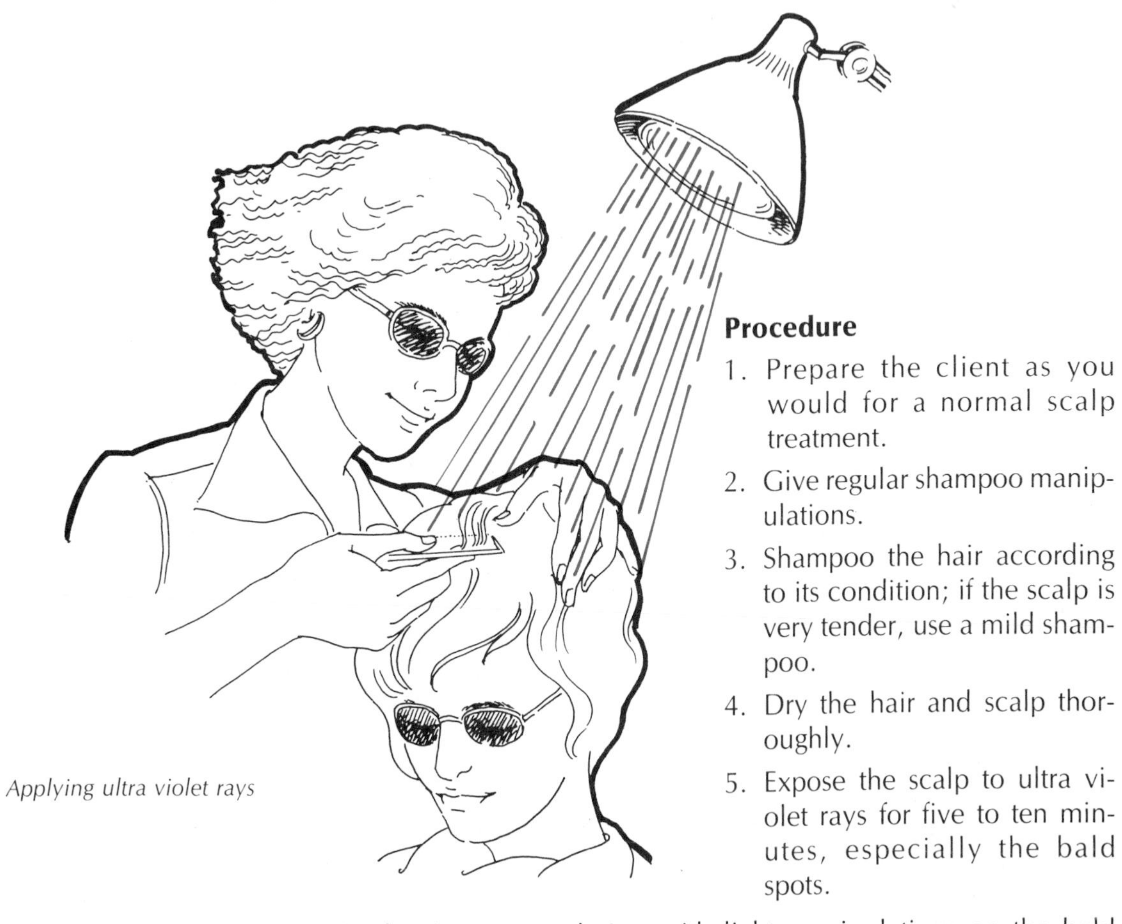

Applying ultra violet rays

Procedure

1. Prepare the client as you would for a normal scalp treatment.
2. Give regular shampoo manipulations.
3. Shampoo the hair according to its condition; if the scalp is very tender, use a mild shampoo.
4. Dry the hair and scalp thoroughly.
5. Expose the scalp to ultra violet rays for five to ten minutes, especially the bald spots.
6. Apply ointment or lotion with light manipulations on the bald spots.
7. Apply high-frequency current for about five minutes. If an ointment is used, apply direct current; if a lotion is used, apply indirect current.
8. Style the hair, using a comb only.
9. Clean up your workstation.

REMINDERS AND HINTS ON SCALP AND HAIR CARE

1. An abnormal scalp and hair condition requires very careful analysis in order to give the appropriate scalp and hair treatment.
2. Some scalp conditions might be infectious. Therefore, use only sanitized implements on clients.

REVIEW QUESTIONS

Scalp and Hair Care

1. *What is the purpose of proper scalp care and treatment?*
2. *Why is regular scalp manipulation important?*
3. *Name the normal and abnormal conditions of the scalp and hair.*
4. *How can dandruff be identified and what is its treatment?*
5. *How is a dry hair and scalp condition determined and what is its treatment?*
6. *How is an oily hair and scalp condition determined and what is its treatment?*
7. *When should corrective hair treatments be used?*
8. *What is alopecia areata and what is its treatment?*

Chapter 10

HAIR SHAPING

LEARNING OBJECTIVES

The student successfully mastering this chapter will be able to:

1. *Describe how hair shaping serves as a foundation for other professional cosmetology services.*
2. *Demonstrate the correct usage of scissors, thinning shears, razor, clippers and other implements.*
3. *Demonstrate the correct method of sectioning taught by the school.*
4. *Demonstrate the correct way to hold hair shaping implements.*
5. *Demonstrate thinning techniques with shears, razor and thinning shears.*
6. *Demonstrate basic cutting techniques with shears and razor.*
7. *Demonstrate the cutting techniques of hair tapering or shingling.*
8. *Discuss the use of clippers in hair shaping.*
9. *Demonstrate and discuss the use of the razor in hair shaping.*
10. *Gain an understanding of how to treat children and young clients.*
11. *Explain the procedure for cutting over-curly hair.*

The art and technique of hair shaping must be mastered by the student of cosmetology before he or she can be qualified to work in the better salons. Thorough instruction is required in the proper way to shape the hair, using regular scissors, thinning shears, clippers or razor. Instruction must be followed by practice under the guidance of the instructor. A good hair shaping serves as a foundation for beautiful styles. The cosmetologist's education is not complete until he or she has acquired this artistic skill and the judgment necessary for successful hair shaping.

Modern hairstyles are designed to accentuate the client's good points while minimizing the poor features. The cosmetologist must be guided by the client's wishes as well as by what is best for the client's personality. In selecting the proper hairstyle, the cosmetologist should take into consideration the person's head shape, facial contour, neckline, and hair texture as well as height, crown size, ear size, and neck length.

IMPLEMENTS USED IN HAIR SHAPING

A cosmetologist will find that the quality of the implements selected and used in hair shaping is important. To do work, the cosmetologist should buy and use only superior implements from a reliable manufacturer.

Improper use will quickly destroy the efficiency of any implement, however perfectly it might be made at the factory.

The following are the implements used in hair shaping:

Regular hair shaping scissors

Thinning shears (single- or double-notched blades)

Razors (shapers)

Hair clippers

Combs

HAIR SHAPING IMPLEMENTS

Haircutting Scissors

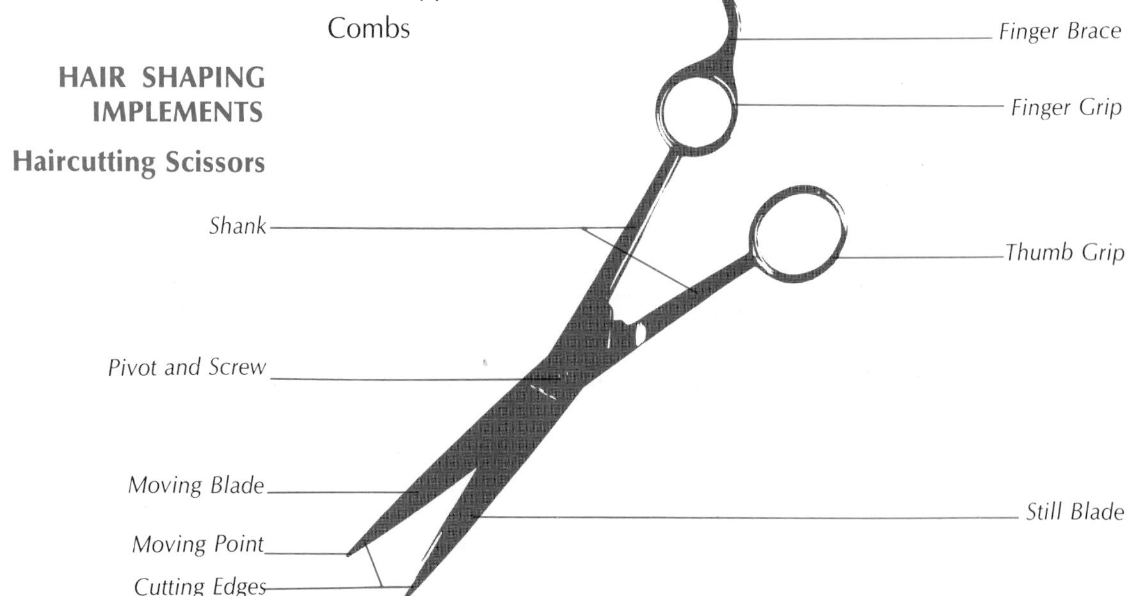

Thinning Shears

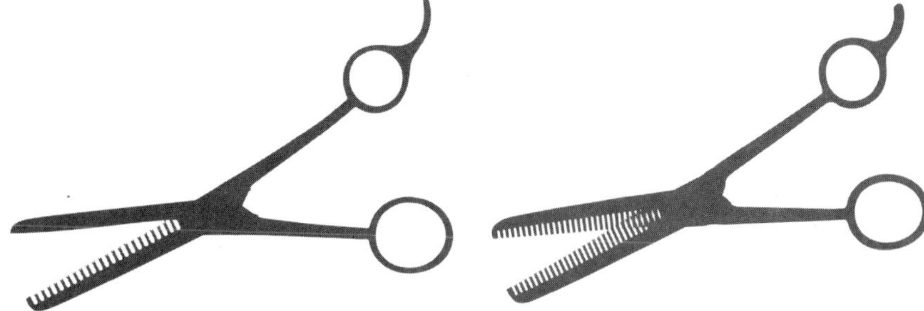

Thinning Shears—One Blade Notched   Thinning Shears—Both Blades Notched

Straight Razor

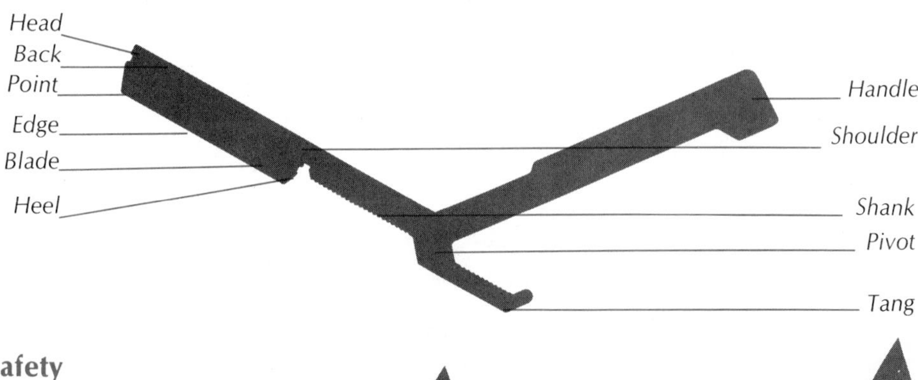

Razors with Safety Guards

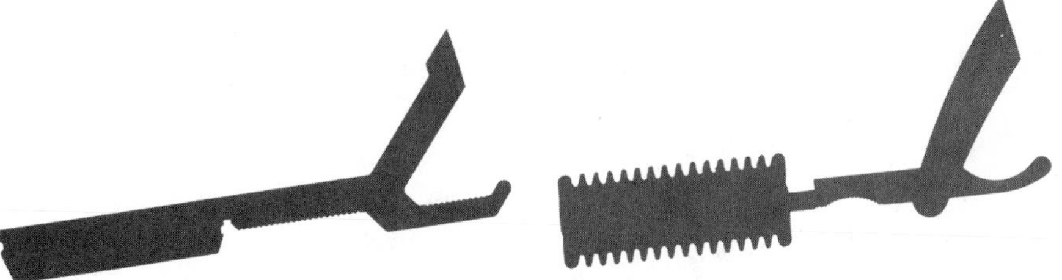

Single Edge Razor with Safety Guard   Double Edge Razor with Safety Guard

Popular Combs

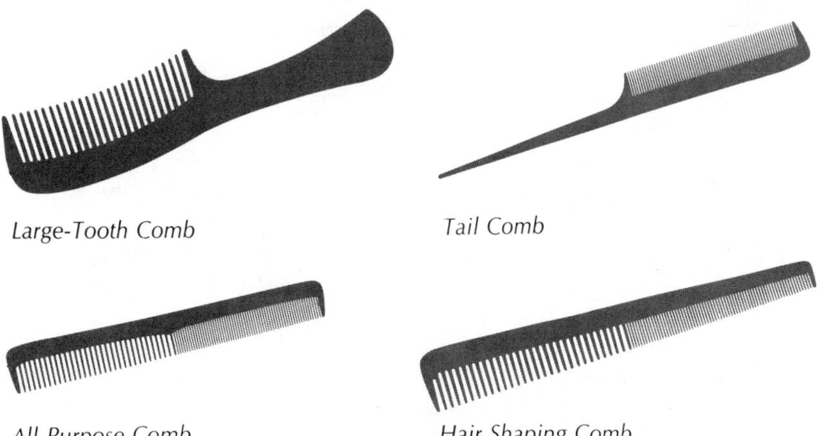

Large-Tooth Comb   Tail Comb

All-Purpose Comb   Hair Shaping Comb

SECTIONING FOR HAIR SHAPING

By following a step-by-step practical procedure, the student will soon learn how to perform a professional hair shaping. The first step is to section the hair properly. Sectioning provides a method of control and allows the natural growth patterns to show.

The following illustrations cover the practical and accepted methods for dividing the hair into either four or five sections. In any case, follow your instructor's methods for dry or wet hair shaping.

Four Section and Guideline Parting

Part hair down the center from the forehead to nape and also across the top of the head from ear to ear. Pin up the four sections and leave nape hair to use as a guide for length.

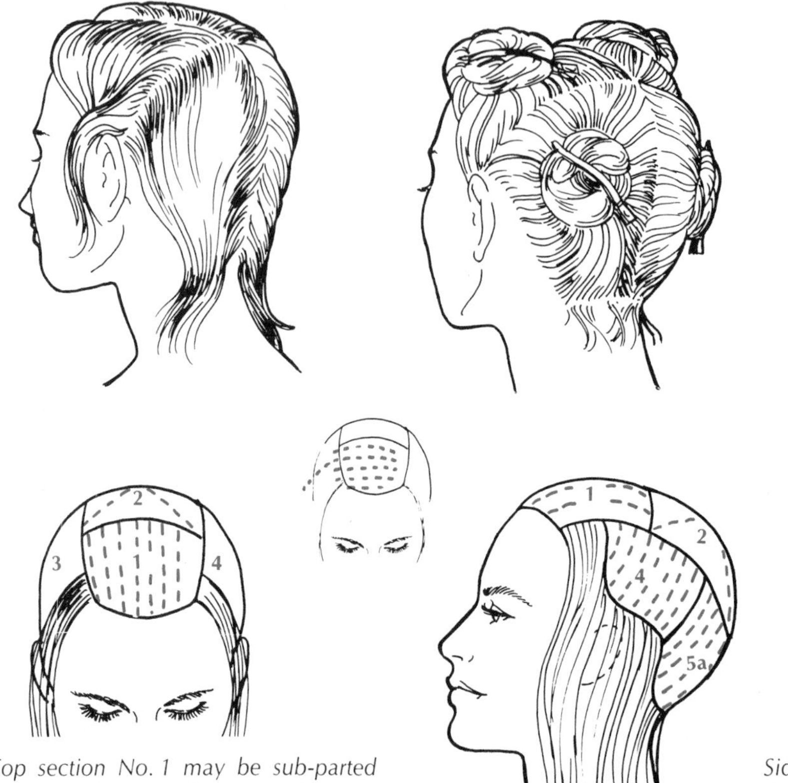

Five Section and Guideline Parting

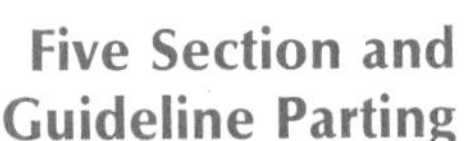

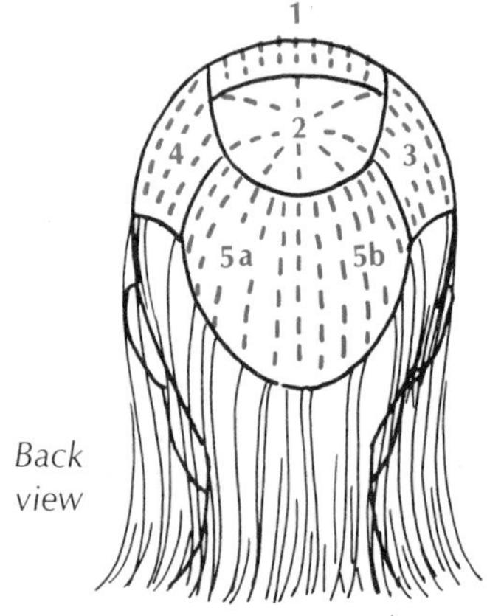

Back view

Top section No. 1 may be sub-parted either in a horizontal or vertical direction.

Side view

Five section parting, with sub-parting panels. Section and pin up the hair in the order shown in the illustrations.

The back section (No. 5) may be divided into sections No. 5a and No. 5b for easier handling.

Alternate Five Section and Guideline Method

Another way to divide the hair into five sections is to part the hair across the crown from ear to ear, then subdivide the hair in the same order as shown in the illustration.

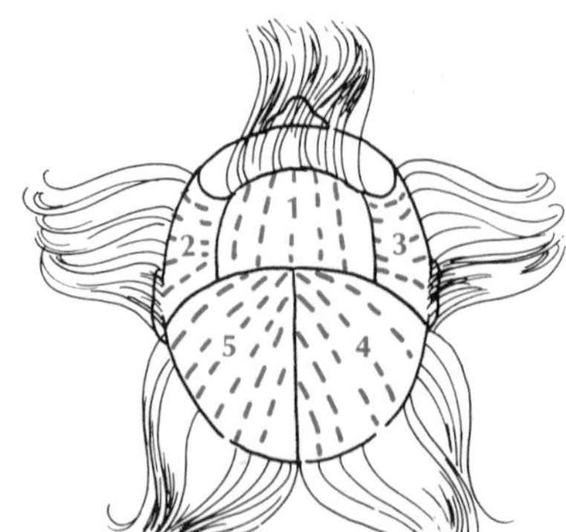

Hair divided into five sections with center back parting

HOLDING HAIR SHAPING IMPLEMENTS

Scissors

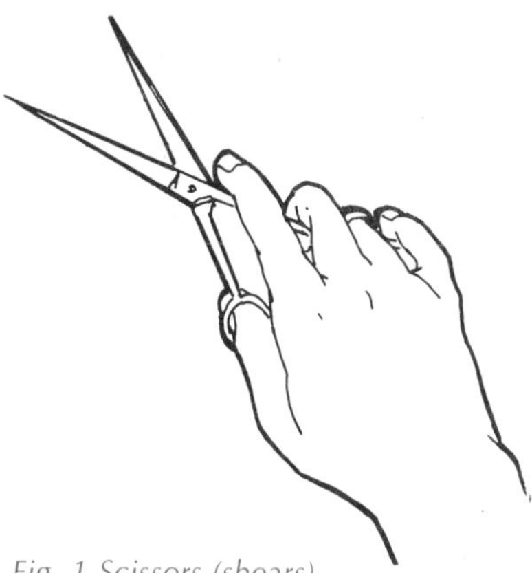

Fig. 1 Scissors (shears)

Hair shaping scissors are correctly handled by inserting the third (ring) finger into the ring of the still blade and placing the little finger on the finger brace. The thumb is inserted into the ring of the movable blade. The tip of the index finger is braced near the pivot of the scissors in order to have better control (fig. 1).

Thinning Shears

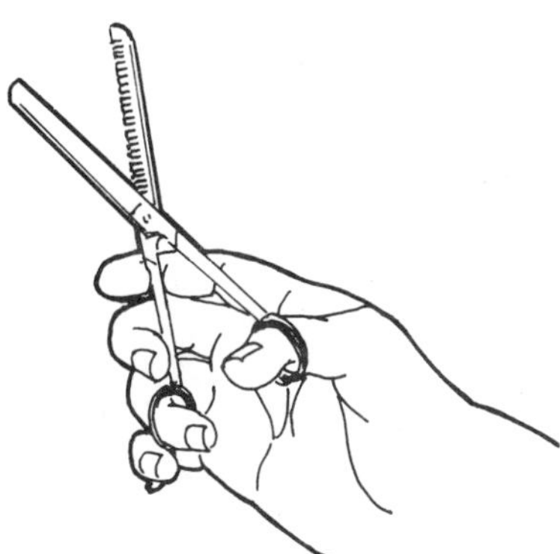

Fig. 2 Thinning shears with one blade notched

Excess bulk is removed from the hair by the use of thinning shears. As can be seen in the accompanying illustration (fig. 2), they are quite similar to hair shaping scissors, except they have one or both blades notched or serrated. The single notched edge cuts more hair. Which one is used depends on the preference of the cosmetologist. The notches help the cosmetologist control the amount of hair that is removed. Both thinning shears and shaping scissors are held in the same way.

Comb and Scissors

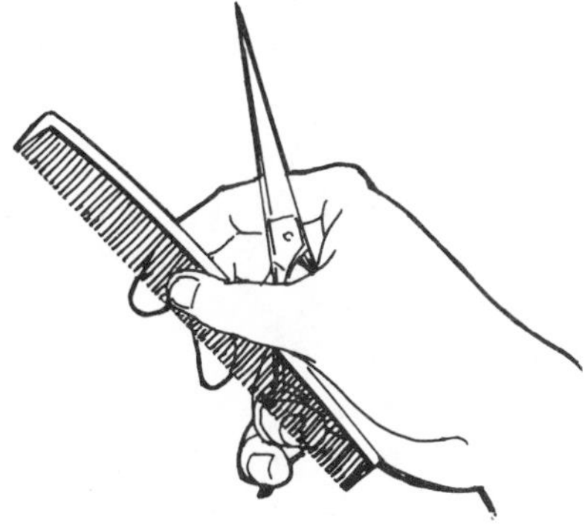

Fig. 3 Holding comb and scissors

Whenever it is necessary to use the comb during hair shaping, close the blades of the scissors, remove the thumb from the ring and rest scissors in the palm. Hold the scissors securely with the ring finger. The comb is held with thumb and fingers (fig. 3).

Note When combing the hair, hold comb and scissors in the right hand, as shown in fig. 3. When shaping (cutting) the hair, hold the comb in the left hand. To speed up hair shaping, do not lay down comb or scissors.

HAIR THINNING

The purpose of thinning the hair is to remove excess bulk without shortening the hair length. For best results, follow these suggestions:

1. When using a razor for thinning or shaping, first dampen the hair.
2. When using thinning razors or regular scissors, the hair may be either either dry or damp.

The **hair texture** determines the point where thinning should start on the hair strand. As a rule, fine hair may be thinned closer to the scalp than coarse hair, because if coarse hair is thinned too close to the scalp, the short, stubby ends will protrude through the top layer. On the other hand, fine hair is softer and more pliable and when cut very short, it will lay flatter on the head.

How much to thin depends on the particular hairstyle to be created and the amount of bulk to be removed. As a guide, start thinning different textures of hair as follows:

1. Fine hair—1/2″ to 1″ (1.25 to 2.5 cm) from the scalp.
2. Medium hair—1″ to 1 1/2″ (2.5 cm to 3.75 cm) from the scalp.
3. Coarse hair—1 1/2″ to 2″ (3.75 to 5 cm) from the scalp.

Hair Thinning Areas

There are several areas where it is not advisable to thin the hair:

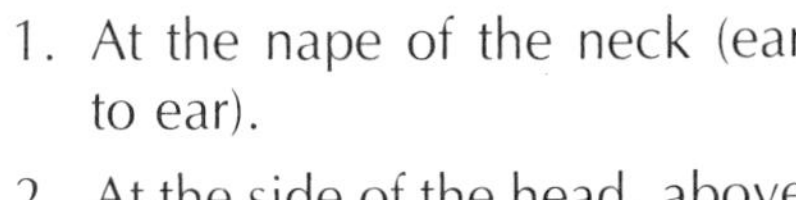

1. At the nape of the neck (ear to ear).
2. At the side of the head, above the ears.
3. Around facial hairline. Usually hair is not heavy at hairline.
4. In the hair part. The cut ends would be seen in the finished hairstyle.

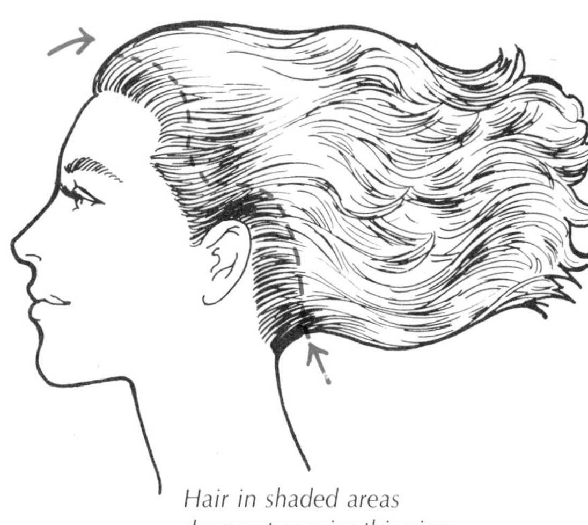

Hair in shaded areas does not require thinning

Note

Never thin the hair near the ends of a strand; to do so will render the hair shapeless. Do not thin hair prior to a permanent wave because hair will be difficult to wrap and the perm may damage unprotected ends.

Caution

Greater care must be exercised to avoid removing too much hair in the thinning process. Once the hair has been cut, it is impossible to replace it and it is probable that it might become impossible to develop the desired hairstyle.

Thinning with Thinning Shears

When using the thinning shears, grip the hair firmly between the middle and index finger.

Procedure

1. Pick up a strand of hair from 1/2″ to 1″ (1.25 to 2.5 cm) wide by 2″ to 3″ (5 to 7.5 cm) long, depending on its texture.
2. Hold the strand straight out from the scalp between the middle and index fingers.
3. Place thinning shears 1″ to 2″ (2.5 to 5 cm) from the scalp, depending upon texture.
4. Cut the strand by partly closing the thinning shears 3/4″ through the strand (fig. 4).
5. Move out another 1 1/2″ (3.75 cm) and cut again.
6. Repeat again if the hair is long enough.

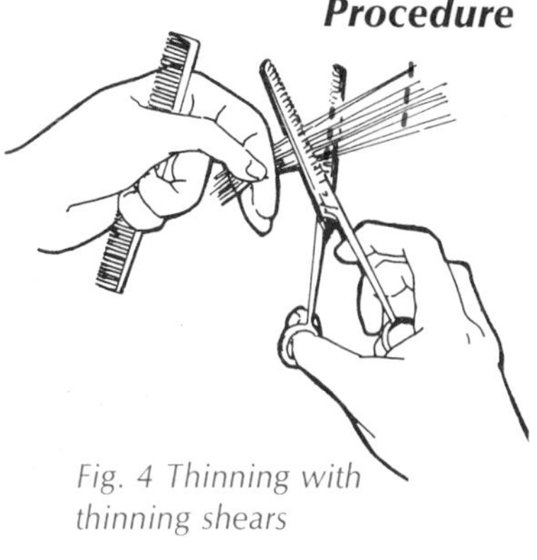

Fig. 4 Thinning with thinning shears

Note It is advisable to avoid thinning the top part of the strand so that the longer style length will provide a smooth finished surface.

Thinning with Haircutting Scissors (Shears)

When using regular haircutting scissors to thin the hair, pick up smaller sections of hair than when using the thinning shears. The technique also changes. This process of thinning with scissors is known as **slithering.**

Procedure

1. Hold a strand of hair straight out between the middle and index finger.
2. Place the hair in the scissors so that only the underneath hair will be cut.
3. Start with the scissors about 1″ to 1 1/2″ (2.5 to 3.75 cm) from the scalp and close scissors lightly as they are moved toward the scalp (fig. 5).
4. Repeat this procedure twice on each strand.

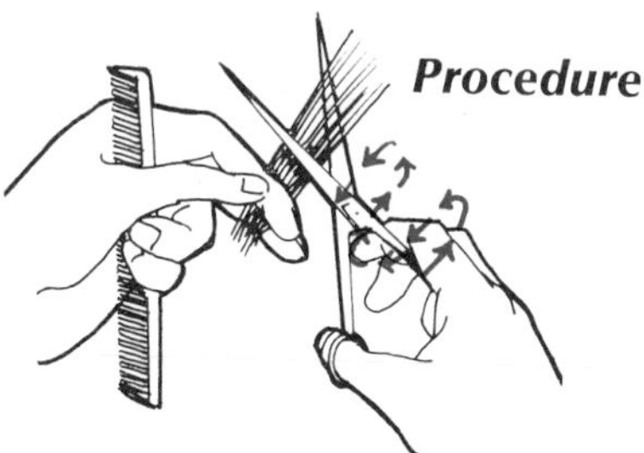

Fig. 5 Thinning with haircutting scissors (shears)

Note Alternate method of holding the hair is with the thumb and index finger (fig. 6).

Back combing. The short hair may be back combed and then slithered as shown in fig. 7. This removes the least amount of bulk.

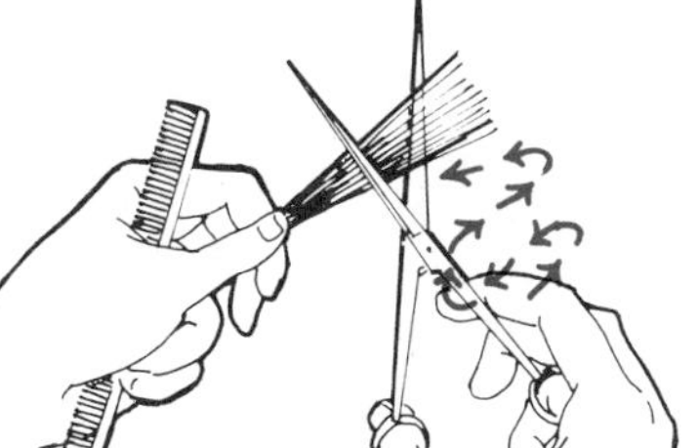

Fig. 6 Holding the hair with thumb and index finger

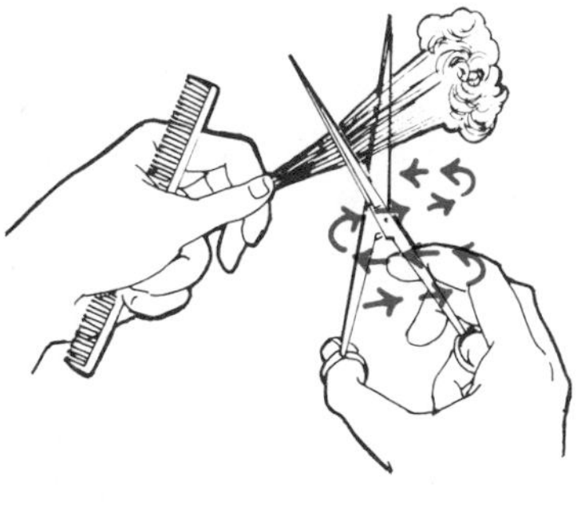

Fig. 7 Slithering the hair after back combing

HAIR SHAPING WITH SCISSORS

Scissors hair shaping may be done on either wet or dry hair.

Wet shaping. The hair may be shaped immediately after it has been shampooed. Most hair is shaped in this manner.

Dry shaping. If the hair is shaped while dry, it is usually shampooed after the shape is completed.

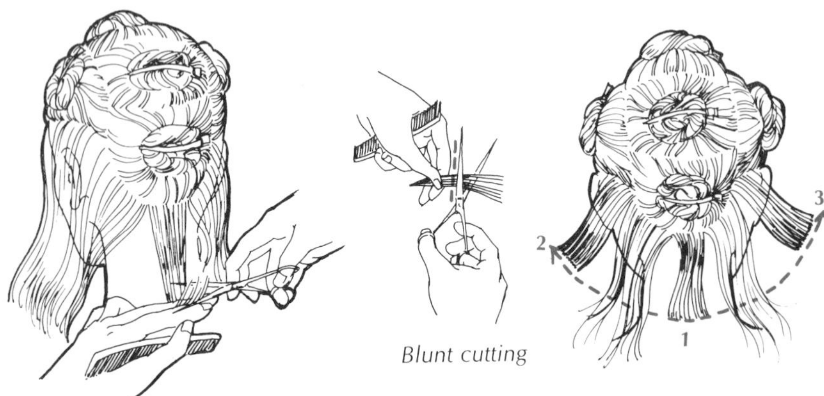

Fig. 8 Blunt cutting strand at center nape to desired length

Fig. 9 Following up by cutting all remaining guideline hair

Preparation

1. Seat the client; adjust the neck strip and plastic cape.
2. Examine the head shape, facial features and hair texture.
3. Comb and brush the hair free of tangles.
4. Shaping may be done on dry or damp hair.

Procedure

1. Divide the hair into four or five sections.
2. Determine the length of the nape guideline hair.
3. Blunt cut the guideline strand of nape hair (fig. 8).
   a) Blunt cut the strand on the left side, using the earlobe as a guide at 0° or 45° angle (fig. 9).
   b) Blunt cut the strand on the right side to match the left side (fig. 9).
   c) Blunt cut from the back center to the left front.
   d) Blunt cut from the back center to the right front. For a completed guideline, see fig. 10.

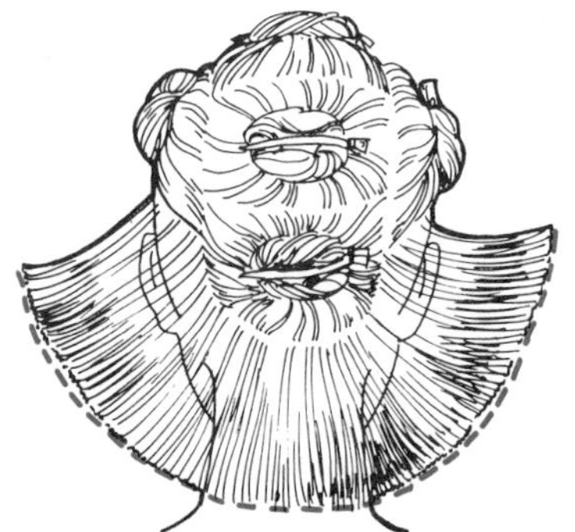

Fig. 10 Properly cut guideline hair

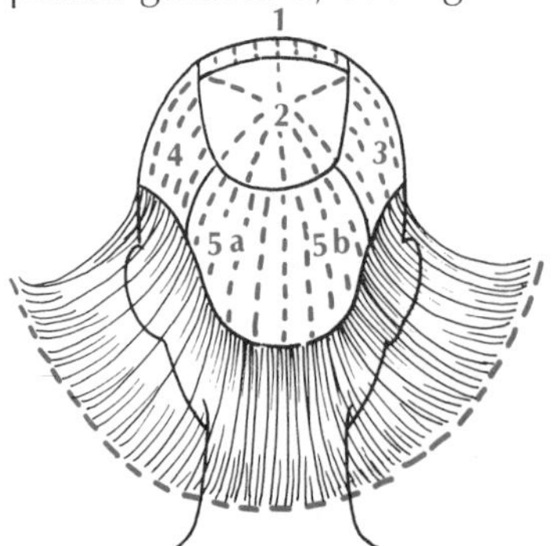

Fig. 11 Divide section No. 5 into two equal parts

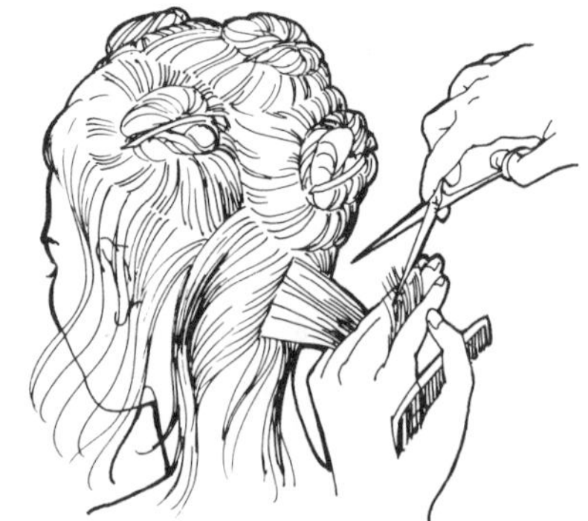

Fig. 12 Blunt cutting section No. 5b

Let down section No. 5 and divide it into two equal parts (No. 5a and No. 5b). Match the length with the guideline hair. Either the left or right side may be done first (fig. 11). Hold the hair out from the head while blunt shaping (fig. 12). Continue cutting sections No. 3 and No. 4 in the same manner.

Crown Section

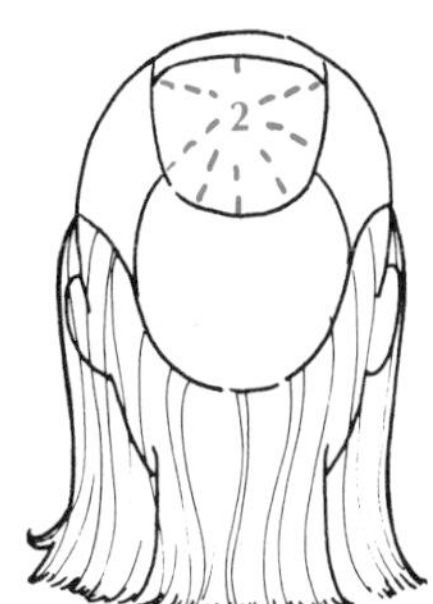

Fig. 13 Crown section

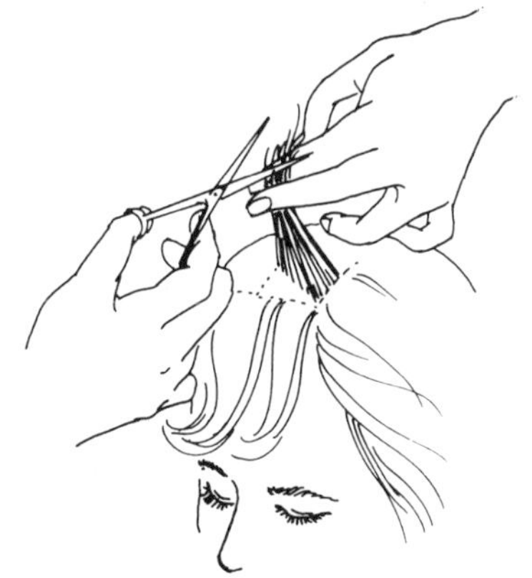

Fig. 14 Shaping crown section

Crown Section No. 2. Hold a pie-shaped section out from the head; match the length by picking up the strands from the section already cut. Continue around the head, matching the length with the side and back hair (figs. 13 & 14).

Top Section

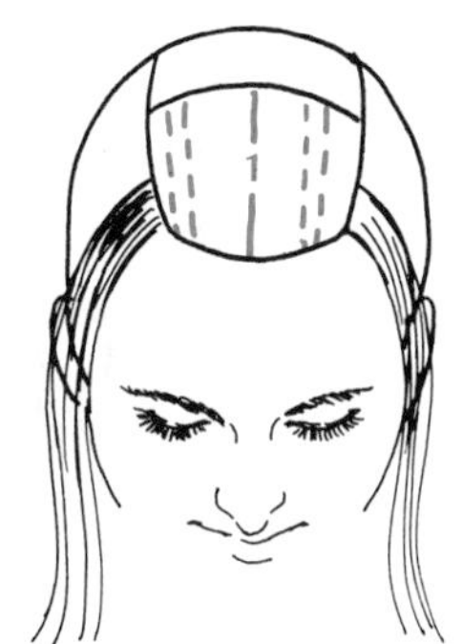

Fig. 15 Top view. Section No. 1 with vertical partings

Divide section No. 1 into two parts. Pick up the hair from the middle of the section, using the previously cut hair as a guide. Maintain the hand movement in a 45° (.785 rad.) arc. Cut both parts of section No. 1 in the prescribed manner (figs. 15 & 16).

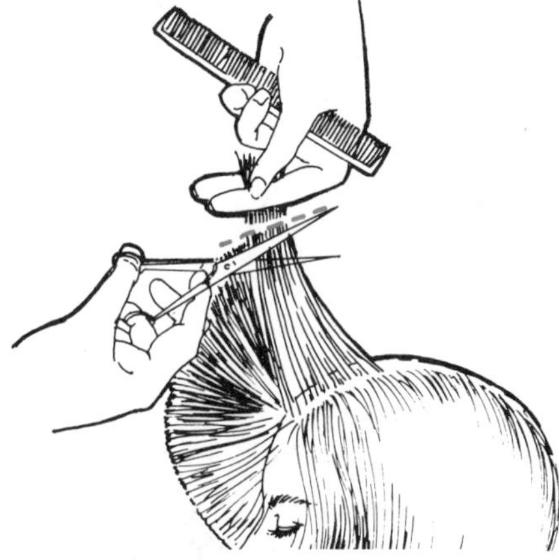

Fig. 16 Shaping top section

If **bangs** are to be cut, move from the side to directly in front of the client for even cutting. Test the hair for bounce (elasticity), then determine the desired length. If the bangs are to be short, use the bridge of the nose as a guide and hold the hair without too much tension. If the style is to be long, shape the strands to blend into the length of the sides.

Reducing bulk. To complete the hair shaping, remove excess bulk by thinning or texturizing with a razor, thinning shears or scissors. It is recommended that all hair be checked for proper length.

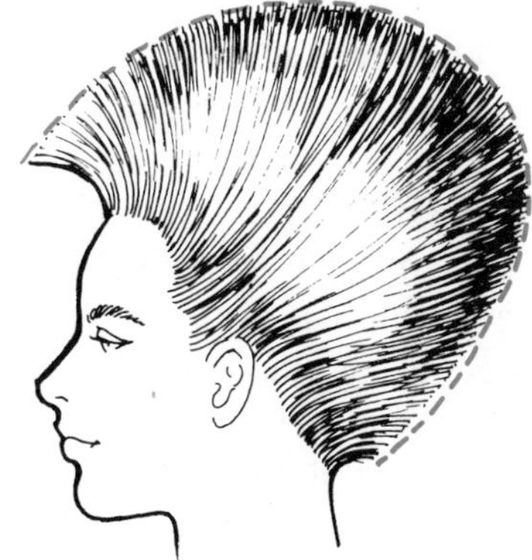

Correct uniform shaping

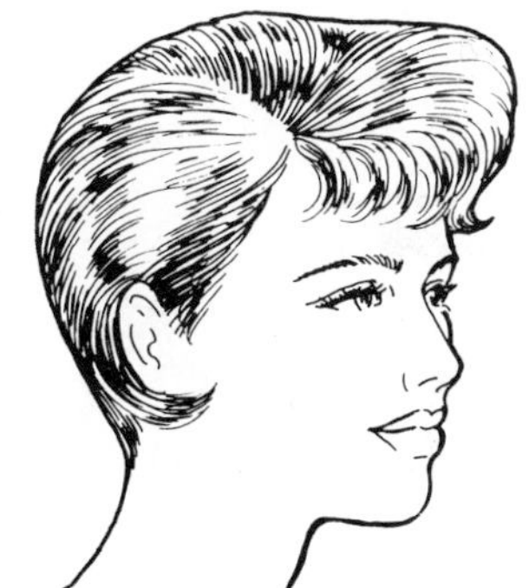

Completed shaping with bang effect and/or off-face style

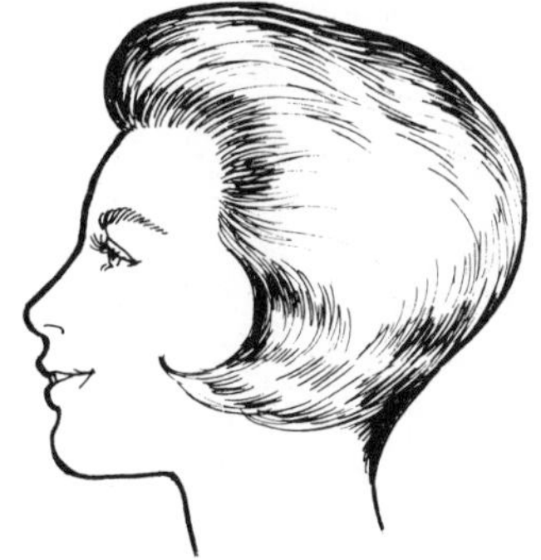

Hair shaping for straight back style

Completion

Remove the neck strip and plastic cape. Thoroughly clean all hair clippings from the cape, the client's clothing and the work area. You may then proceed with the next service.

TAPERING (SHINGLING)

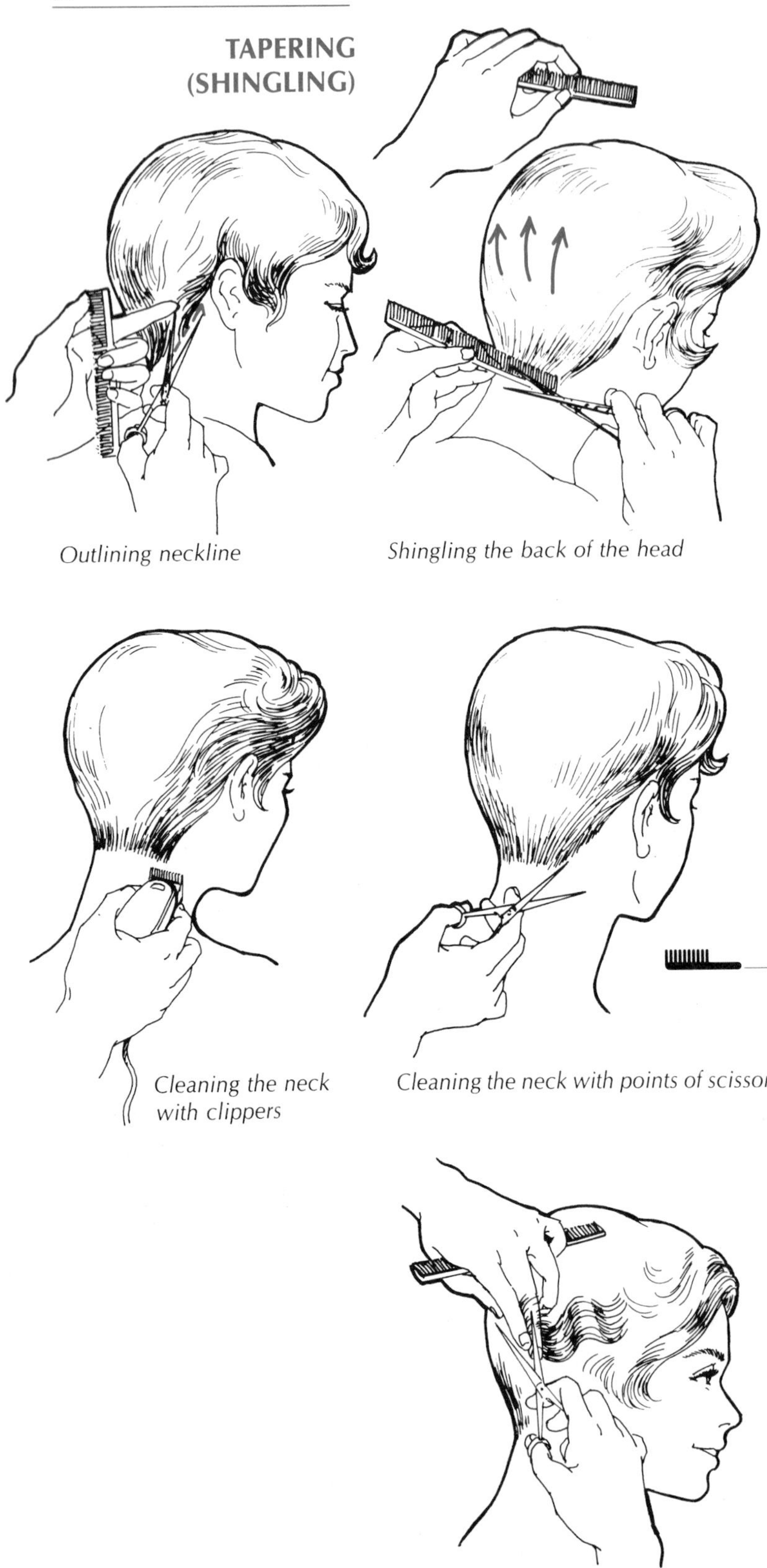

Outlining neckline

Shingling the back of the head

Cleaning the neck with clippers

Cleaning the neck with points of scissors

Removing hair ends

Regardless of the prevailing hair fashion, there always will be a number of clients who want their hair cut short. To satisfy these clients, you must know how to taper (shingle) the hair. **Tapering** (shingling) is cutting the hair close at the nape and gradually allowing it to get longer toward the crown without showing a definite line. The accompanying illustrations show how tapering (shingling) is accomplished with the use of shears and comb.

Procedure

Tapering or shingling should be done at eye level. Starting at the napeline, cut the hair upward in a graduated effect. After reaching the tip of the section being tapered or shingled, turn the comb downward and comb the hair. Proceed, section by section, until the entire back of the head is tapered or shingled in a smooth, uniform manner.

Note

In tapering or shingling, the blades of the scissors are held parallel with the comb; only the top blade moves and does the cutting.

USING CLIPPERS

There is a mistaken notion that the use of clippers to clean the neckline has a tendency to make the hair grow thicker on the neck. This is not true, because the amount of human hair can only be as great as the number of follicles in the area, and these do not increase in number with the use of clippers or any other implements.

USING A RAZOR

The successful cosmetologist must be able to handle all implements efficiently, including the straight razor.

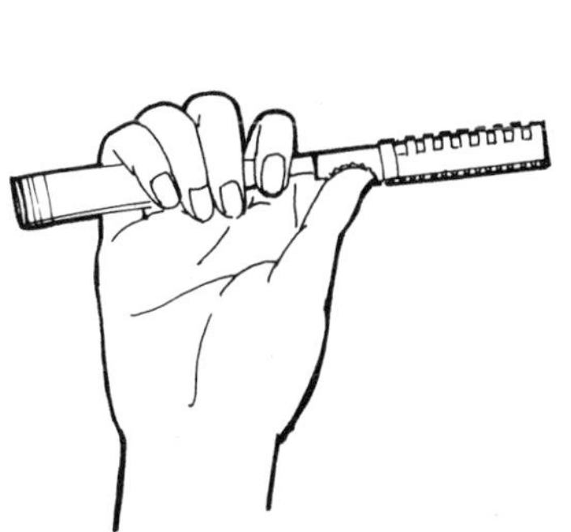
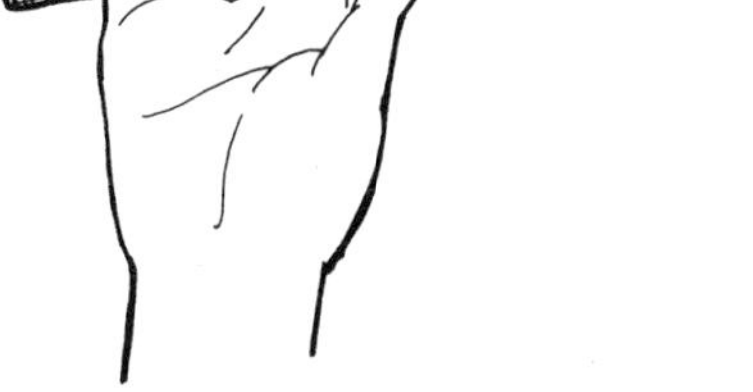
Fig. 17 Finger wrap hold

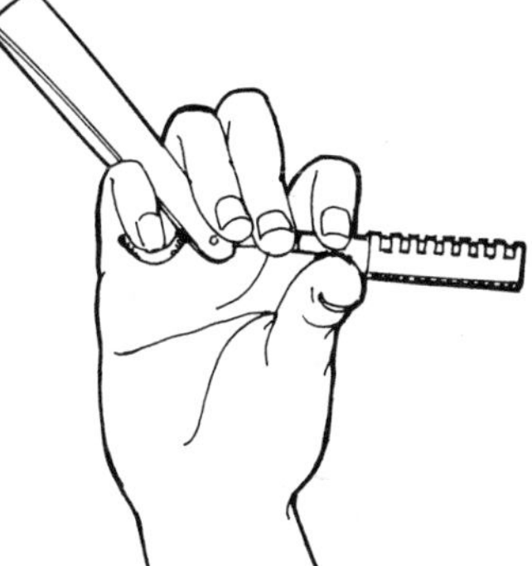
Fig. 18 Three finger hold

Fig. 19 Holding razor and comb

How to Hold the Razor

Finger wrap hold. Place the thumb in the groove of the shank and fold the fingers over the handle of the razor. The guard faces the cosmetologist while working (fig. 17).

Three finger hold. Place three fingers over the shank, the thumb in the groove of the shank and the little finger in the hollow part of the tang (fig. 18).

Note

When combing the hair, hold the razor and comb in the right hand (fig. 19). When shaping the hair with a razor, hold the comb in the left hand. Do not put the comb or razor down.

When using the razor, keep the hair damp to avoid pulling the hair and prevent dulling the razor.

Changing Blades

Removing old blade. Remove the guard. With the left hand, hold the shaper firmly above the joint. Catch the blade in the teeth of the upper part of the guard and push out the blade (fig. 20).

Inserting new blade. Slide the blade into the groove, pushing the end with your fingers. Place the tooth end of the guard into the blade notch and slide in the blade until it clicks into position (fig. 21).

Slide the guard over the blade, making sure the free or open end is over the cutting edge of the blade (fig. 22).

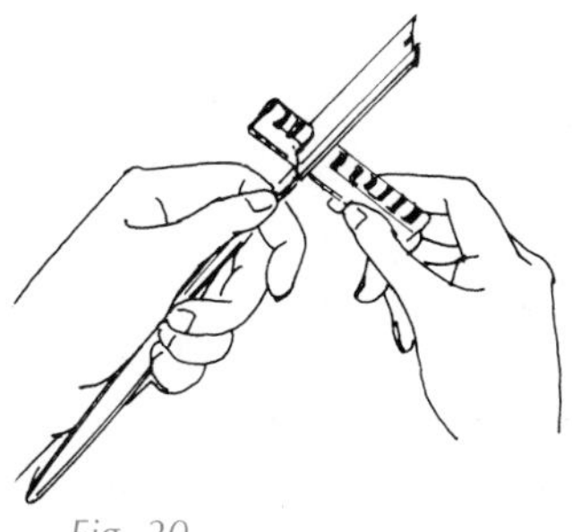
Fig. 20

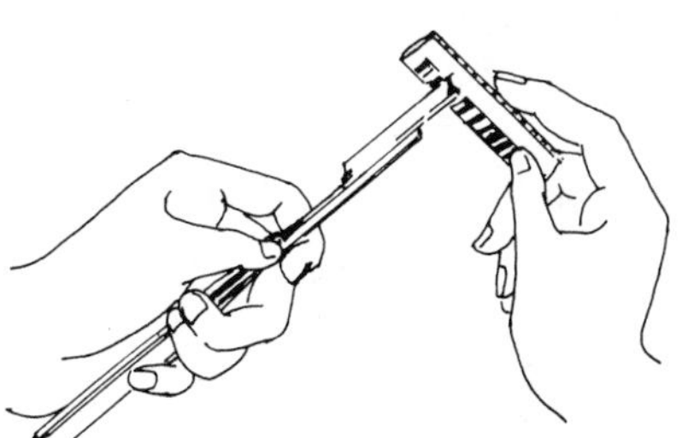
Fig. 21

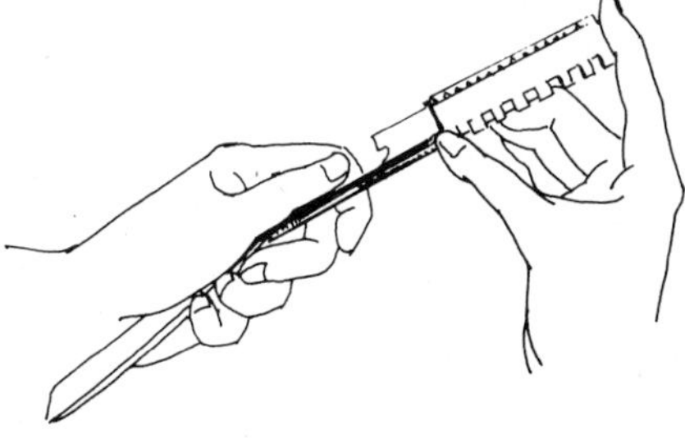
Fig. 22

THINNING WITH RAZOR

Hold out a strand of wet hair between the middle and index fingers. Place the razor flat, **not erect,** about 1″ to 2″ (2.5 to 5 cm) from the scalp (depending on the hair texture), and use short, light, steady strokes toward the hair ends.

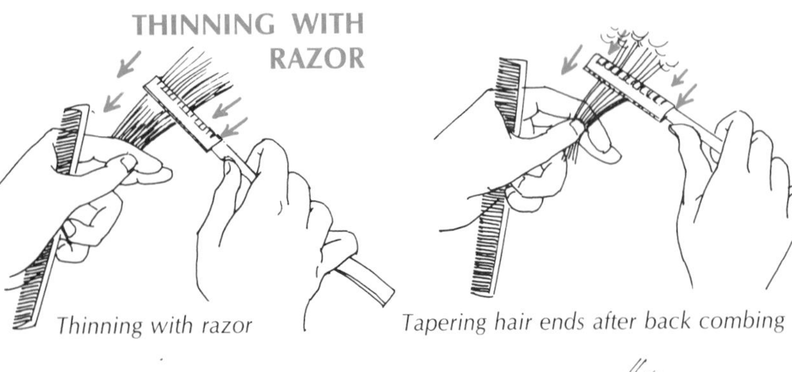

Thinning with razor *Tapering hair ends after back combing*

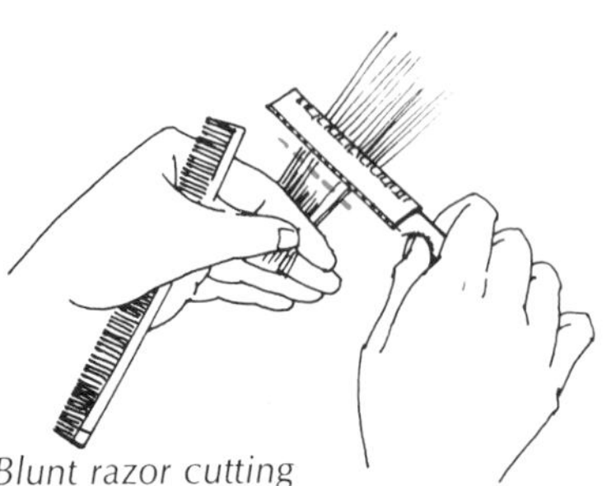

Blunt razor cutting

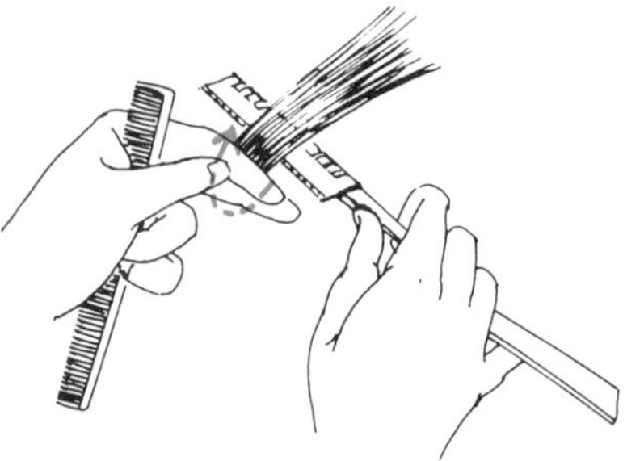

Razor under cutting with upward stroke

HAIR SHAPING WITH RAZOR

Preparation

1. Seat the client; adjust the neck strip and plastic cape.
2. Examine the head shape, facial features and hair texture.
3. Comb and brush the hair free of tangles.
4. Shampoo or wet the hair.

Procedure

1. Divide the hair into five sections.
2. Determine the length of the nape guideline hair.
3. Blunt cut the guideline of nape hair (fig. 23).
   a) Blunt cut on the left side; use the earlobe as guide (fig. 24).
   b) Blunt cut on the right side to match the left side (fig. 24).
   c) Use the guideline hair to cut from the back center to the left front and back center to the right front (fig. 24).
   d) Completed guideline (fig. 25).

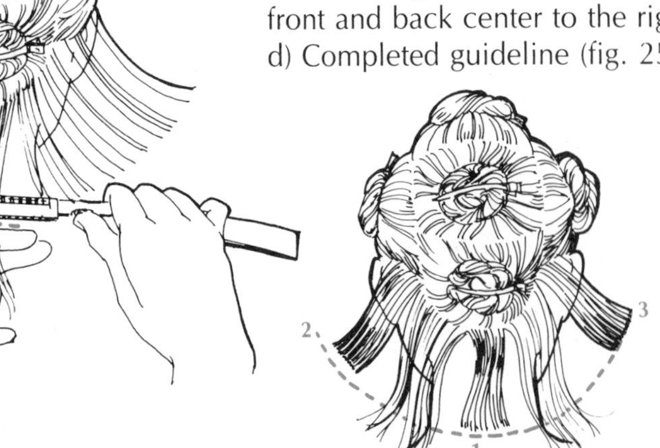

Fig. 23 Blunt cutting a strand at the center nape for desired hair length

Fig. 24 Following up by cutting all remaining guideline hair

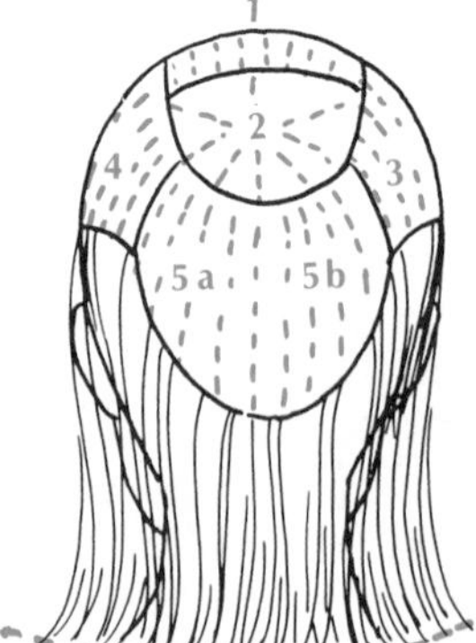

Fig. 25 Completed guideline

Shaping back section (5a, 5b). Divide section No. 5 into two parts (sections No. 5a and No. 5b). From the center of section No. 5a, pick horizontal strands. Pick up a guideline strand for length. When the guideline hair falls away, cut the hair, moving the hands out and upward into a 45° (.785 rad.) angle.

Shaping section 4. Proceed to cut to the left into section No. 4 in the same manner.

Shaping section 3. Return to section No. 5b and cut this section, moving to the right into section No. 3, always lifting hands in an upward 45° (.785 rad.) arc as the hair is cut. **Measure carefully with the guideline hair.**

Shaping section 2. Next, proceed to cut section No. 2 (crown), using previously cut hair as a guide.

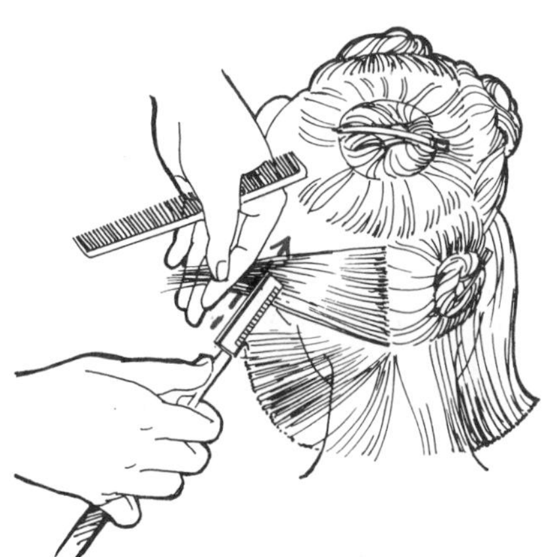

Sections 5A and 5B

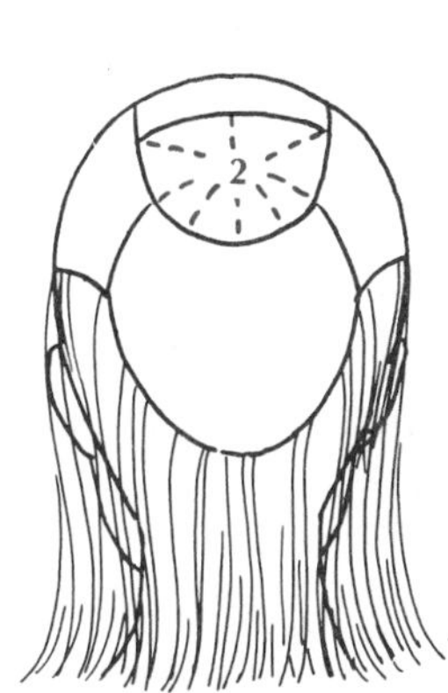

Section No. 2

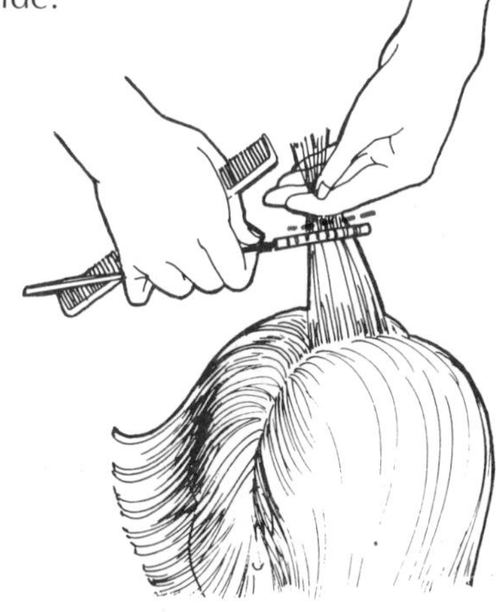

Shaping section No. 2

Shaping section 1. Divide section No. 1 into two parts. Pick up hair from the middle of the section, using previously cut hair as a guide. Maintain the hand movement in a 45° (.785 rad.) arc. Proceed to cut both parts of section No. 1 in the prescribed manner.

Bangs. To cut bangs evenly, move your position from the side to directly in front of the client. Test hair for bounce (elasticity), then determine the desired length. If the bangs are to be short, use the bridge of the nose as a guide. If the style is to be long, shape bangs to blend into the length of the sides.

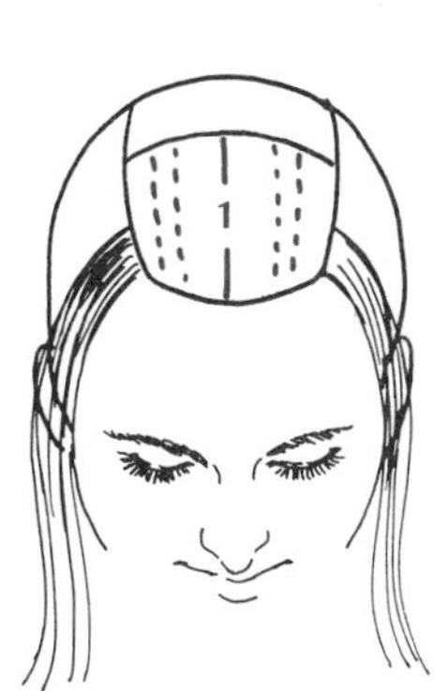

Section No. 1 shown with vertical parting

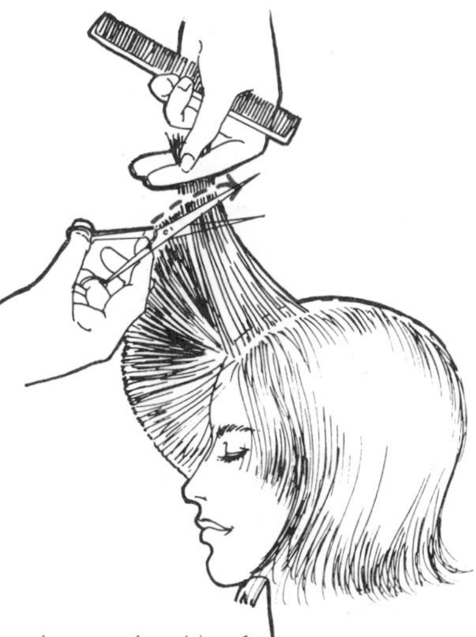

Shaping section No. 1

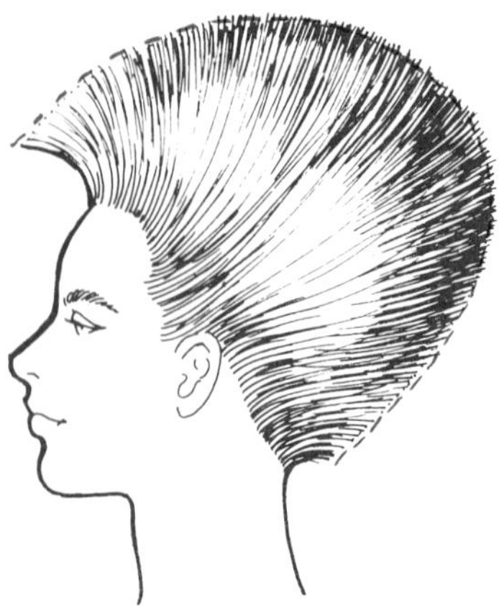

Correct uniform shaping

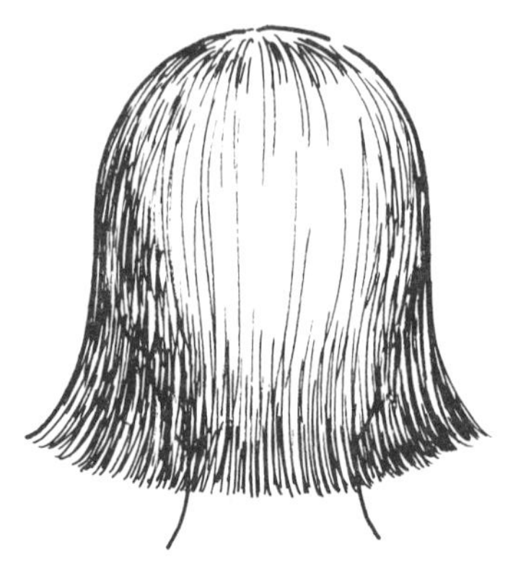

Back view—uniform shaping

Reducing bulk. To complete shaping the hair, remove excess bulk by thinning with a razor, thinning shears or scissors. It is recommended that all hair be checked for proper length.

Completion. Remove the neck strip and plastic cape. Thoroughly clean all hair clippings from the cape, client's clothing and work area. You may then proceed with the next professional service desired by the client.

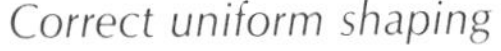

Note Cutting the hair properly serves as a foundation for a variety of beautiful hairstyles.

LEARN HOW TO HANDLE CHILDREN

Special consideration should be given to children and teenagers. Hairstylists who know how to handle children usually will attract the mothers to their salons for their own hairstyling.

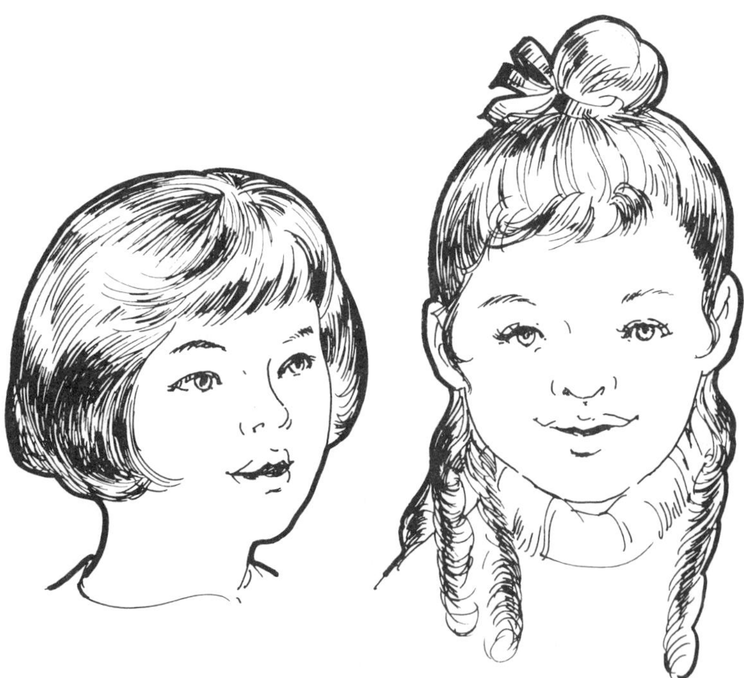

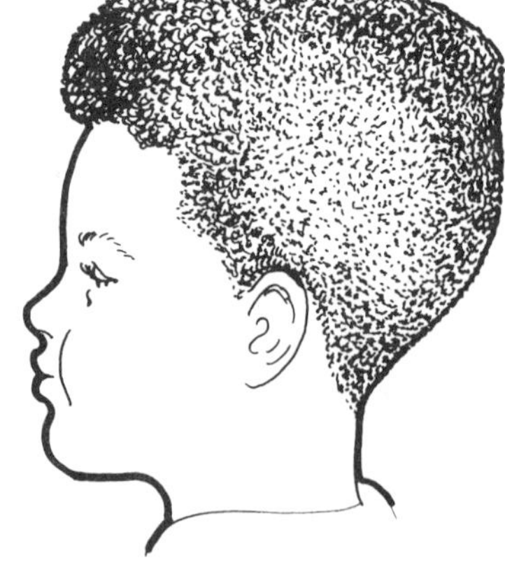

Popular hairstyles for youngsters

SHAPING OVER-CURLY HAIR

Over-curly hair has its own particular characteristics, as have the other types of hair, which require special techniques for styling. Of prime importance to the hairstylist is the ability to create a hairstyle that will enhance the appearance of the client and to visualize how the finished hairstyle will look. Knowing the correct shaping and styling techniques and using common sense in their application are basic to the success of the hairstylist.

The steps outlined below represent one method of shaping and styling over-curly hair. Where your instructor's methods differ, follow those techniques.

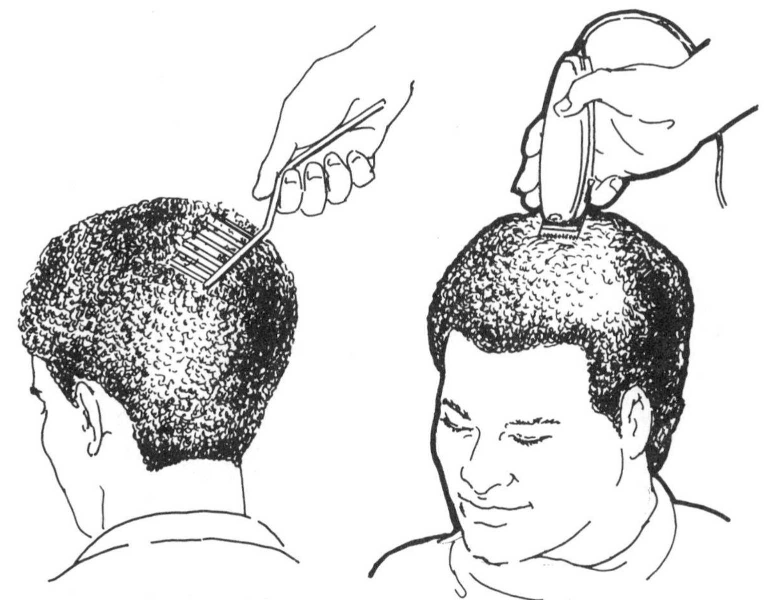

Combing hair upward with hair lifter *Shaping hair to desired length*

Procedure

1. Drape the client for hair shaping.
2. Shampoo and dry the hair thoroughly.
3. Apply an emollient product lightly to the scalp and hair to replace lost oil.
4. Using a wide-tooth comb or hair lifter, comb the hair upward and slightly forward, making the hair as long as possible. Start at the crown and continue until all hair has been combed out from the scalp and distributed evenly around the head. Combing in a circular pattern will usually help avoid splits.
5. Shape the hair. Visualize the style and length desired. Start by tapering the sides and cut in the direction the hair will be combed.

6. Taper the back part of the hair to blend with the sides.
7. Trim extreme hair ends of the crown and top areas to the desired length.
8. For an off-the-face hairstyle, comb the hair up and backward. For forward movement, comb the hair up and forward.
9. Blend the side hair with the top, crown and back hair.
10. Outline the hairstyle at the sides, around the ears and in the nape area, using either scissors or a trimmer (clipper).
11. Give a finishing touch. Fluff the hair slightly with a hair lifter, wherever needed. Spray the hair lightly to give it a natural, lustrous sheen.

POPULAR HAIRSTYLES

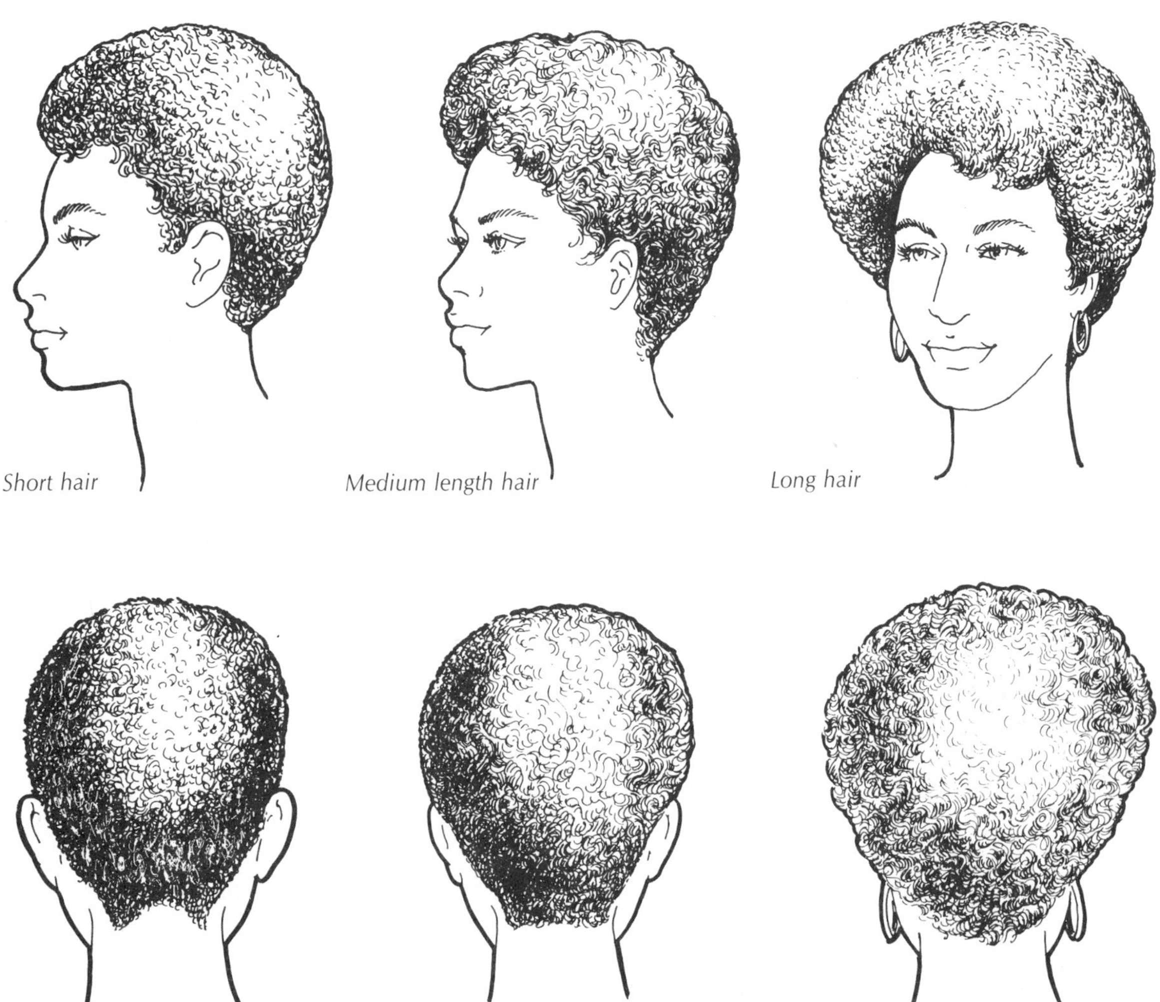

Short hair — *Medium length hair* — *Long hair*

Back view — *Back view* — *Back view*

DEFINITIONS PERTAINING TO HAIR SHAPING

Back combing: Combing the short hairs of a strand toward the scalp. Other terms used for back combing are **teasing, ratting, matting** and **French lacing.**

Basic hair shaping: Shaping the hair to a length that is not too long or too short so that it properly fits many different hairstyles.

Blunt cutting: Cutting the hair straight off, without tapering.

Dry cutting: Shaping the hair with scissors while it is dry.

Effilating: A French term for **slithering.**

Featheredge: When the hair at the nape is tapered (shingled) in a graceful upward effect and the neck is cleaned with scissors, razor or clippers.

Guideline: A strand of hair at the nape or sides of the head that is cut to a precise length. This cut strand establishes a guideline to be followed in shaping the balance of the head and helps to establish the general shaping pattern.

Hair shaping: The process of thinning, tapering and shortening the hair using comb, scissors, thinning shears or razor to mold the hair into a becoming shape; also known as **haircutting.**

Hairstyling: Arranging the hair in various attractive shapes or styles. The contour of the face, shape of the head and the season's current styles must be considered when styling hair.

Hairstylist: One who has the artistic ability to suggest and create an attractive new hair fashion.

Layer cutting: Tapering and thinning the hair by dividing it into many thin layers.

Natural hairline: Where no artificial hairline is created in short hairstyles, the hair at the nape is left in its natural hairline.

Neck trim: Cutting and shaping the hair at the nape into a "V", oval or round shape or shingling the hair into a featheredge effect.

Razor cutting: The use of the razor in thinning or cutting wet hair.

Scissors cutting: Shaping the hair with the scissors.

Shingling: Cutting the hair close to the nape with the hair becoming gradually longer toward the crown, without showing a definite line.

Slithering: The process used in thinning and tapering the hair at the same time with the scissors.

Tapering: Shortening the hair in a graduated effect; also known as **feathering.**

Thinning: Decreasing the thickness of the hair where it is too heavy.

Trimming or **clipping:** Removing split hair ends or cutting the extreme ends of the hair with the scissors.

REVIEW QUESTIONS Hair Shaping

1. *How does hair shaping serve as a foundation for other professional cosmetology services?*
2. *What is the correct usage of scissors, thinning shears, razor and clippers?*
3. *What is the correct method of sectioning taught by the school?*
4. *What is the correct way to hold scissors, thinning shears, razor and clippers?*
5. *How can thinning techniques be done using the scissors, razor or thinning shears?*
6. *Show the basic techniques for cutting with shears and razor.*
7. *Show how to taper or shingle cut the hair.*
8. *How are clippers used in hair shaping?*
9. *How is the razor used in hair shaping?*
10. *What is the advantage of being able to service children and young adults?*
11. *What is the procedure for cutting over-curly hair?*

Chapter 11

FINGER WAVING

LEARNING OBJECTIVES

The student successfully mastering this chapter will be able to:

1. *List the reasons for studying finger waving.*
2. *Identify horizontal finger waves and how they are accomplished.*
3. *Recognize alternate methods of finger waving.*
4. *Complete the technique required for vertical finger waving.*
5. *Recognize the purpose of shadow waving and how it is used.*
6. *List at least five suggestions or hints for better finger waving.*

Training in finger waving is important because it teaches the technique of moving and directing the hair. It also helps to develop the dexterity, coordination and finger strength required for professional hairstyling. In addition, it provides valuable training in creating hairstyles and in molding hair to the curved surface of the head.

PREPARATION

Always wash your hands before giving your client any salon service. Make sure all necessary implements have been sanitized and towels and other supplies are clean and fresh. Prepare the client in the same manner as you would for a shampoo.

Shampoo the client's hair at the shampoo bowl, towel blot the hair and seat the client comfortably at the station.

Soft natural waves are more easily obtained if the hair has a natural wave or has been permanently waved. A finger wave, correctly done, complements the client's head and individual features.

FINGER WAVING LOTION

Waving lotion makes the hair pliable and keeps it in place during the finger waving procedure. The proper choice of waving lotion is governed by the texture and condition of the client's hair. A good waving lotion is harmless to the hair and does not flake when dry.

Application of Lotion

Waving lotion is applied to the hair while it is damp. This permits the lotion to be distributed smoothly and evenly.

Use an applicator to apply the waving lotion and a comb to distribute it through the hair. Avoid the use of an excessive amount of waving lotion.

Part the hair down to the scalp, comb smooth and mold it into the planned style. The hair will move much easier if you use the coarse teeth of the comb. Follow the natural growth pattern when combing and parting the hair. You will find the hair easier to mold, and it will not buckle or separate in the crown area.

Note Apply lotion to one side of the head at a time; this prevents it from drying and requiring an additional application.

To locate the natural hair growth, comb the hair away from the face and push hair forward with the palm of your hand.

The finger wave may be started on either side of the head. However, in this presentation, the hair is parted on the left side and the wave is started on the right (heavy) side.

HORIZONTAL FINGER WAVING

Shaping the Top Area

Using the index finger of your left hand as a guide, shape the top hair with a comb using a circular movement. Starting at the hairline, work toward the crown in 1 1/2" to 2" (3.75 to 5 cm.) sections at a time until the crown has been reached (fig. 1).

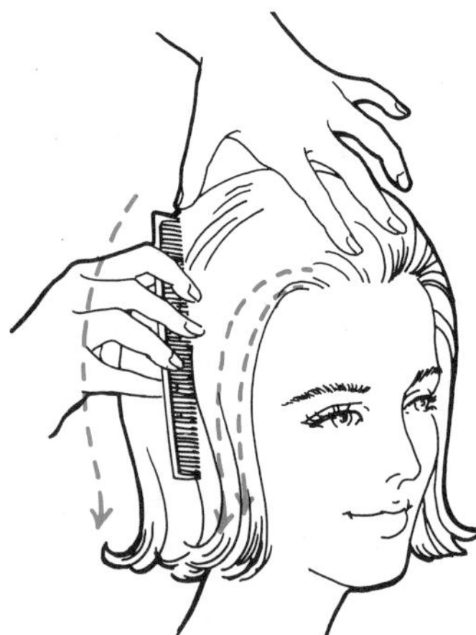

Fig. 1 Shaping the top area

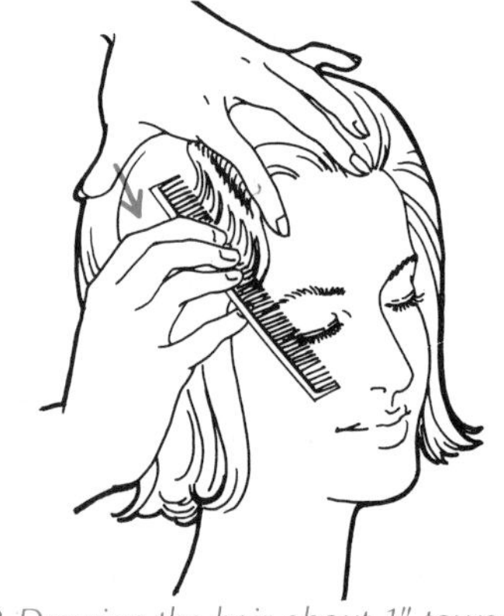

Fig. 2 Drawing the hair about 1" toward fingertip

Forming the first ridge. Place the index finger of the left hand directly above the position for the first ridge. With the teeth of the comb pointing slightly upward, insert the comb directly under the index finger. Draw the comb forward about 1" (2.5 cm.) along the fingertip (fig. 2).

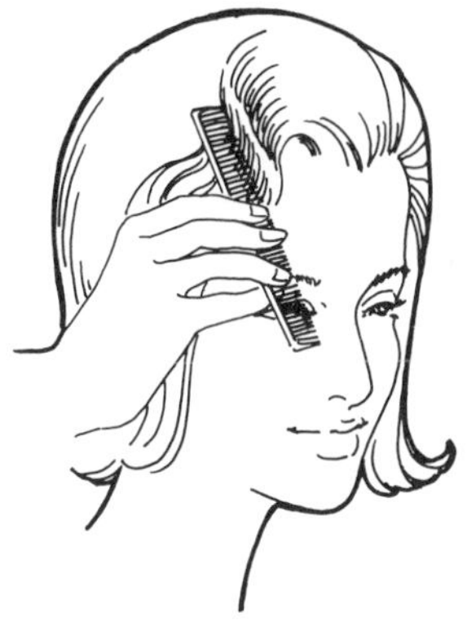

Fig. 3 Flattening the comb against head

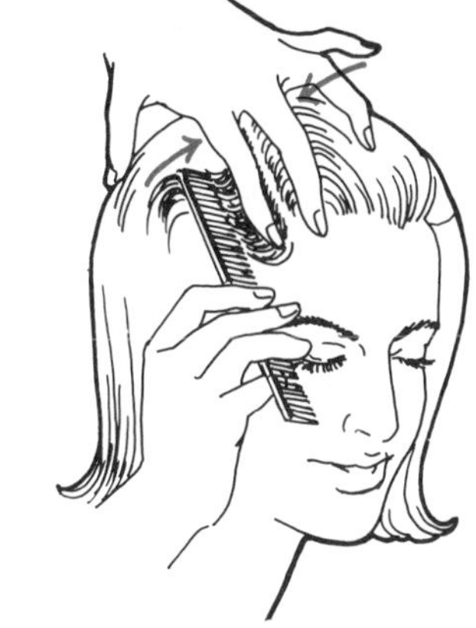

Fig. 4 Emphasizing ridge

With the teeth still inserted in the ridge, flatten the comb against the head to hold the ridge in place (fig. 3).

Remove the left hand from the head and place the middle finger above the ridge and the index finger on the teeth of the comb. Emphasize the ridge by closing the two fingers and applying pressure to the head (fig. 4).

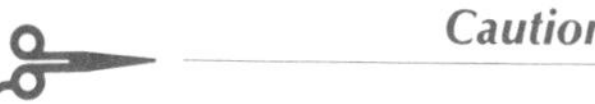

Caution Do not try to increase the height of the ridge by pushing or lifting it up with the fingers. Such movement will distort and move the ridge formation off its base.

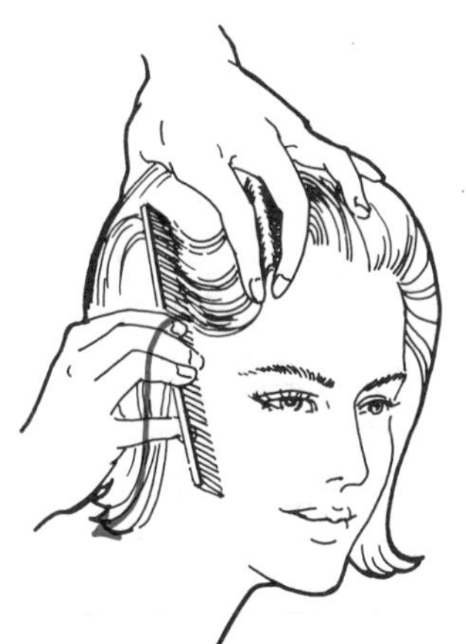

Fig. 5 Combing hair in semi-circle direction

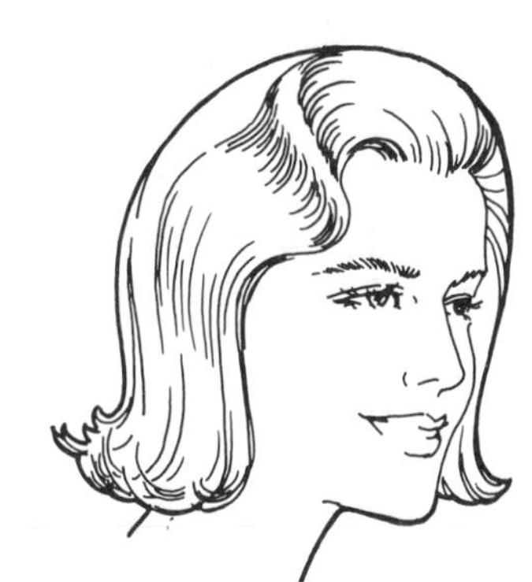

Fig. 6 Completed first ridge at the crown

Without removing the comb, turn the teeth downward and comb the hair into a right, semi-circular direction to form a dip in the hollow part of the wave (fig. 5).

Follow this procedure, section by section, until the crown has been reached, where the ridge phases out (fig. 6).

The ridge and wave of each section should match evenly, without showing separations in the ridge and hollow part of the wave.

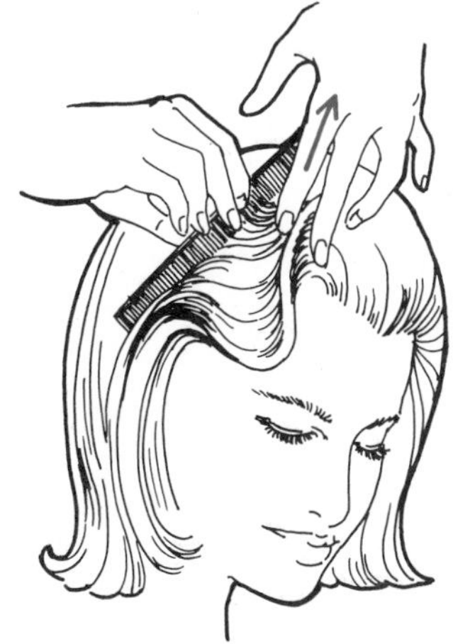

Fig. 7 Starting the second ridge

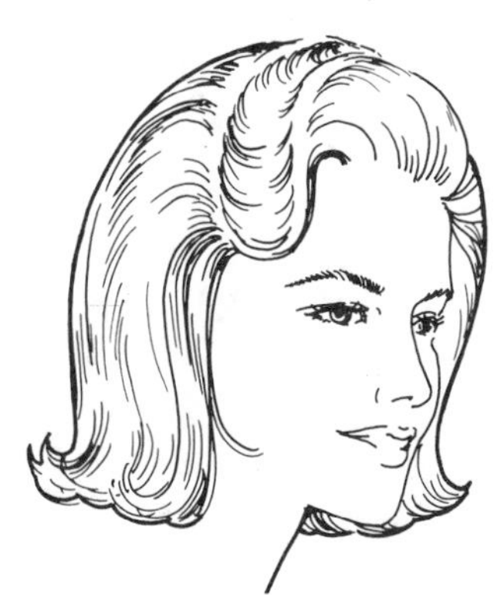

Fig. 8 Completing second ridge

Forming the second ridge. Begin at the crown area (fig. 7). The movements are the reverse of those followed in forming the first ridge. The comb is drawn from the tip of the index finger toward the base of the index finger, thus directing formation of the second ridge. All movements are followed in a reverse pattern until the hairline is reached, thus completing the second ridge (fig. 8).

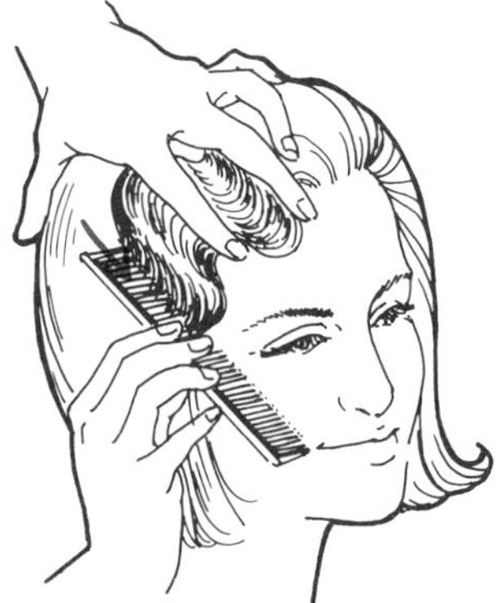
Fig. 9 Starting the third ridge

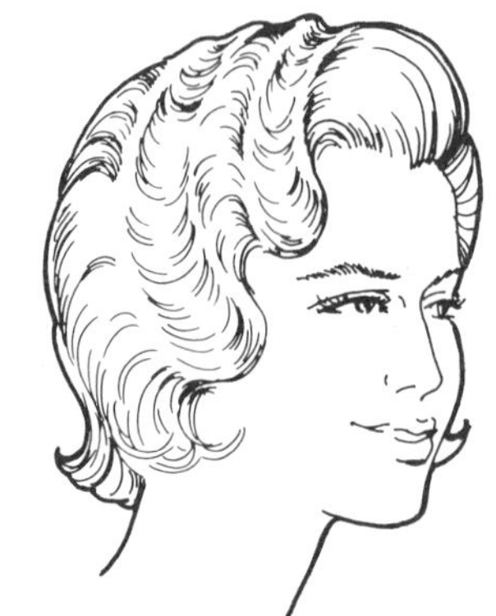
Fig. 10 Completed right side

Forming the third ridge. Movements for the third ridge closely follow those used in creating the first ridge. However, the third ridge is started at the hairline and extended toward the back of the head (fig. 9).

Continue alternating directions until the side of the head has been completed (fig. 10).

Shaping the Left Side of the Head

Procedure

Use the same procedure for the left (light) side of the head as you used for finger waving the right (heavy) side of the head.

1. Shape the hair as shown in fig. 11.
2. Starting at the hairline, form the first ridge, section by section, until the second ridge of the opposite side is reached (fig. 12).
3. Both the ridge and the wave must blend without splits or breaks with the ridge and wave on the right side of the head (fig. 13).
4. Start with the ridge and wave in the back of the head and proceed, section by section, toward the left side of the face.
5. Continue working back and forth until the entire side is completed (fig. 14).

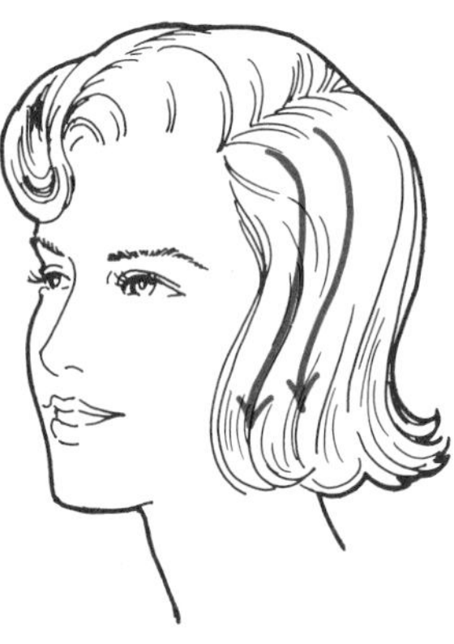
Fig. 11 Shaping for the left side

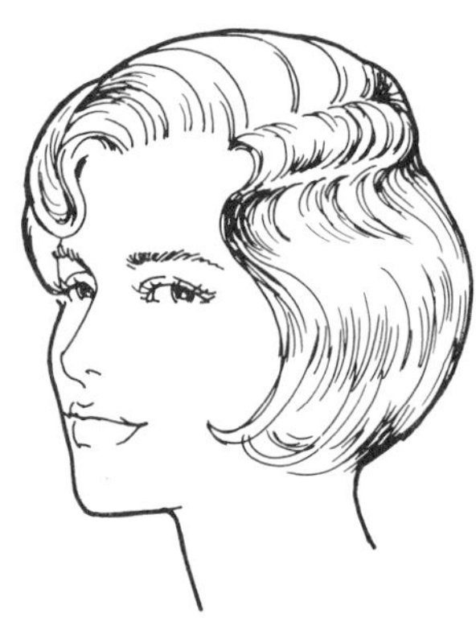
Fig. 12 First ridge starts at the hairline

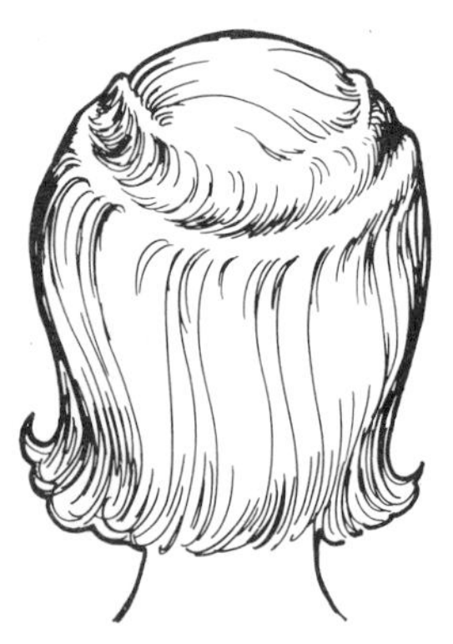
Fig. 13 Ridge and wave matched in the crown area

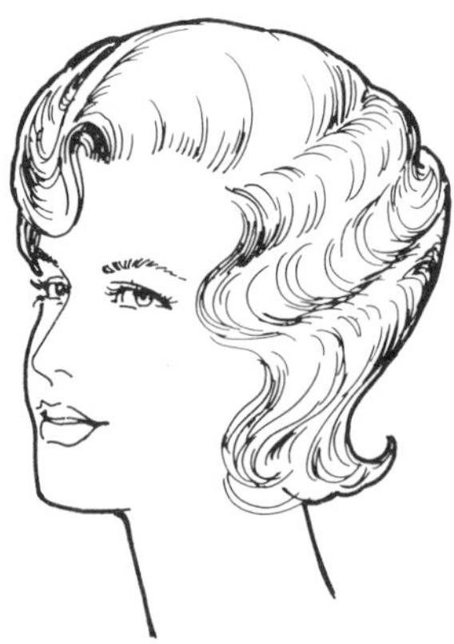
Fig. 14 Left side completed

Completion

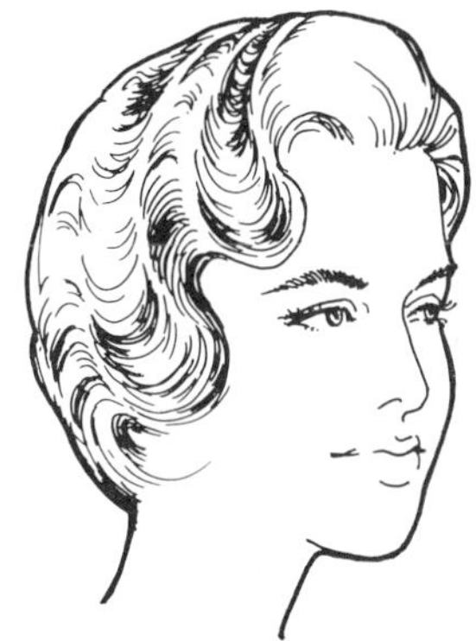
Fig. 15 Full side view

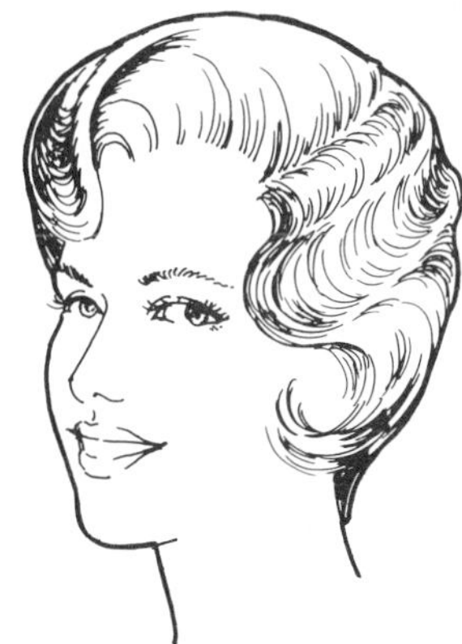
Fig. 16 Left side view

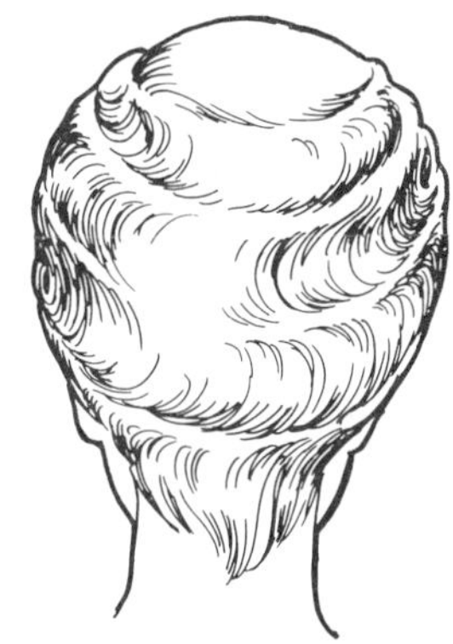
Fig. 17 Full back view

1. Secure the style with hairpins or clips, if needed, and safeguard the client's forehead and ears while under the dryer with cotton, gauze or paper protectors.
2. Adjust the dryer to medium heat and allow the hair to dry thoroughly.
3. Remove the client from under the dryer.
4. Remove the clips or pins from the hair.
5. Comb out the waves into a soft coiffure.
6. Clean up the styling area.
7. Sanitize combs, hairpins and clips after each use.

ALTERNATE METHOD OF FINGER WAVING

Hair parted on the left side. The following is an alternate method in performing finger waving.

1. Shape the top right (heavy) side.
2. Phase out the first ridge starting at the front **right** side, and working around to the crown.
3. Start a ridge on the **left** front side and go all around the head, finishing on the right front hairline.
4. Start another ridge on the front right hairline and finish on the left front side. Continue, left to right and right to left, until the entire head is completed.

This method eliminates the matching or ridges and waves at the back part of the head. (Completion is the same as it is for the previous method of finger waving.)

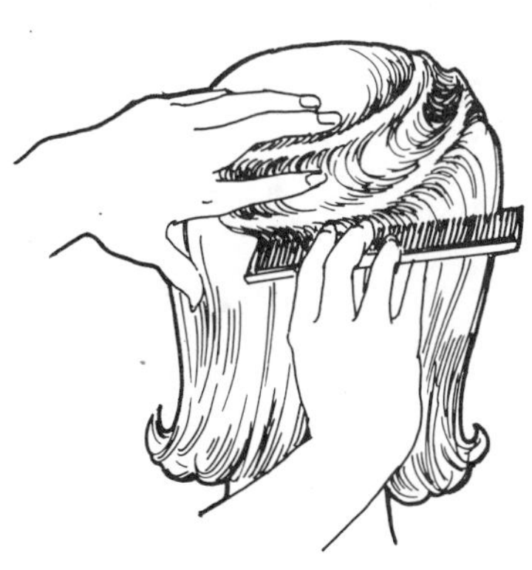
Fig. 18 Finger waving around the head

VERTICAL FINGER WAVING

Vertical finger waving differs from horizontal waving in that the ridges and waves run up and down the head. In horizontal finger waving they go parallel around the head.

The procedure for making vertical ridges and waves is the same as that for horizontal finger waving.

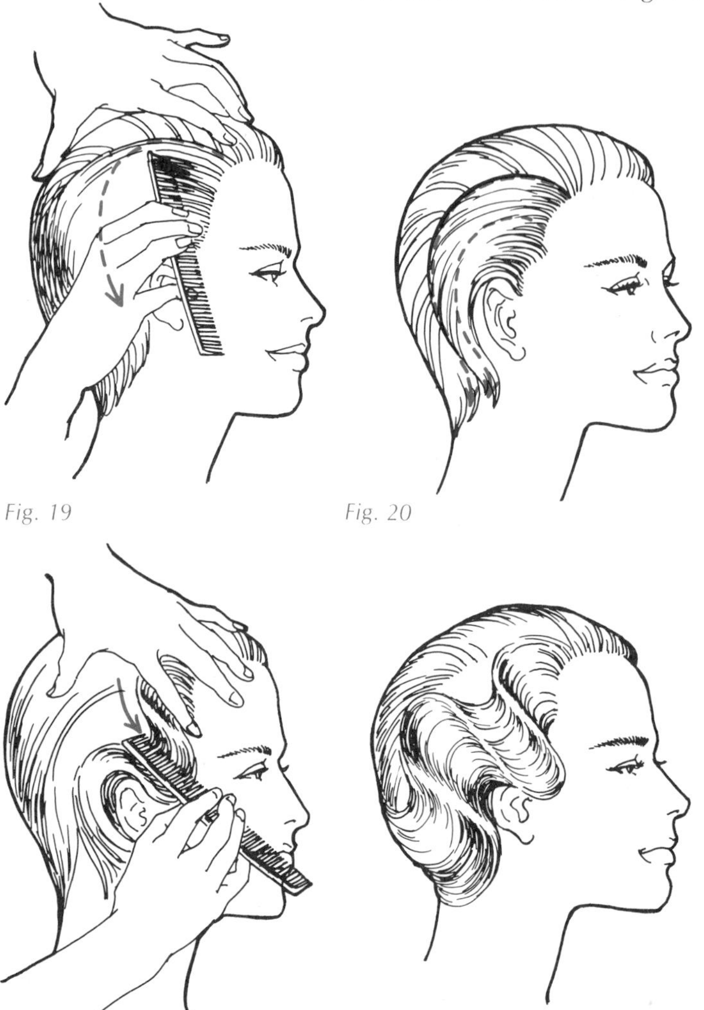

Fig. 19 Fig. 20 Fig. 21 Fig. 22

Procedure

1. Make a side part, extending from the forehead to crown.
2. Form shaping in a semicircular effect (figs. 19 & 20).
3. Make the first section of the ridge and wave (fig. 21).
4. Continue with additional sections until the part is reached.

Start the second ridge at the hair part. Start the third ridge at the hairline. A completed side is shown in fig. 22. (Completion is the same as it is for horizontal finger waving.)

Since finger waving is the art of directing and molding hair into waves and patterns with the finger and comb, it is an excellent introduction to hairstyling.

SHADOW WAVE

A shadow wave is a shallow wave with low ridges that are not very sharp. The waves are formed in the regular manner, but the comb does not penetrate to the scalp. The hair layers underneath are not waved.

This type of wave is sometimes desirable for a client who wishes to dress the hair very close to the head.

REMINDERS AND HINTS ON FINGER WAVING

1. Wash the hands and have sanitized implements and supplies available.
2. Avoid using excessive waving lotion.
3. Use hard rubber combs with both fine and coarse teeth.
4. Before finger waving, locate the natural or permanent wave in the hair.
5. To emphasize the ridges of a finger wave, press the ridge between the fingers, holding the fingers against the head.
6. To wave the underneath hair, insert the comb through the hair to the scalp.
7. For a longer-lasting finger wave, mold the waves in the direction of the natural growth.
8. To safeguard the client's forehead and ears from intense heat while under the dryer, use cotton, gauze or paper protectors.
9. Secure the hair with clips or hairpins to protect the setting while it is being dried.
10. Thoroughly dry the hair before combing it out.
11. Prolonged drying under heat will dry the natural oils of the hair and scalp.
12. Finger waves will not remain in place if the hair is combed out before it has been completely dried.
13. Lightened or tinted hair that tangles is easier to comb if a cream rinse is used.
14. Lightly spraying the hair with lacquer will hold the finger wave and give the hair a sheen.

REVIEW QUESTIONS

Finger Waving

1. *Why is the study of finger waving important to cosmetologists?*
2. *What are horizontal finger waves and how are they accomplished?*
3. *Name alternate methods of finger waving.*
4. *What is the technique required for vertical finger waving?*
5. *What is shadow waving? How is it used?*
6. *Name at least five suggestions or hints for better finger waving.*

Chapter 12

HAIRSTYLING

LEARNING OBJECTIVES

The student successfully mastering this chapter will be able to:

1. *Explain why styling hair is an important part of cosmetology.*
2. *List the implements and materials used in hairstyling.*
3. *Describe the procedure for removing tangles from the hair.*
4. *Demonstrate the correct technique for making a part.*
5. *Describe how to find the natural part.*
6. *Identify the parts of a pin curl and describe the functions of each.*
7. *Explain the difference between "clockwise curls" and "counterclockwise curls."*
8. *Demonstrate the formation of shapings for pin curl placement, explaining how curl and stem direction are determined from the shaping.*
9. *Name four types of pin curl bases.*
10. *Demonstrate pin curl techniques for the right and left side of the head.*
11. *Explain why the anchoring of pin curls is an important technique.*

12. *Describe six effects of pin curl settings.*
13. *Explain the effects and demonstrate the formation of ridge and skip waves.*
14. *Explain the effects and demonstrate the formation of stand-up and semi-stand-up curls.*
15. *Explain the effects and demonstrate proper technique with rollers.*
16. *Explain the effects and demonstrate the formation of barrel curls.*
17. *Demonstrate the techniques to achieve volume and indentation in setting.*
18. *Explain the effects achieved by cylinder and tapered rollers.*
19. *Give suggestions for hair partings depending on the client's face shape.*
20. *Demonstrate comb-out techniques including back combing and back brushing.*
21. *Cite examples applying artistry to hairstyling in adapting for facial types, head shapes, glasses, nose structures and eyes.*
22. *Explain how hairstyling artistry makes it possible for cosmetologists to style hair that will most complement the client.*
23. *Demonstrate braiding techniques.*

The cosmetologist of today must have a basic knowledge of hairstyling to keep up with the ever-changing fashions. The successful cosmetologist is capable of giving a personal touch to each coiffure so that it is suitable to the individual.

It is always advisable to examine the client's hair before starting the shampoo. This gives the cosmetologist the opportunity to do a rough combing and to decide how the hair should be worn to produce the most flattering results. It also affords the chance to visualize the desired hairstyle and to plan the proper hair shaping.

The cosmetologist who hopes to become a proficient hairstylist must understand hair structure and the overall importance of hair shaping, permanent waving, hair straightening, thermal waving and curling, hair coloring, hair chemistry and the action of hair conditioners.

Better styling results can be obtained when the hair is in good condition.

IMPLEMENTS AND MATERIALS USED IN HAIRSTYLING

CLIPS

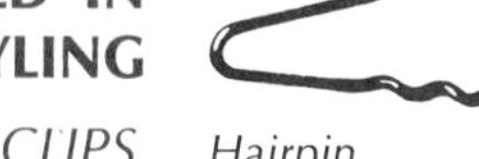

Hairpin

Single Prong Clip

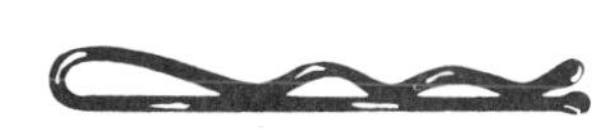

Bobby Pin

Double Prong Clip

Roller Pin

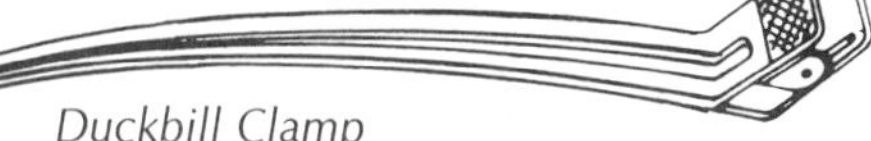

Duckbill Clamp

CYLINDER SHAPED ROLLERS

One Half Size

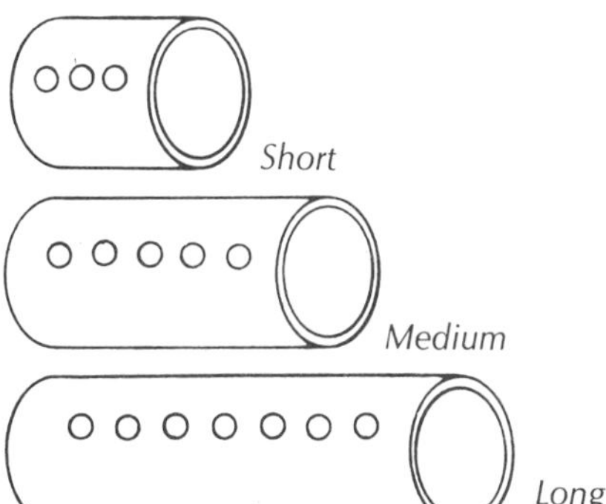

Short

Medium

Long

BOTTLES

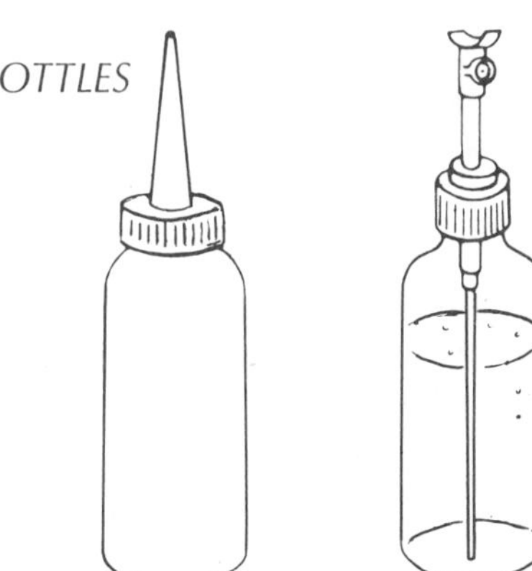

Spout Plastic Bottle Dispenser

Press-Spray Plastic Dispenser Bottle

POPULAR COMBS

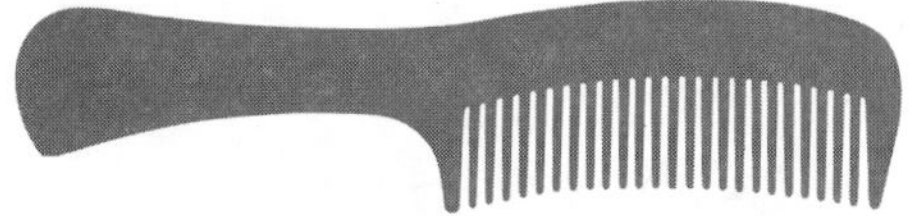

Large-Tooth Comb

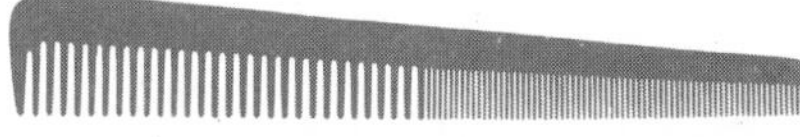

Haircutting Comb

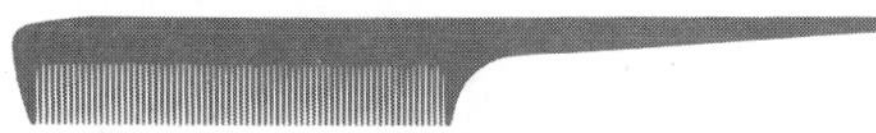

Tail Comb

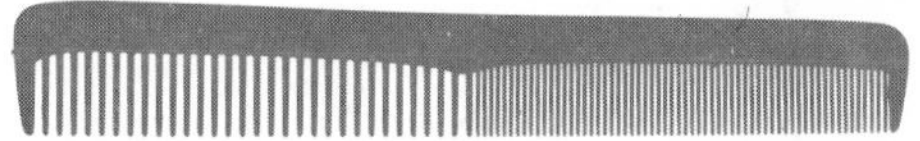

All-Purpose Comb

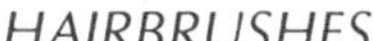

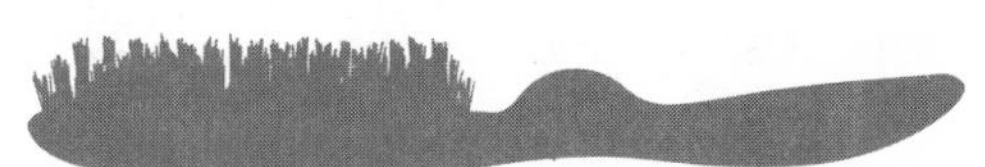

HAIRBRUSHES —*Natural Bristles. Brushes made from natural boar bristles are used for brushing out a setting, removing tangles or giving a scalp treatment.*

—*Synthetic Bristles. Brushes made from synthetic bristles are used to smooth and style hair.*

REMOVING TANGLES FROM HAIR

Removing tangles from the hair is very important for successful hairstyling. To prevent damage, tangles must be removed in a systematic manner.

Always begin in the nape area. With the coarse teeth of a comb, section off a small part of hair and comb across and down each strand (fig. 1). Work across the back sections in steps, going up to the crown. The size of the sections picked up depends on hair elasticity; for fine or lightened hair, pick up smaller sections.

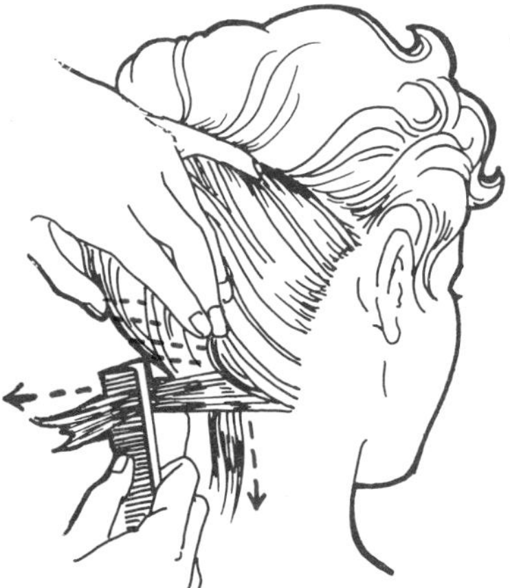

Fig. 1 Removing tangles from the nape area

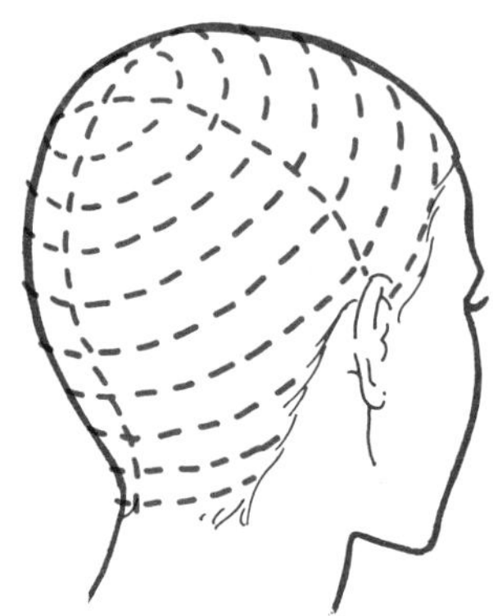

Fig. 2 Combing pattern for removing tangles

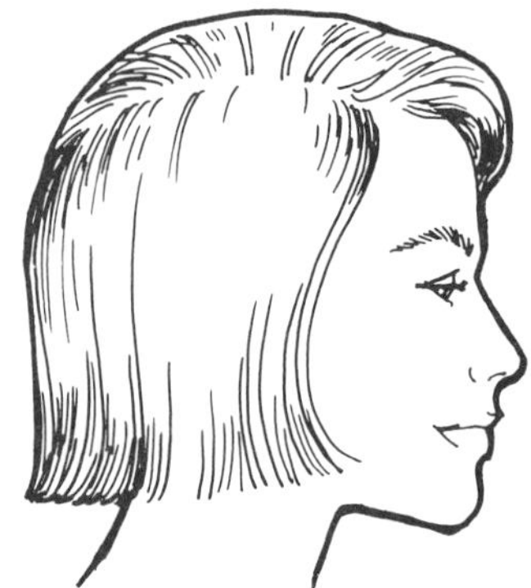

Fig. 3 Tangles removed

Fig. 2 shows combing pattern for removing tangles from hair. After tangles are removed, the hair is ready for setting or other service (fig. 3).

MAKING A PART

Clean partings are essential to good hairstyling. Comb the hair straight back. Hold the comb slightly angled and place it slightly in front of the hairline. Draw the comb in an even line toward the back until the length of the part is reached (fig. 4).

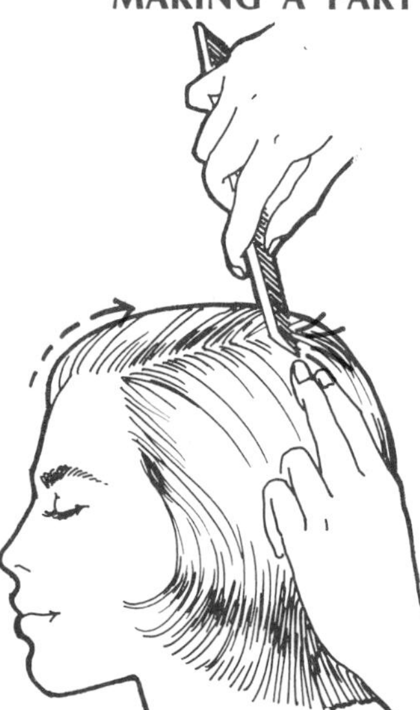

Fig. 4 Drawing the comb back full length

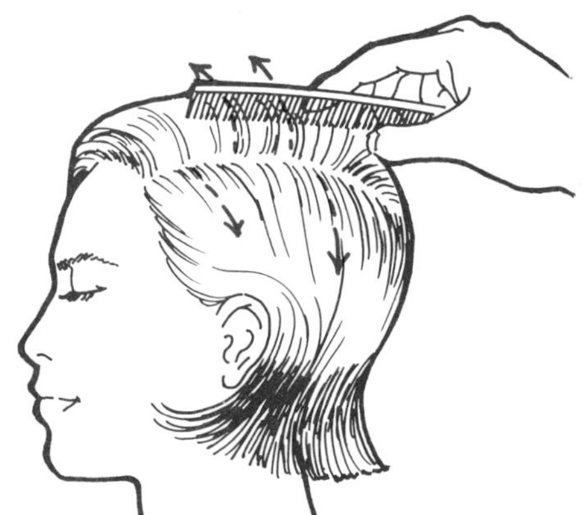

Fig. 5 Combing the hair above and below the part

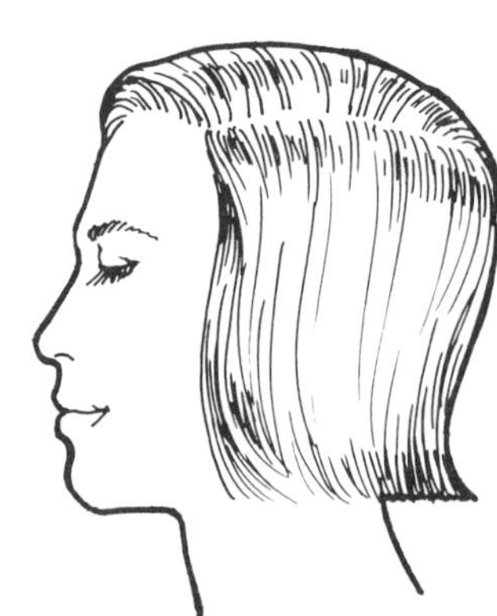

Fig. 6 Hair combed with straight part

Hold the lower side of the part with the left hand while combing hair toward the right; then comb the hair down below the part (fig. 5). A clean, straight part is illustrated in fig. 6.

FINDING THE NATURAL PART

If a natural hair part is desired, it can be made in the following manner:

After shampooing and towel drying the hair, comb it straight back. Place the palm of the left hand on the head and push the hair forward. The hair will separate at the natural part (fig. 7). Separate and comb the hair over to the right (fig. 8). Then comb the hair below the part. Fig. 9 illustrates a clean, straight part.

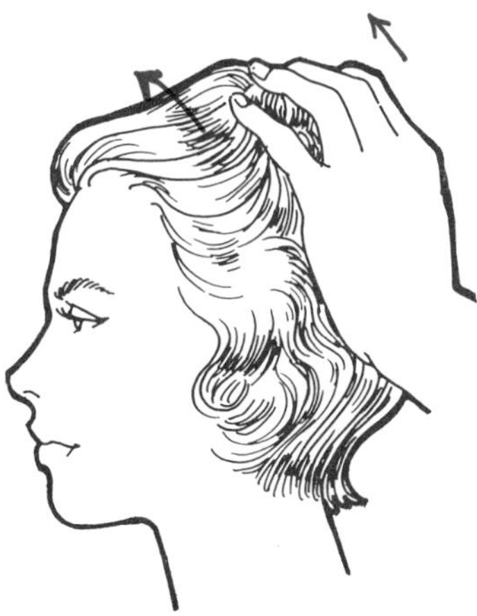

Fig. 7 Finding the natural part

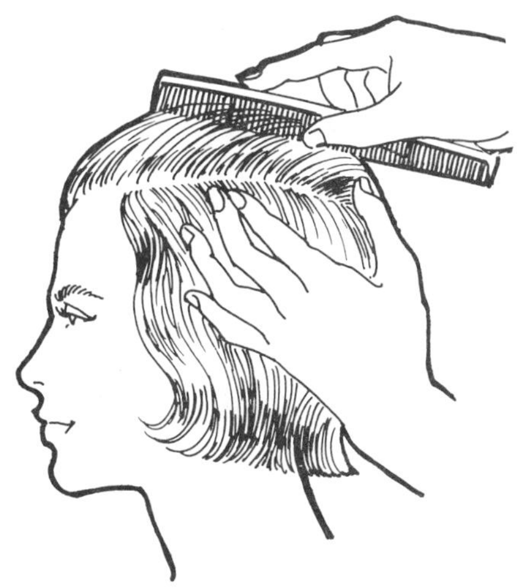

Fig. 8 Combing hair above and below the part

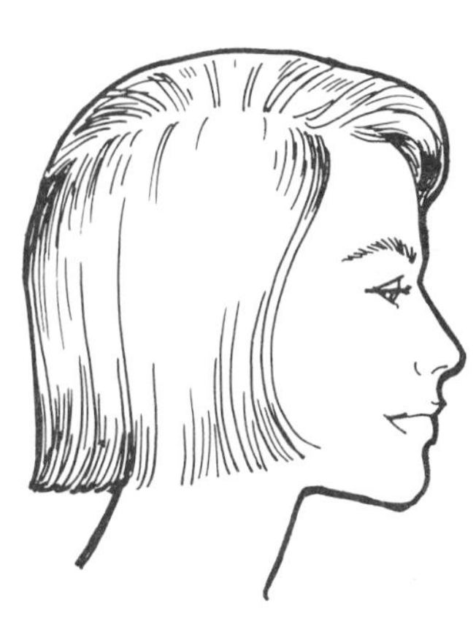

Fig. 9 Hair combed with a straight part

PIN CURLS

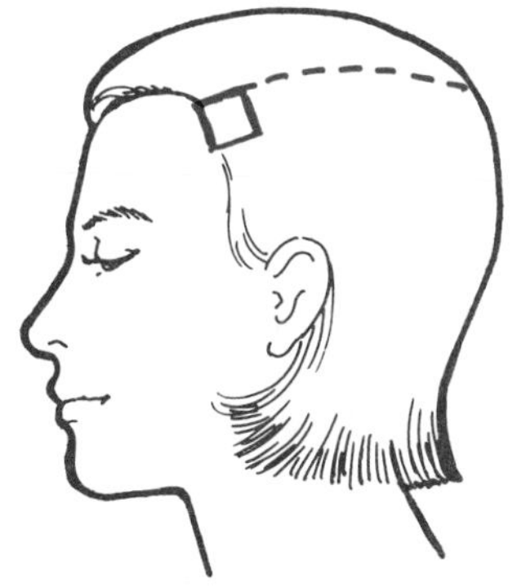

Pin curls (also called sculpture curls), when carefully planned in exact patterns, will result in good lines, ringlets, curls or rolls. Pin curls are suitable for naturally or permanently waved hair. The hair should be properly tapered and pin curls wound smoothly to make them springy and longer lasting.

Parts of a Curl

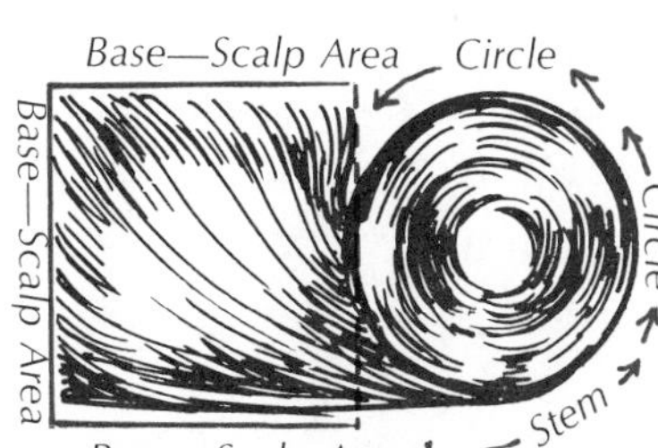

Pin curls are constructed of three principal parts: **base, stem** and **circle**. The **base** is the stationary, or immovable, foundation of the curl, which is attached to the scalp.

The **stem** is the part of the pin curl, between the base and the first arc (turn) of the circle, which gives the circle its direction, action and mobility.

The **circle** is the part of the pin curl that forms a complete circle. The size of the curl governs the width of the wave and its strength.

Mobility of a Pin Curl

The mobility of the curl is determined by the **stem**, depending on the amount of movement that takes place in the stem and circle. Curl mobility is classified as no-stem, half-stem and full-stem.

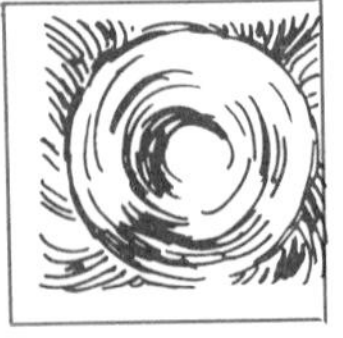

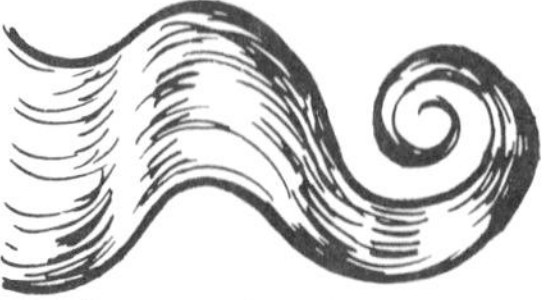

Curl opened out

1. The **no-stem curl** gives the base of the curl a firm, immovable position, permitting only the curl to move. It produces a strong, long-lasting curl. The curl is placed in the center of the base.

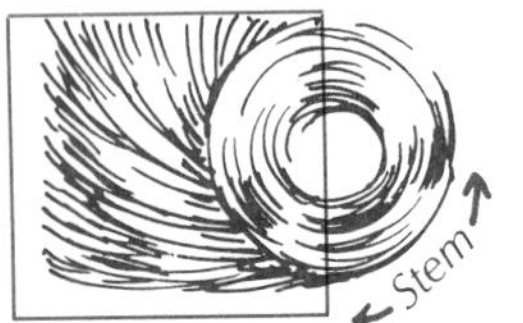

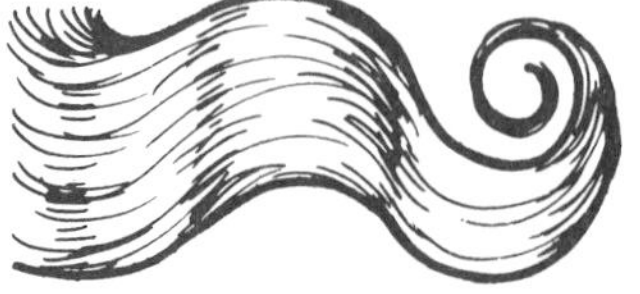

Curl opened out

2. The **half-stem curl** permits freedom of movement, since the half stem allows the circle to move away from its base. It gives good control of the hair and produces softness in the finished wave pattern. The curl is placed on only half of its base.

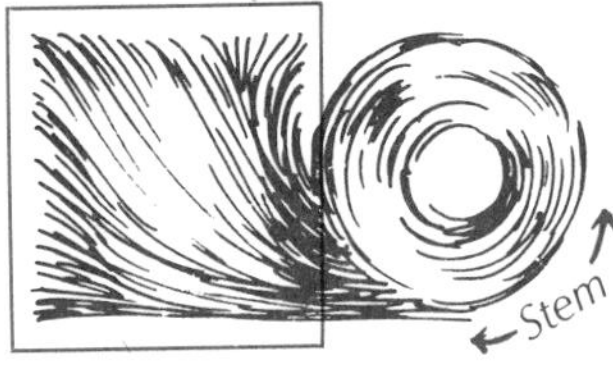

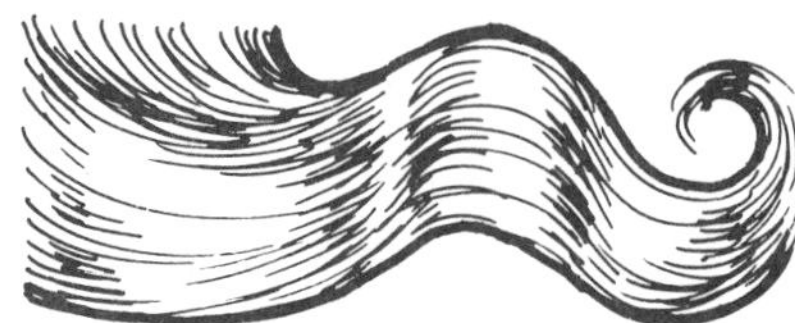

Curl opened out

3. The **full-stem curl** permits the greatest mobility to the curl. It gives the lines and direction as much freedom as the length of the stem will permit. It is used when a strong direction of the hair and a weaker wave pattern is desired. The base can be parted in a square, triangular, half-moon or rectangular section, depending on the area of the head in which the full-stem curls are used. The circle is placed completely off its base.

The type of curl used will determine whether the design is to be close to or away from the head.

Pin Curl Comb-Out

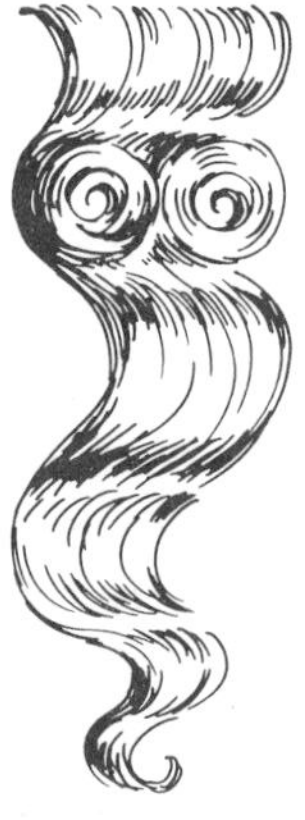

Curl with closed center

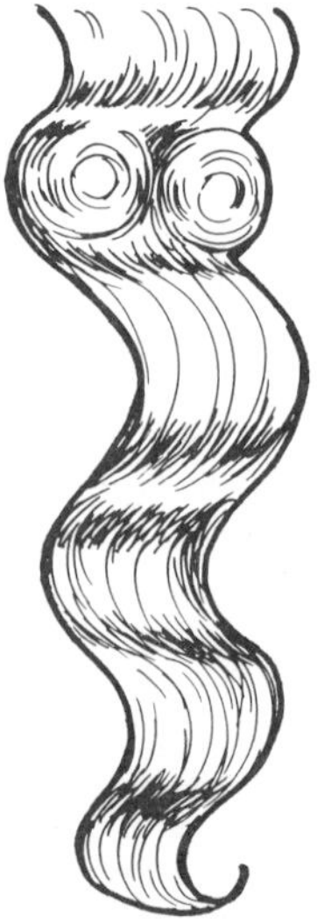

Curl with open center

The size of the curl determines the size of the wave. Note the difference in the size between the combed out wave of a pin curl set with a closed center and that with an open center. To obtain an even, smooth wave and a uniform end curl, the **open center curl** is recommended. A **closed center** is recommended for fine hair if a lot of volume is desired.

Curl and Stem Direction The stem direction may be toward the face, away from the face, upward, downward or diagonal. However, the stem direction is determined by the finished hairstyle needed.

Curl and stem direction in relation to the face is referred to as:

1. **Forward movement**—toward the face.
2. **Reverse (backward) movement**—away from the face.

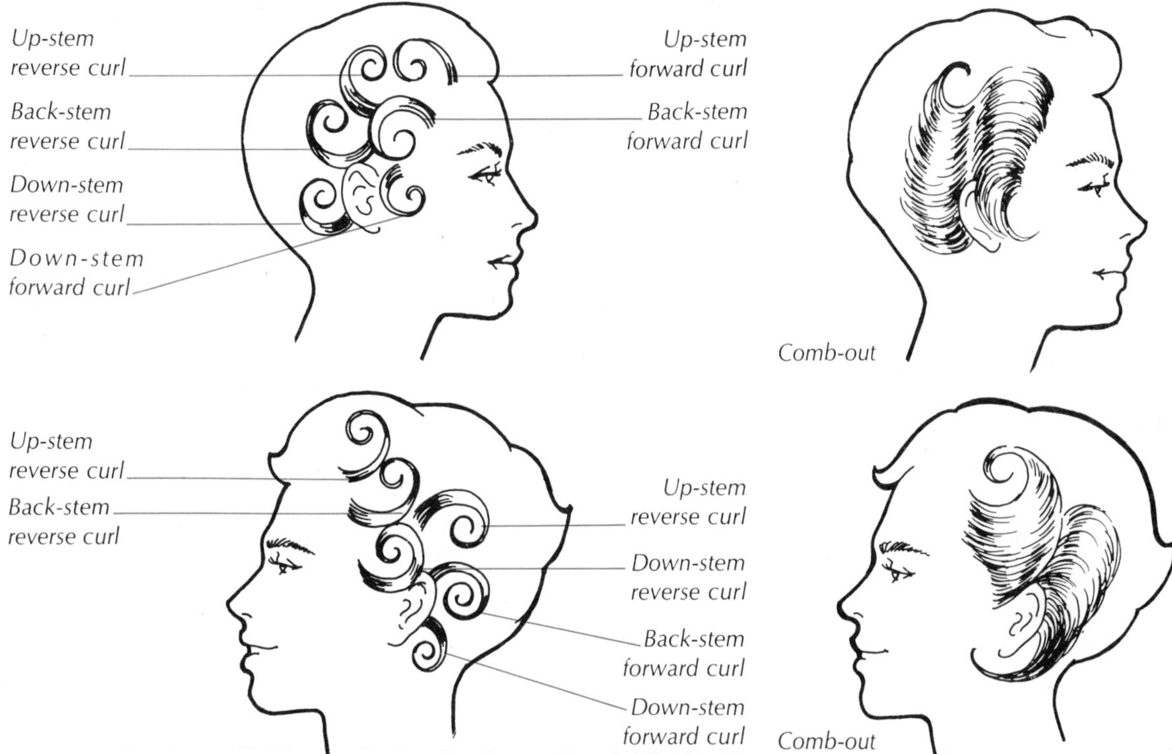

These illustrations are only intended to show stem directions and curl placements and are not intended to be illustrations of pin curl patterns.

CLOCKWISE AND COUNTER CLOCKWISE CURLS

Some hairstylists prefer to use the terms "clockwise curls" and "counter clockwise curls."

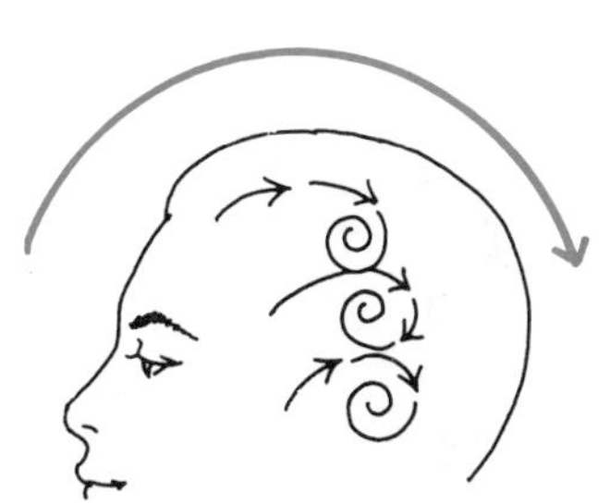
Clockwise curls

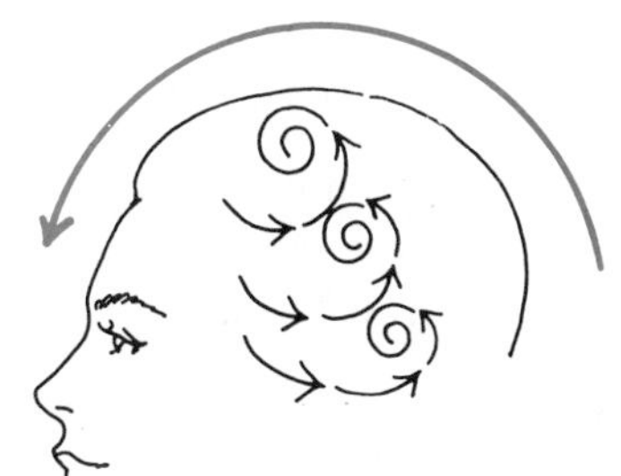
Counter-clockwise curls

Curls formed in the same direction as the movement of the hands of a clock are known as clockwise (C) curls.

Curls formed in the opposite direction to the movement of the hands of a clock are known as counter clockwise (CC) curls.

SHAPING FOR PIN CURL PLACEMENTS

A shaping is a section of hair that has been molded into a design to serve as a base for a curl or wave pattern. The exact point from which the hair is directed in forming a shaping is the **pivot**.

Shapings are classified as **forward** and **reverse**.

Forward Shaping

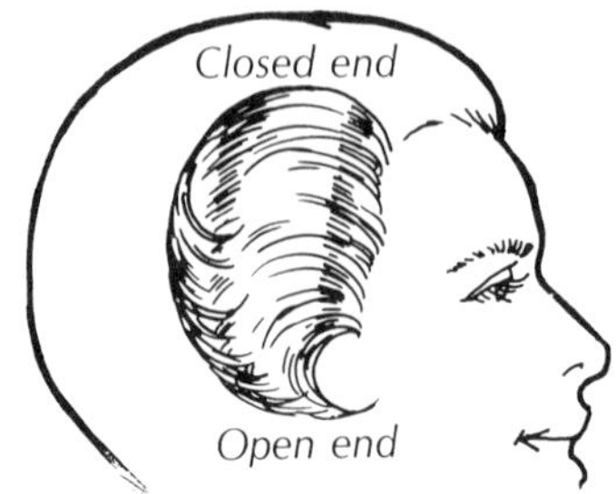

Shaping for right side

A forward shaping is one in which the hair is directed toward the face. This type of shaping is oval in form and larger in size at its **closed end** than at its **open end**.

Side Forward Vertical Shaping

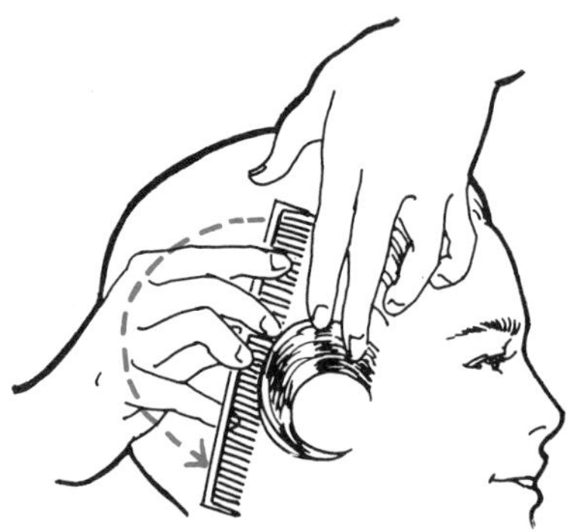

The hair is directed in a circular motion, following the side hair part, downward and toward the face, as shown in the illustration. The size of the shaping depends on the setting for the hairstyle being created.

Top Forward Shaping

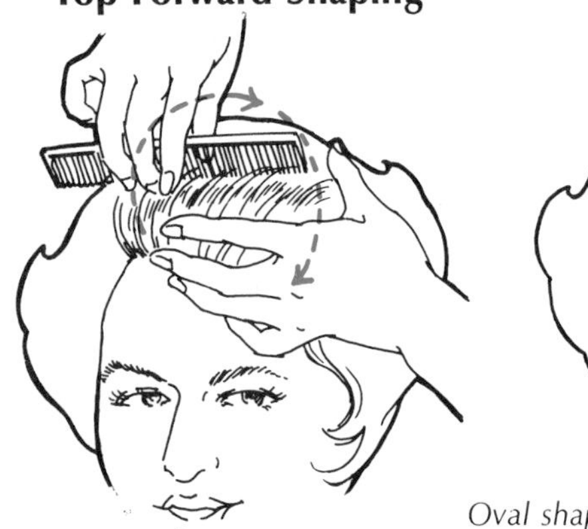

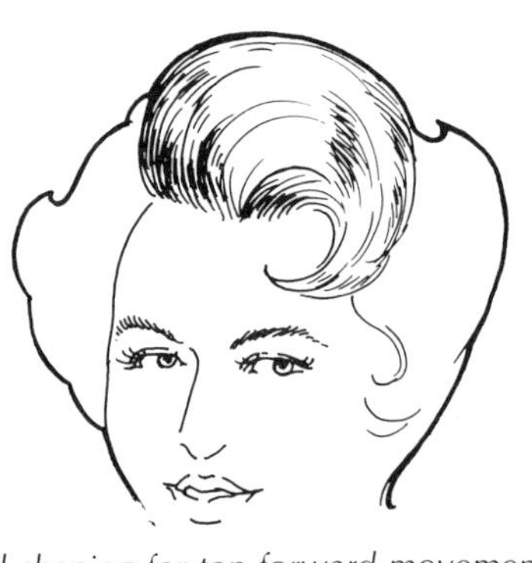

Oval shaping for top forward movement

The hair is comb directed in a circular motion, **away from the forehead**, in a circular effect toward the face.

Diagonal Shaping

This is similar to the side forward shaping, with the exception that the shaping is formed in a diagonal manner to the side of the head.

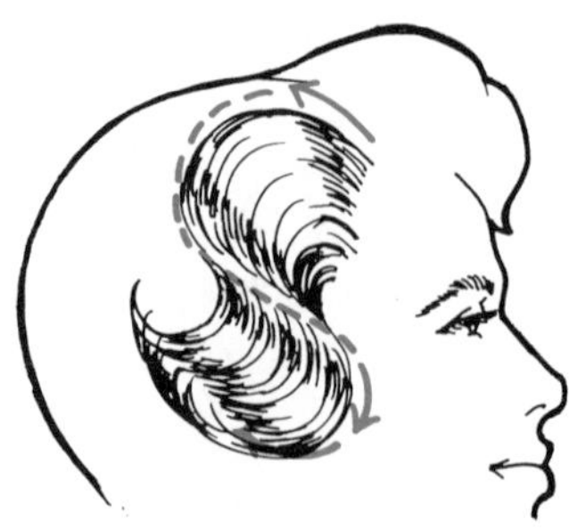

Vertical Shaping

Vertical side shaping is one in which the hair is comb directed in a down-upward circular motion, away from the face.

Left Side Reverse Vertical Shaping

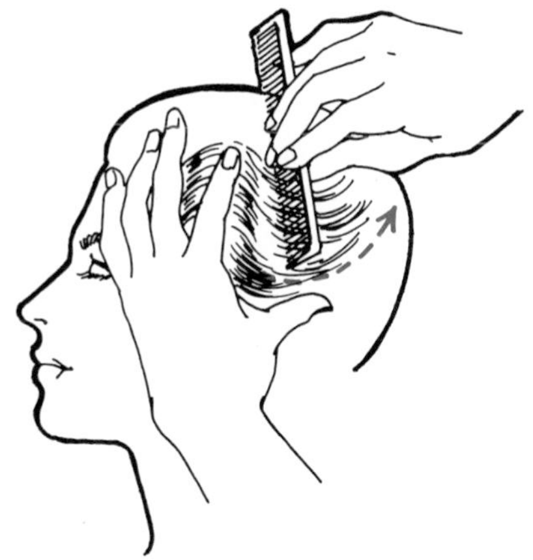

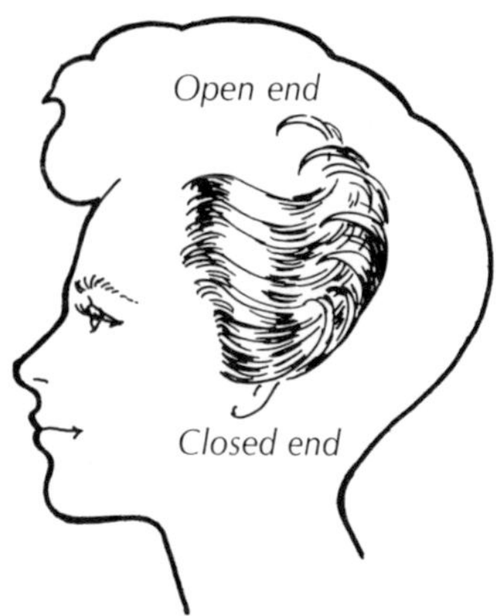

Horizontal Shaping

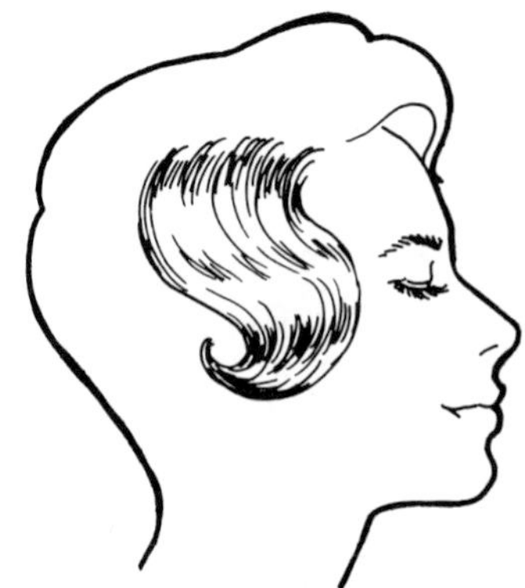

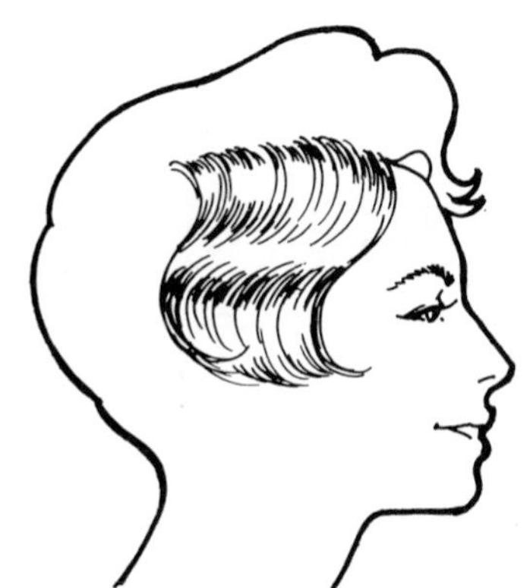

Horizontal oblong shaping is one in which the hair is comb directed parallel with the parting. It is recommended for pin curl parallel construction and may be used for the first movement in finger waving design.

PIN CURL FOUNDATIONS OR BASES

The hair is first divided into sections or panels and then subdivided into the type of foundations or bases required for the various curls. The most common shaped bases in use are rectangular, triangular, arc (half-moon or "C" shape) and square.

To avoid splits in the hair, the hairstylist must use care in the selection and formation of the curl base. Furthermore, uniformity of curl development can be achieved only if the sections of hair are as equal as possible.

It is important to make certain that each curl lies flat and smooth on its base. If extended too far off the base, a loose curl near the scalp will result. The finished curl, however, is not affected by the shape.

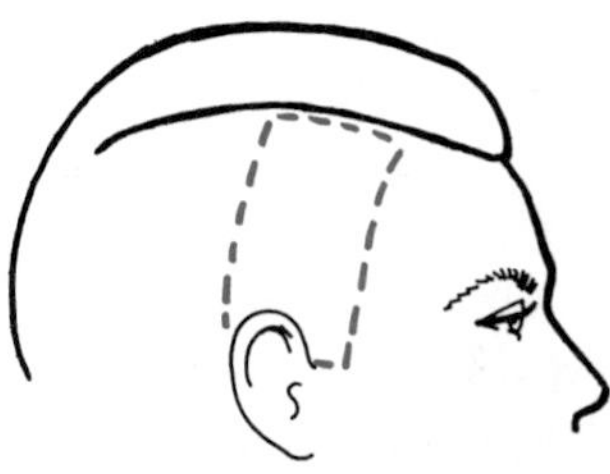

Panel

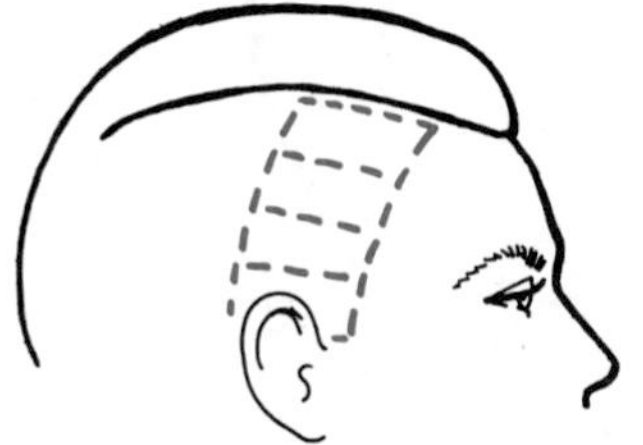

Panel with rectangular bases

Rectangular Base

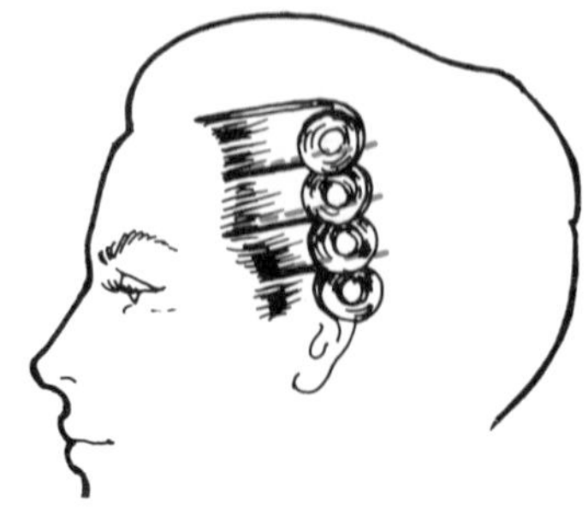

Rectangular base

Rectangular base pin curls are usually recommended at the side front hairline for a smooth, upsweep effect.

To avoid splits in the comb-out, the pin curls must overlap.

Triangular Base

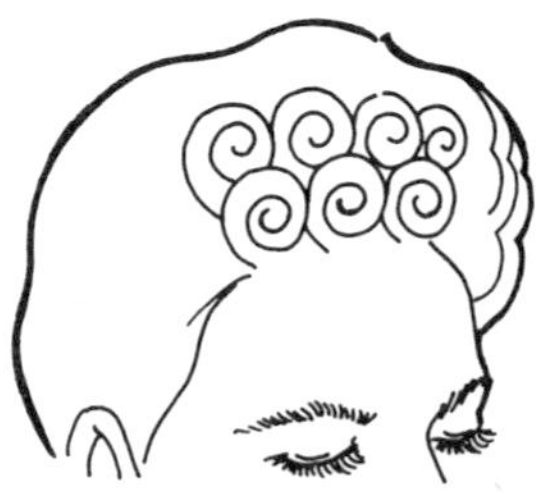

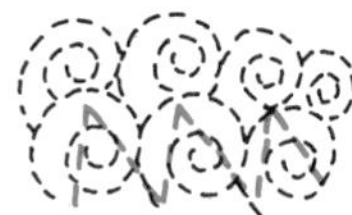

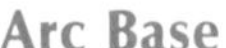

Triangular base

Triangular base pin curls are recommended along the front or facial hairline to prevent breaks or splits in the finished hairstyle. The triangular base allows a portion of hair from each curl to overlap the next and comb into a uniform wave without splits.

Arc Base

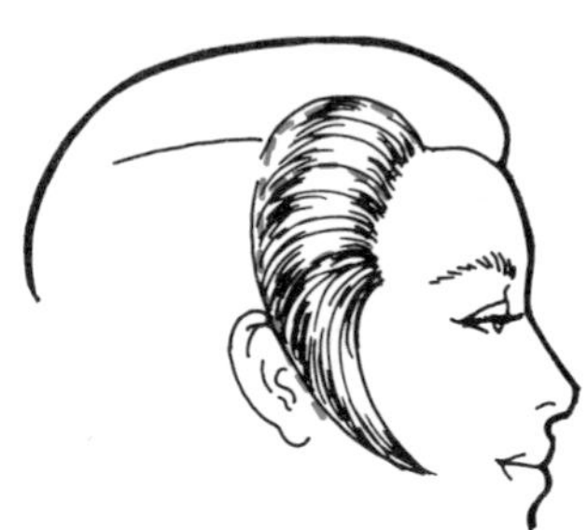

Arc base-side

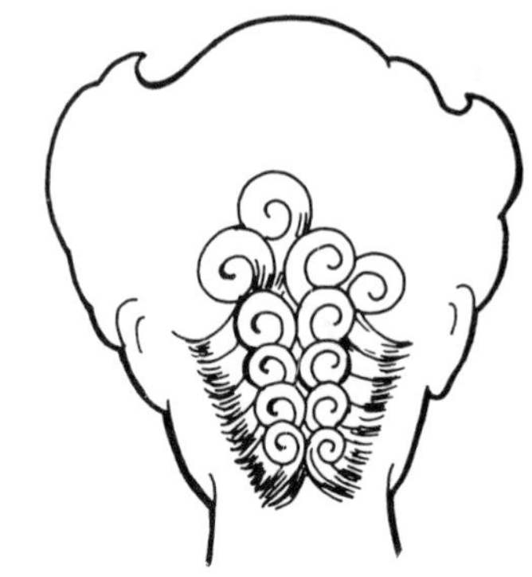

Arc base-back of head

Sides. Arc base pin curls, also known as half-moon or "C" shaped base. Pin curls are carved out of a "C" shaping, thus forming the base shape. Arc bases are used when it is desirable that the curls blend together easily when combed out.

Back of head. Arc base pin curls also may be used for an upsweep effect or French twist at the lower back of the head.

Square Base

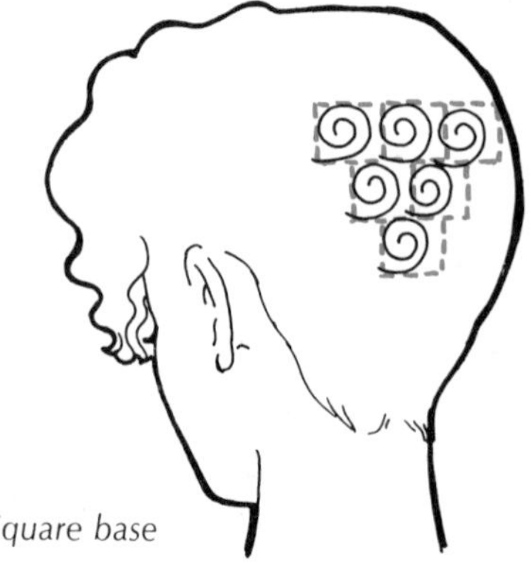

Square base

Square base pin curls are used for even construction suitable for combing and brushing into curls or waves. They can be used on any part of the head and will comb out with lasting results.

To avoid splits, stagger the sectioning as shown in the illustration.

PIN CURL TECHNIQUES

Pin curls can be made in several ways. The following drawings illustrate several methods of forming them. Your instructor may demonstrate other methods which are equally correct.

Pin Curls for Right Side

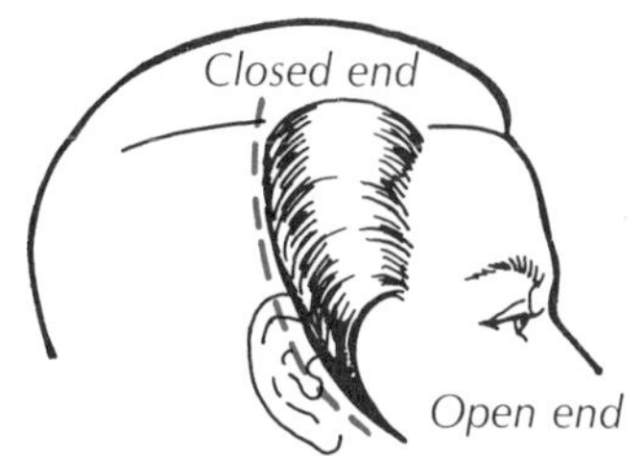

1. Form shaping

Pin curls, carved out of a shaping without disturbing the shaping, are usually referred to as carved curls. To form these curls on the right side of the head follow this procedure:

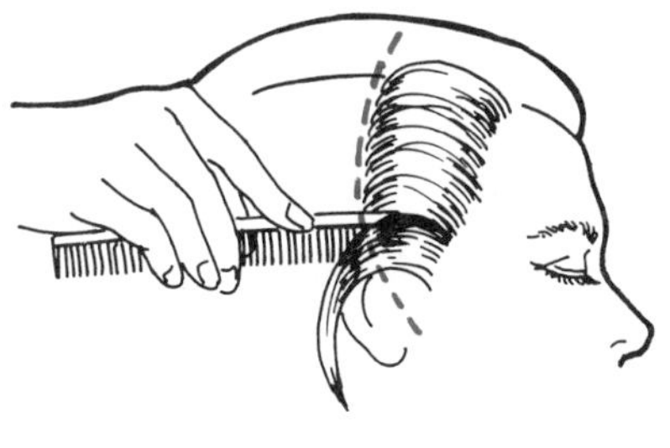

2. Slice the strand for the first curl

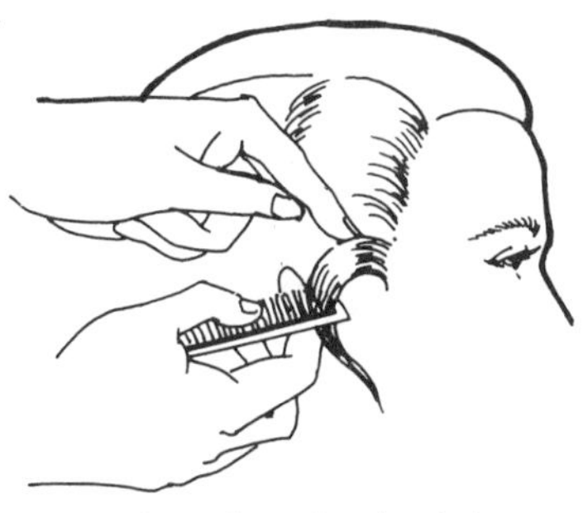

3. Use tip of comb and index finger as a buffer

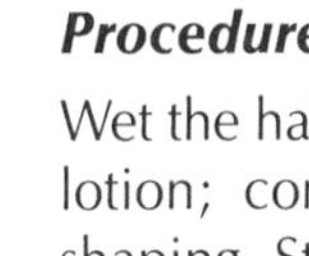

Procedure

Wet the hair with water or setting lotion; comb smooth and form shaping. Start making curls at the open end of the shaping.

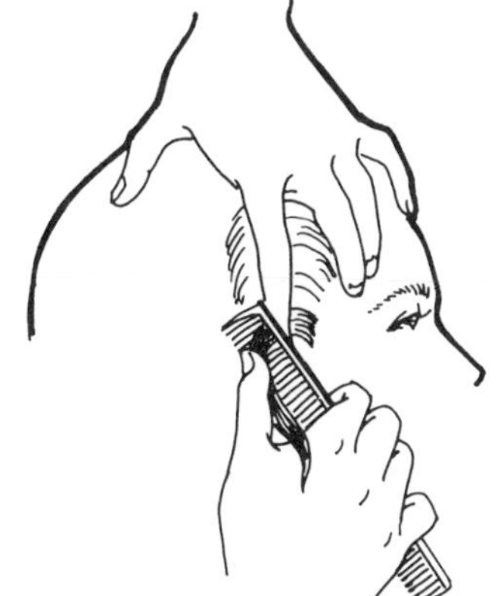

4. Stetch strand by pulling through the back of the comb

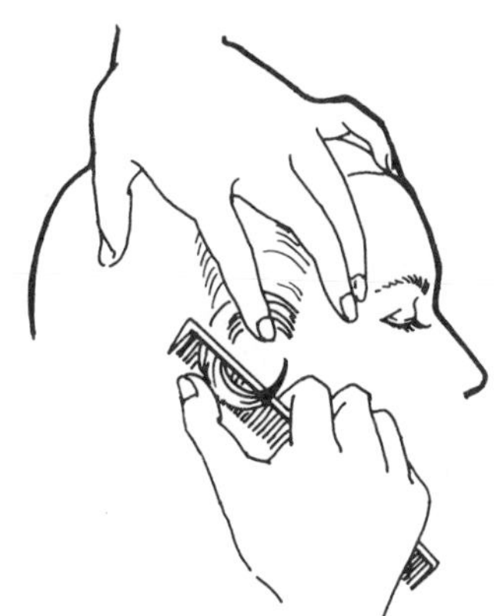

5. Form forward curl

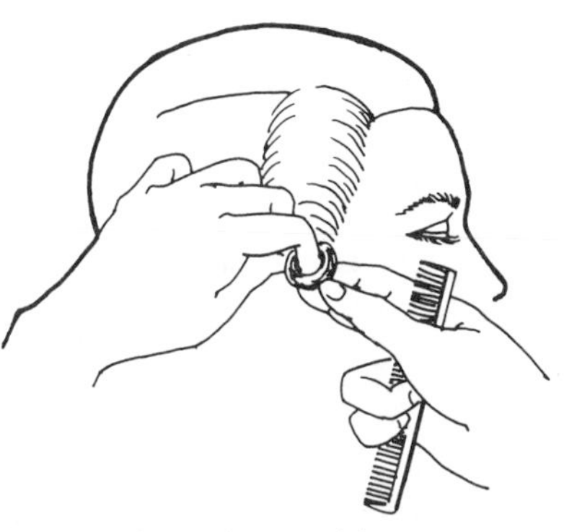

6. Wind the curl around the index finger

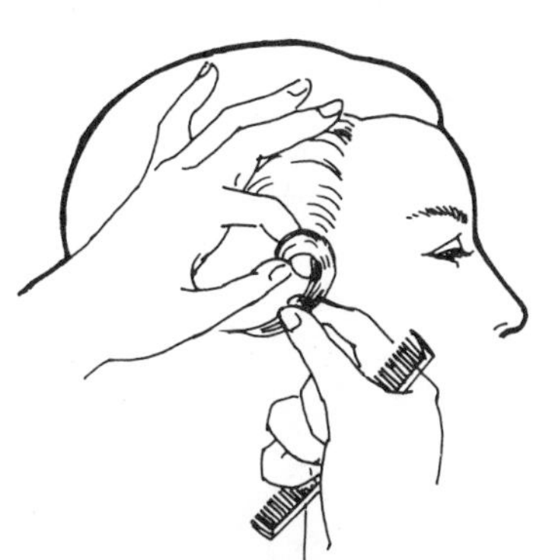

7. Slide curl off the finger, keeping the hair ends in the center of the curl

Note

Whenever a longer-lasting curl movement is desired, the strand should be stretched or tensioned. This is accomplished by ribboning and stretching the strand. Firmly comb it between the spine of the comb and thumb in the direction of the curl movement, as in steps 4 and 5.

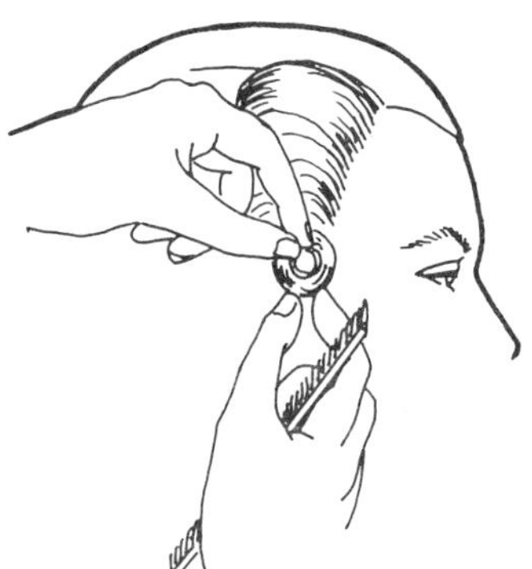

8. *Mold the curl into shaping*

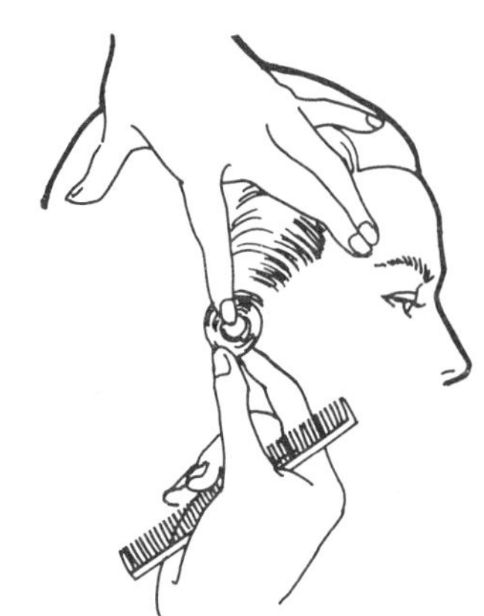

9. *Hold the curl in shaping*

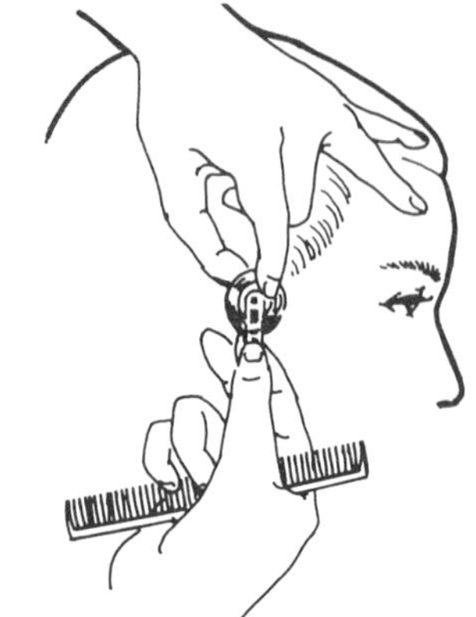

10. *Anchor the curl with a clippie*

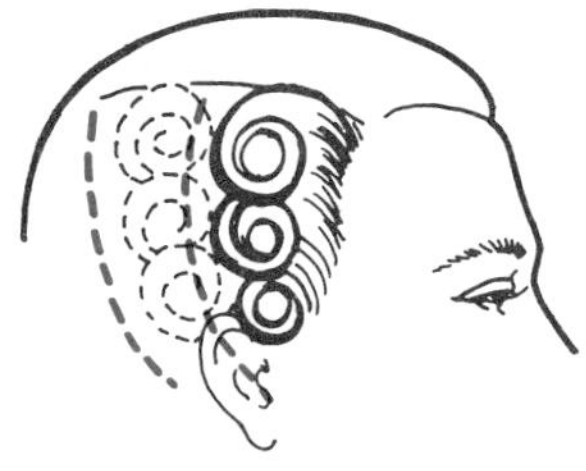

11. *Sculpture the curl arrangement backed up with a second row of curls*

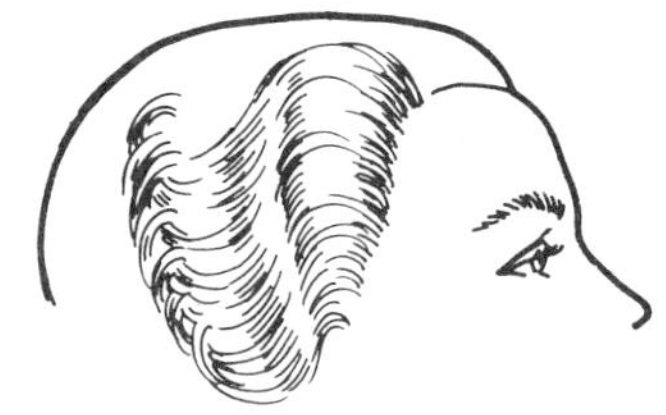

12. *Curls combed into waves with a strong ridge*

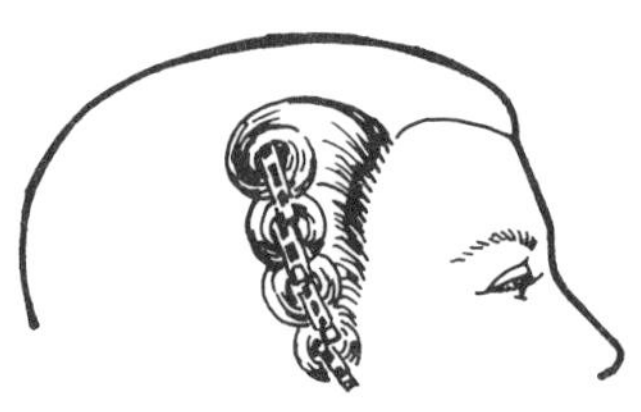

13. *Fine hair usually requires four curls*

Pin Curls for Left Side

Making pin curls on the left side of the head requires a different technique than making them on the right side.

Wet the hair with water or setting lotion, comb smooth and form the shaping. Start at the open end of the shaping.

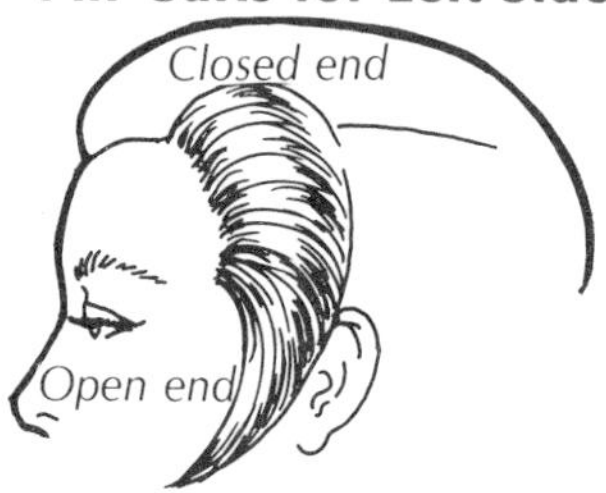

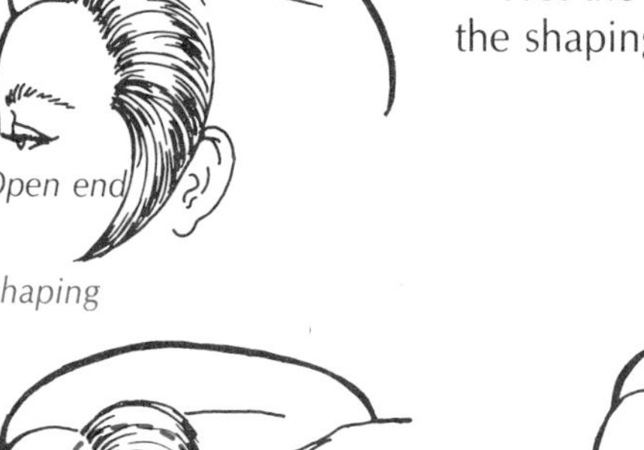

1. *Shaping*

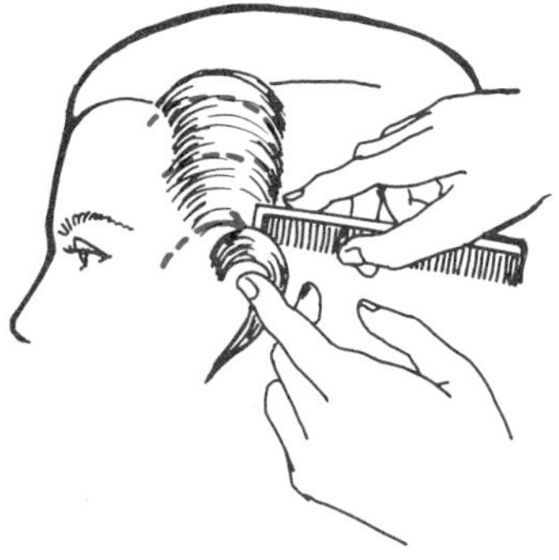

2. *Slicing strand out of shaping*

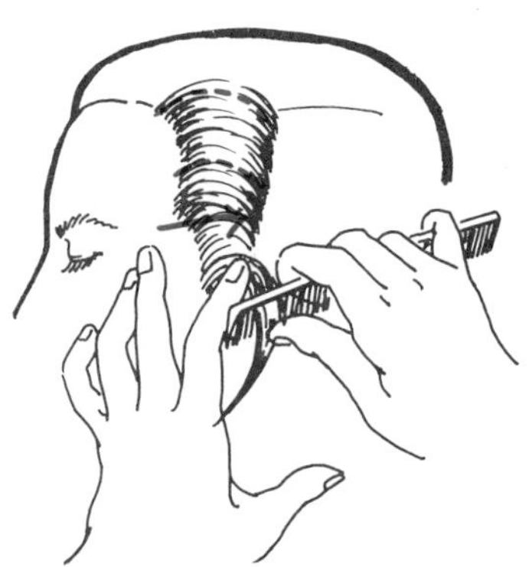

3. *Strand stretched by pulling through backbone of comb*

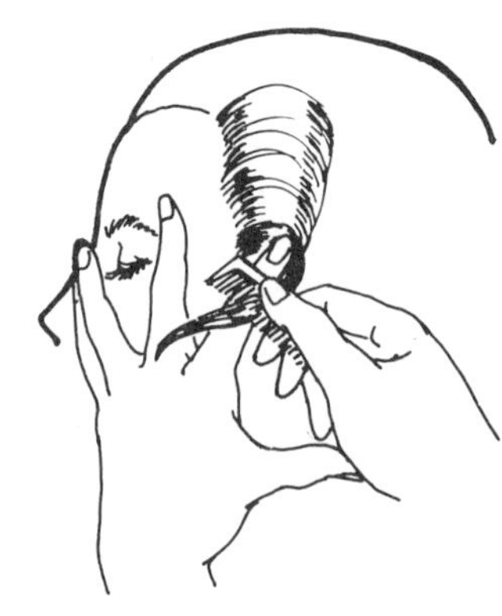

4. *Form forward curl*

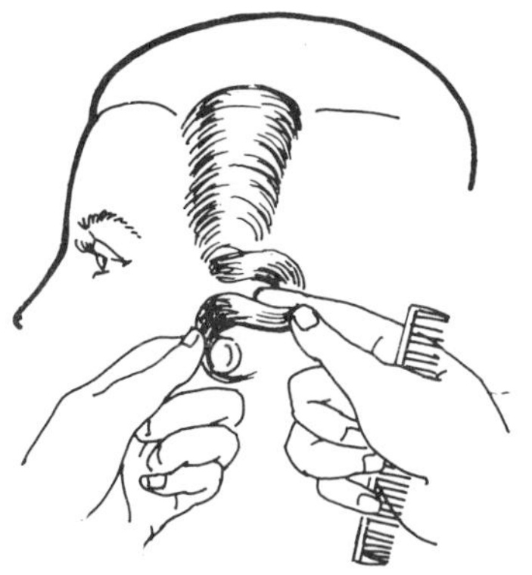
5. Wind strand around the index finger

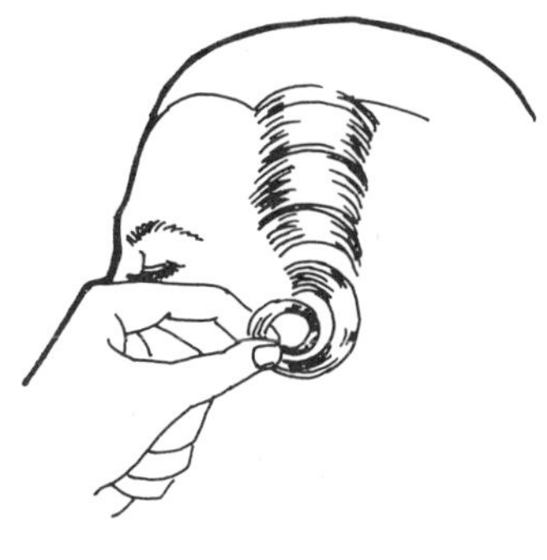
6. Slide the curl off the tip of the finger and mold into shaping

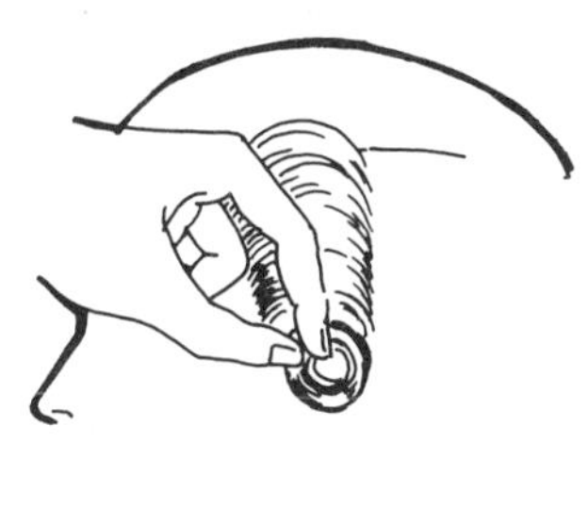
7. Hold curl in shaping

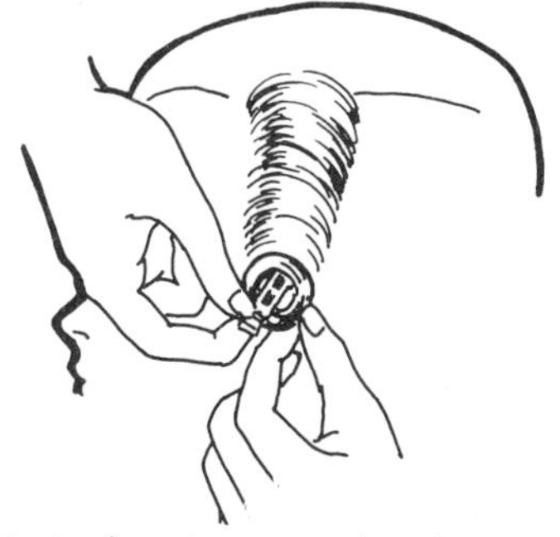
8. Anchor the pin curl with clippie

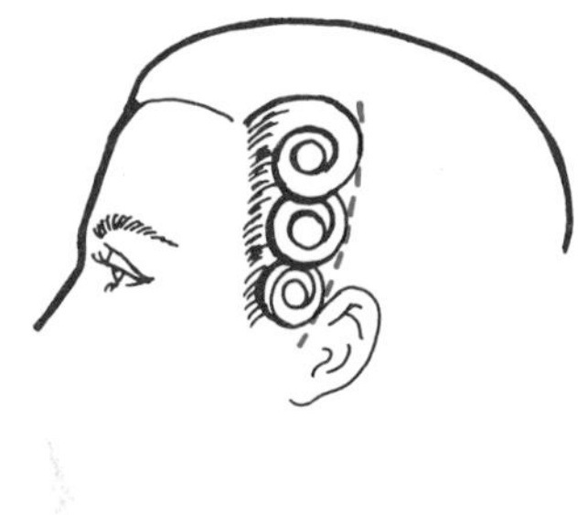
9. Curls fit within curvature of shaping. Curls overlap. Size of curls graduated

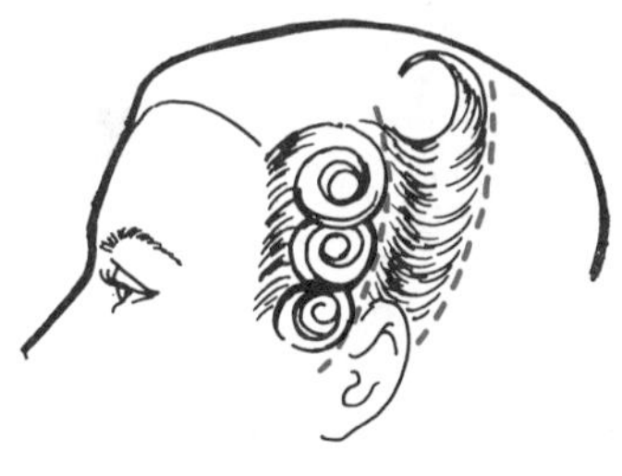
10. Reverse shaping for back-up curls

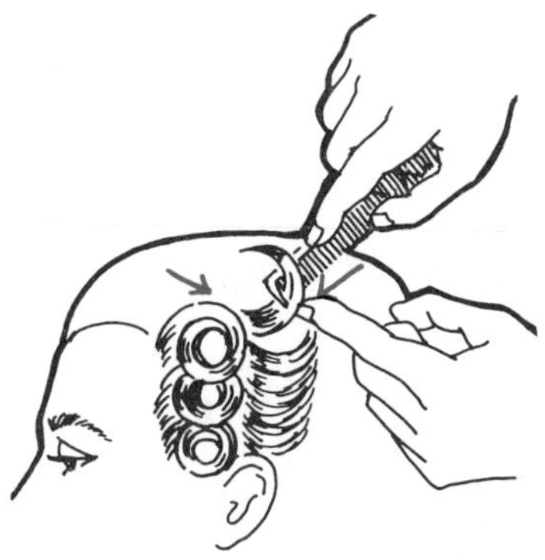
11. To slice a strand, the tip of the comb touches the tip of finger through half the shaping

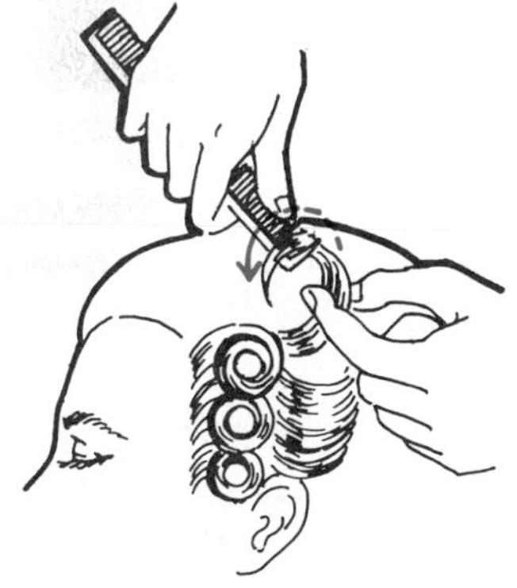
12. Ribbon strand. The use of a coarse or fine tooth comb depends on the texture of the hair.

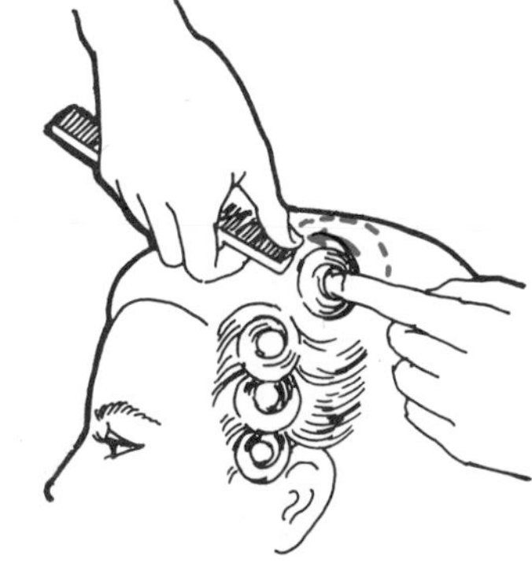
13. Ribbon tip of strand with fine teeth of comb for neat closing of curl

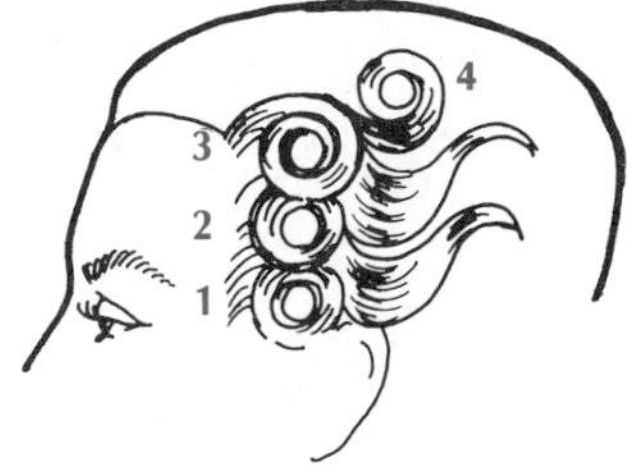

14. Top reverse curl completed and the shaping divided into strands for the next two curls

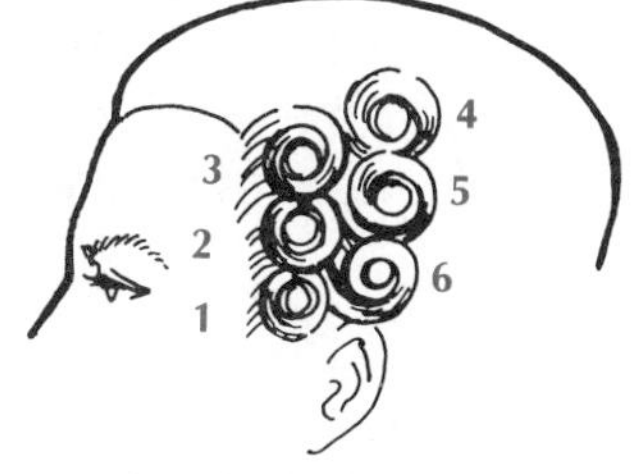

15. Completed second row of curls within curve of shaping

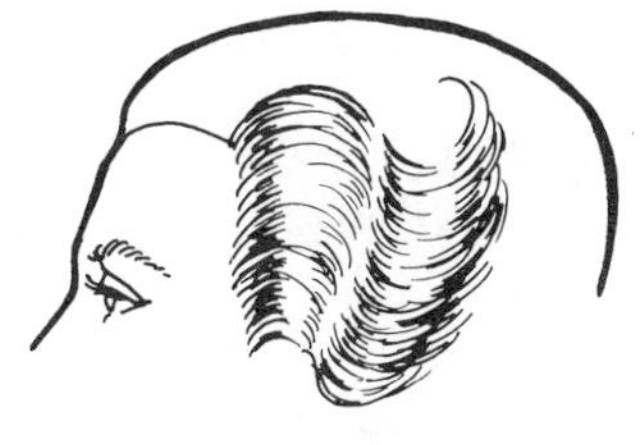
16. Comb-out of forward and reverse pin curl setting into a full, wide wave

Anchoring Pin Curls

Anchoring pin curls is an important technique that must be mastered to achieve success in hairstyling. It is essential that the curls hold firmly as placed, so that the planned pattern can be followed and developed into the desired coiffure.

Every hairstylist or instructor has a favorite method for inserting clips or clippies. Each one of these professional methods can be considered equally correct. However, it is essential that good common sense be used at all times in the insertion of clips or clippies so that pin curls are anchored securely.

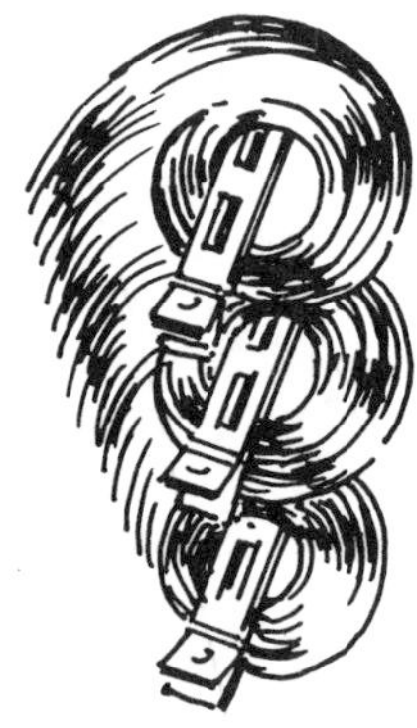

Hairline forward pin curls (clockwise curls)

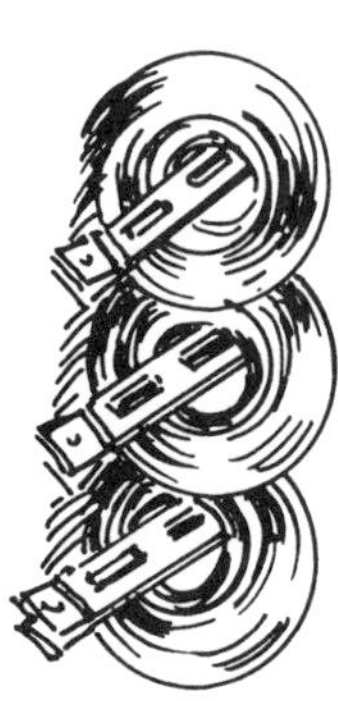

Forward pin curls equal in size. May be used any place on the head.

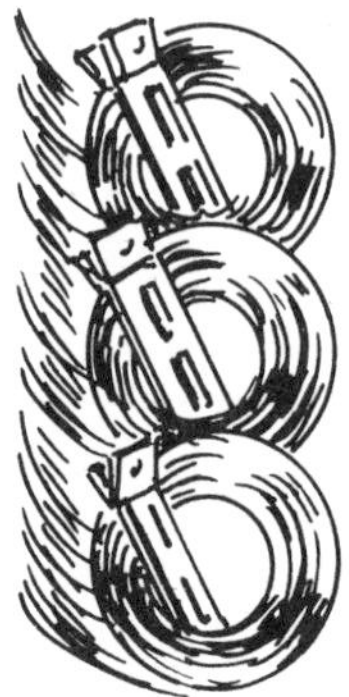

Reverse pin curls (counter-clockwise curls). Equal in size and used any place on the head.

Procedure

To anchor the pin curl correctly, gently slide the clip or clippie through part of the base and/or stem at an angle and across the ends of the curl. This will hold the curl securely without its unfurling, sagging or flipping over.

1. Clips should be anchored in such a manner that they do not interfere with the formation or placement of other curls or with any other step in setting the hair.
2. To avoid indentations or impressions, it is advisable not to pin across the center of the entire curl.
3. The size of clips used should be governed by the size of the curl.
4. To avoid discomfort to the client during the drying process, do not permit the clips to touch the ears, skin or scalp. In the event the clips do touch the skin or ears, place cotton under the part of the clips touching these areas.

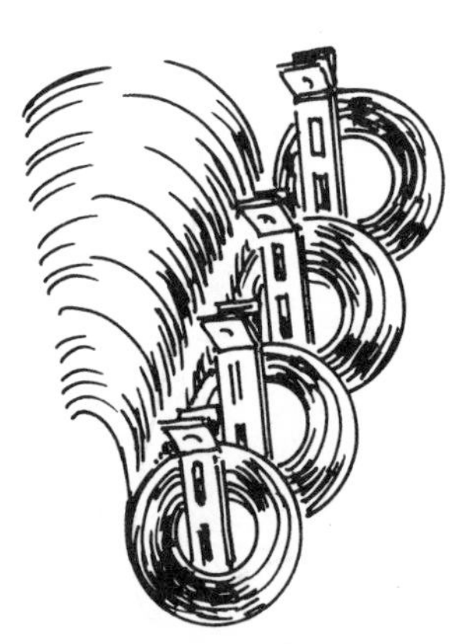

Ridge reverse pin curls (counter-clockwise curls)

EFFECTS OF PIN CURLS

There are a number of pin curl patterns designed to achieve specific effects, several of which are illustrated here.

However, care must be taken that the curls lie evenly and are placed in the direction in which they are intended to be combed; otherwise, a haphazard setting will result, with uneven wave or curl design.

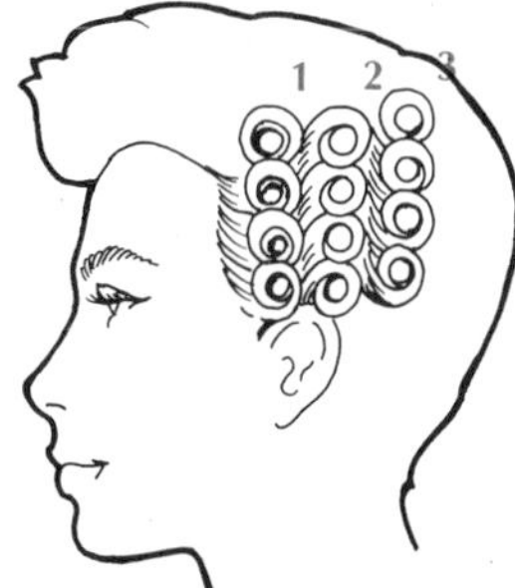

Vertical wave pin curl pattern

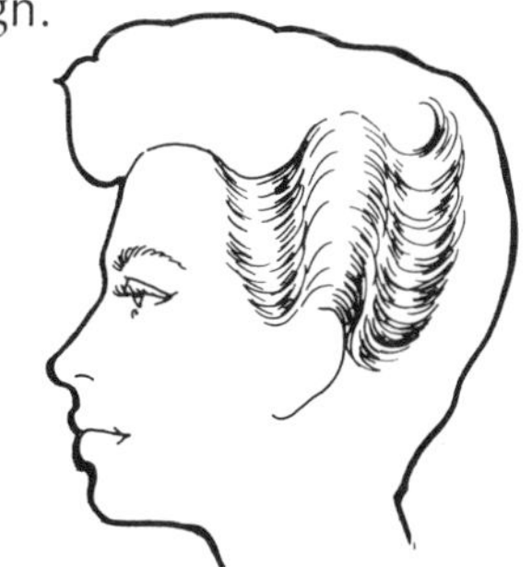
Vertical wave comb-out

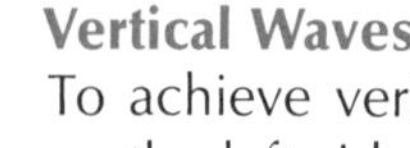

Vertical Waves

To achieve vertical wave effects on the left side of the head, first give a reverse shaping, then follow the pin curl pattern as illustrated.

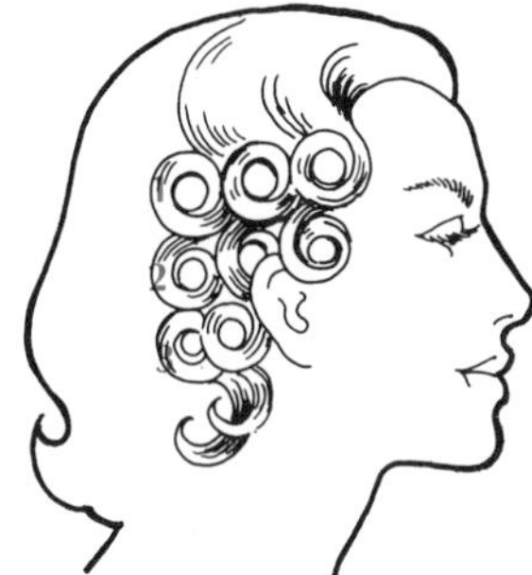
Horizontal wave pin curl pattern

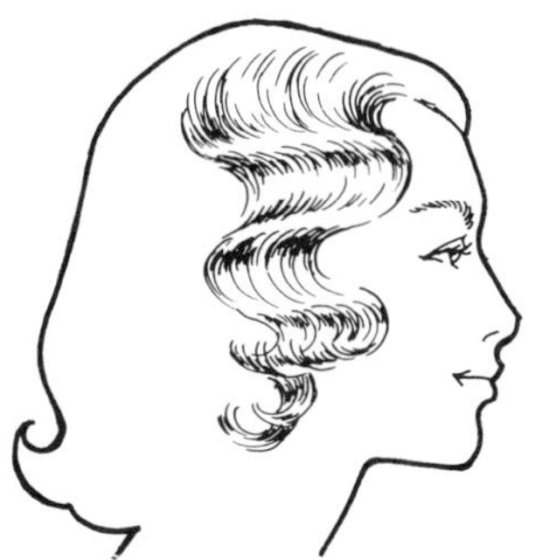
Horizontal wave comb-out

Horizontal Waves

To achieve horizontal waves, the hair is first shaped in a forward semicircular effect from the hair part downward. The pin curls are then set as illustrated. This creates a long-lasting wave close to the head.

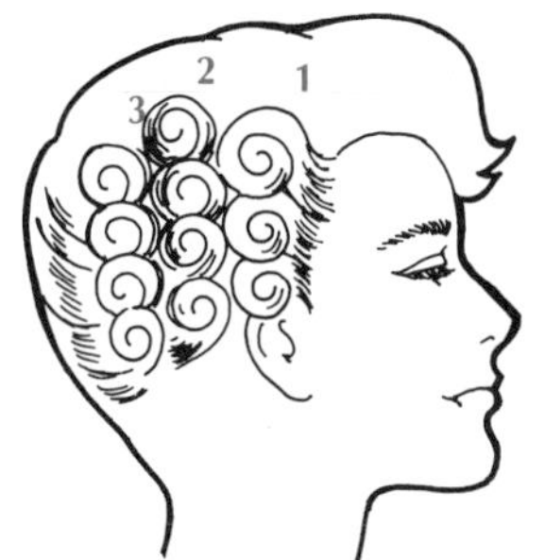

Setting pattern

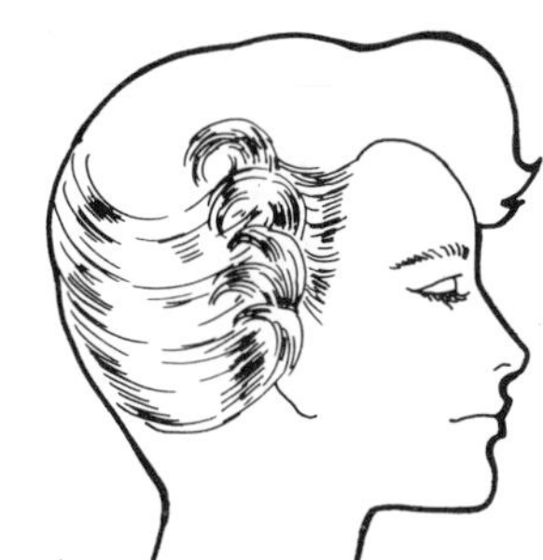
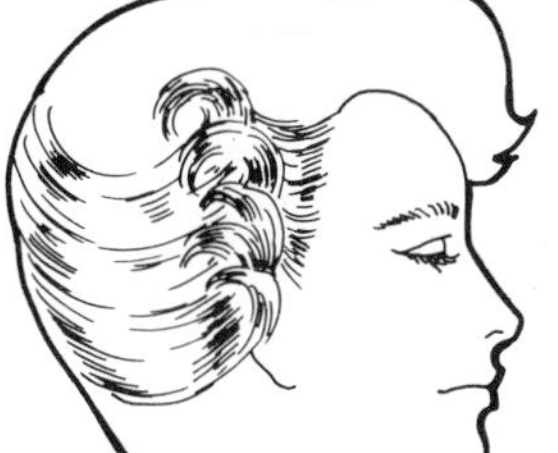
Comb-out

Interlocking Movement

First Row—Back-stem with forward curls

Second and Third Rows—Forward stem with reverse curls

Comb-out—The back curls are combed and interlocked with the front row of curls

Waved Top

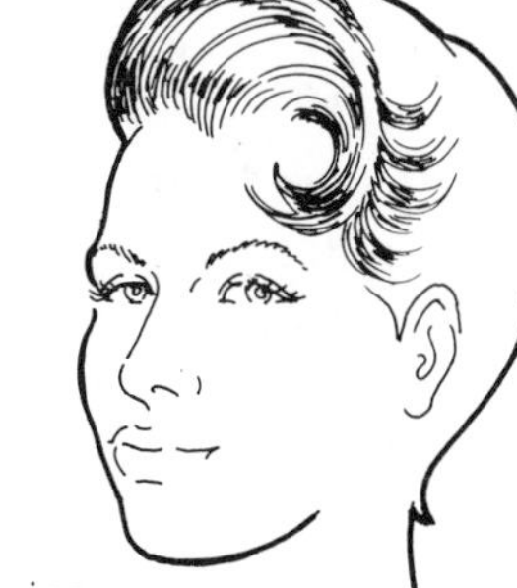
Shaping

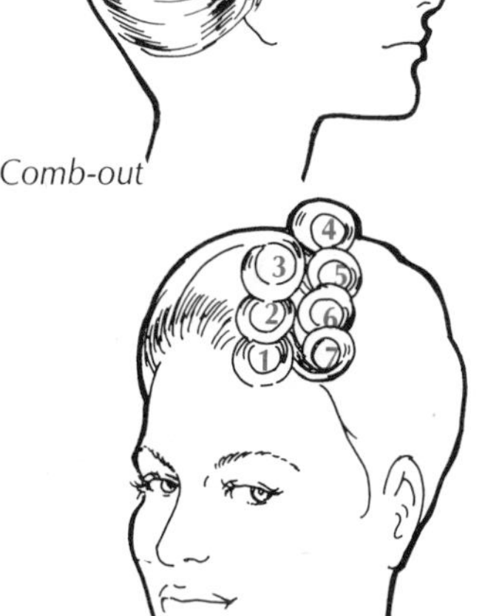

Setting pattern

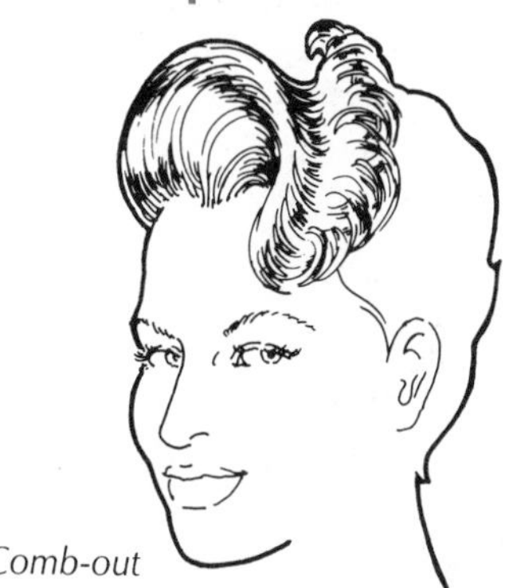
Comb-out

Diagonal Waves

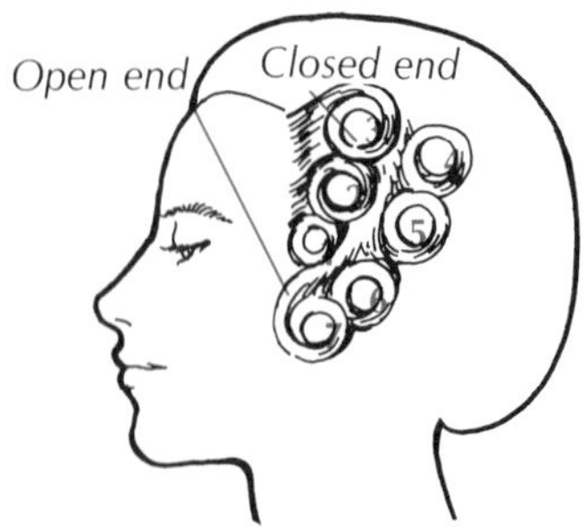

Setting pattern

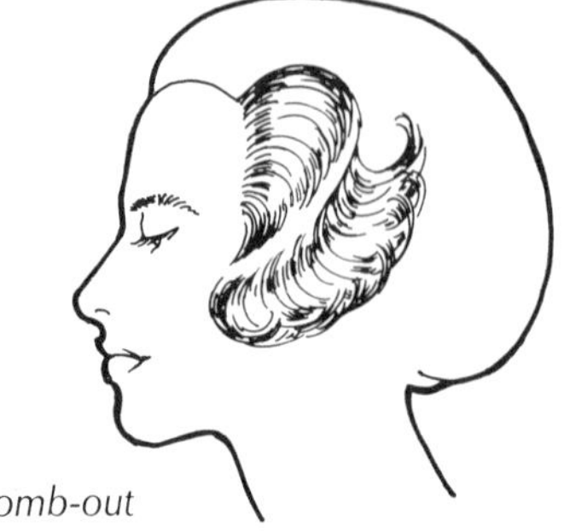
Comb-out

Shape hair—Oval forward shaping
Set—Start at open end
Comb-out—Diagonal waves

Waved Bangs

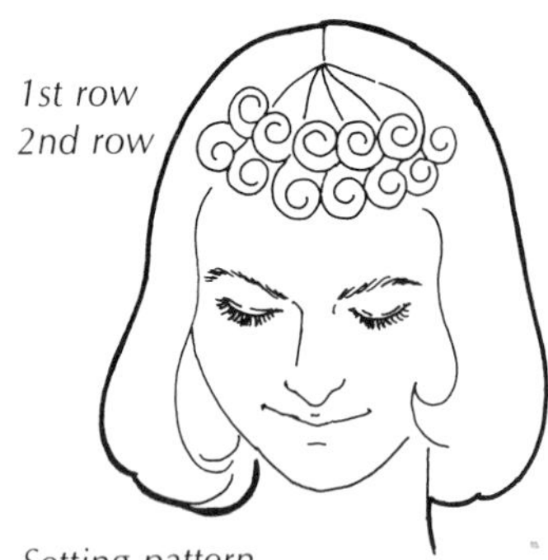

Setting pattern

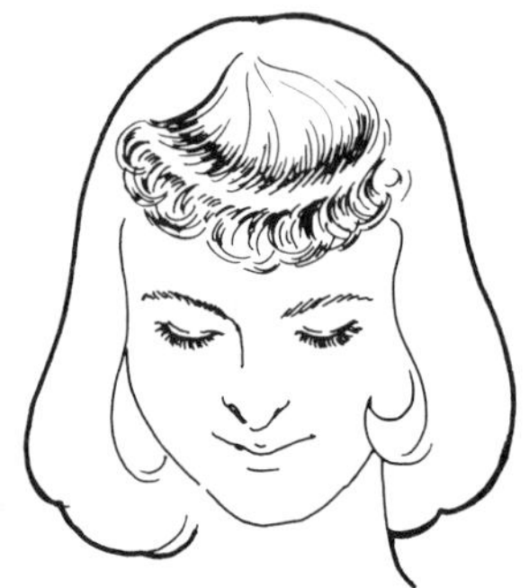
Comb-out

Setting for Fine Hair
Shape hair.
Set—First row
Second row

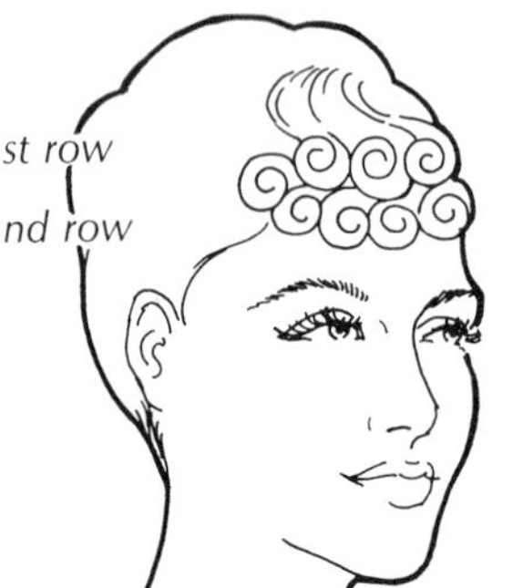

Setting pattern

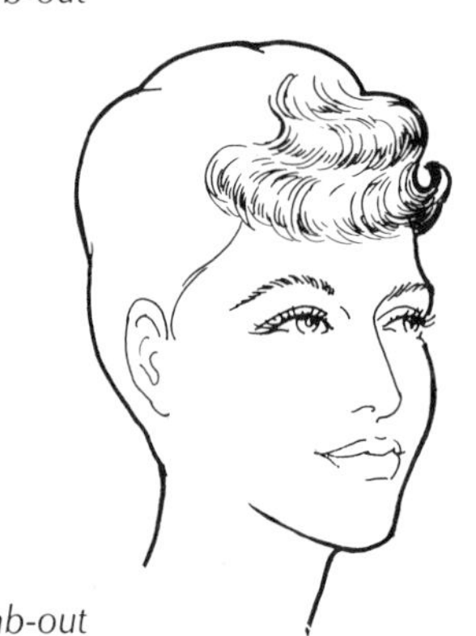
Comb-out

Setting for Normal Hair
Shape hair.
Set—First row
Second row

French Twist

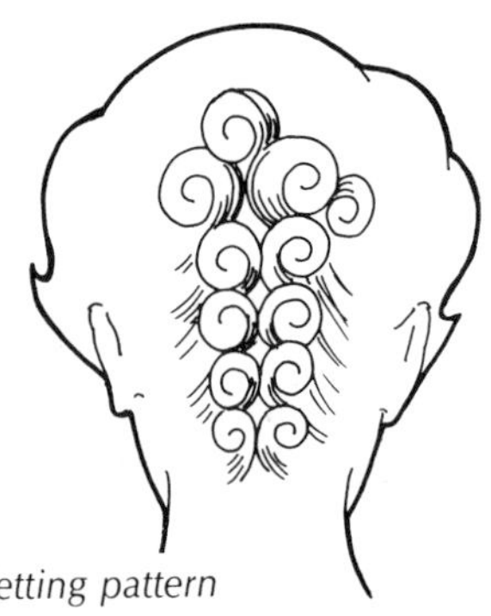
Setting pattern

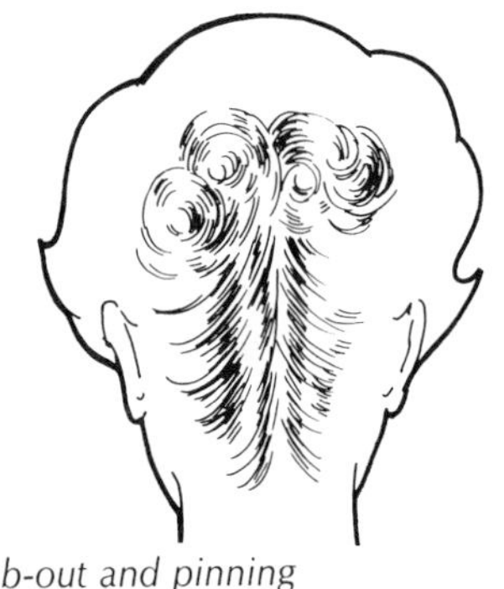
Comb-out and pinning

Setting for Normal Hair
Part off the back area and make vertical center part. Comb both sections toward the center.

Make large, **smooth** pin curls as shown in the illustration.

Brush or comb the other side and fold ends over the first section. Pin hair in herringbone fashion, so ends do not show.

RIDGE CURLS

Ridge curls are pin curls placed behind the ridge of a shaping or finger wave when a loose wave is desired. Care must be taken **not to disturb the ridge** when slicing out the strands for the curls.

Prepare hair. Shape hair and make ridge as for a vertical finger wave. Slice the strand without disturbing the ridge.

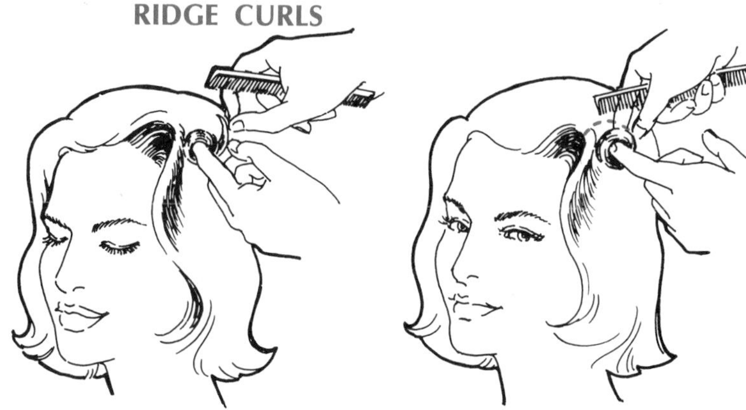

Fig. 10 Wind hair around the fingertip

Fig. 11 Slide strand off the finger and roll it to the base of the ridge

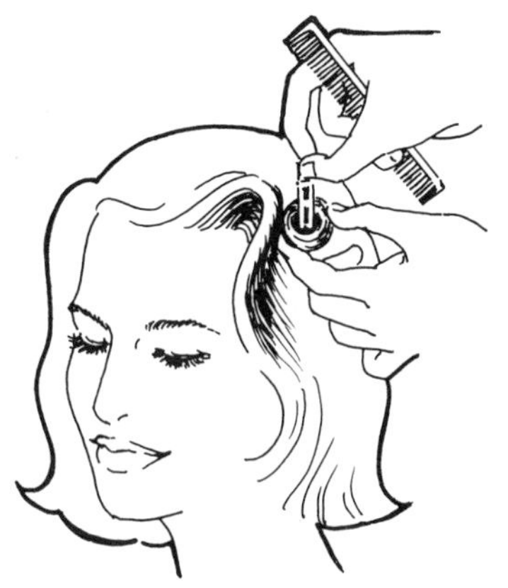

Fig. 12 Anchor curl with clippie

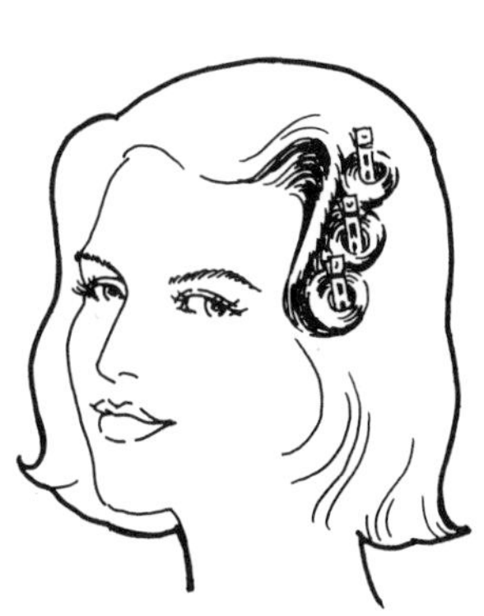

Fig. 13 Completed ridge curl

SKIP WAVE

The skip wave is a combination finger wave and pin curl pattern, the pin curls being placed in alternate finger wave formations. This technique is recommended when wide, smooth-flowing vertical waves are desired.

To obtain best results, the hair should be 3″ to 5″ in length. It is not recommended for hair that has a tight permanent wave or hair that is fine.

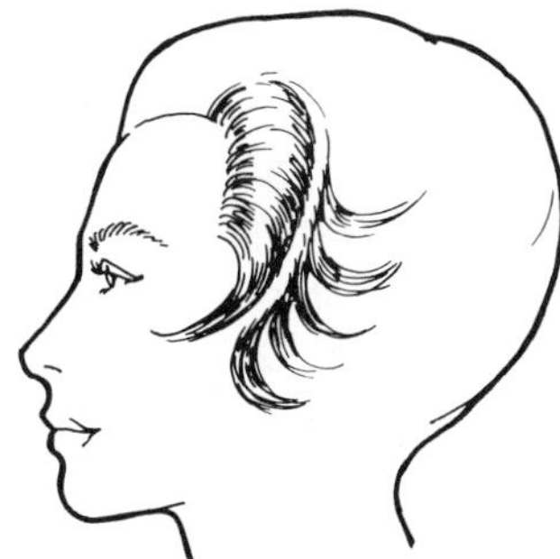

Shaping and ridge for vertical finger wave

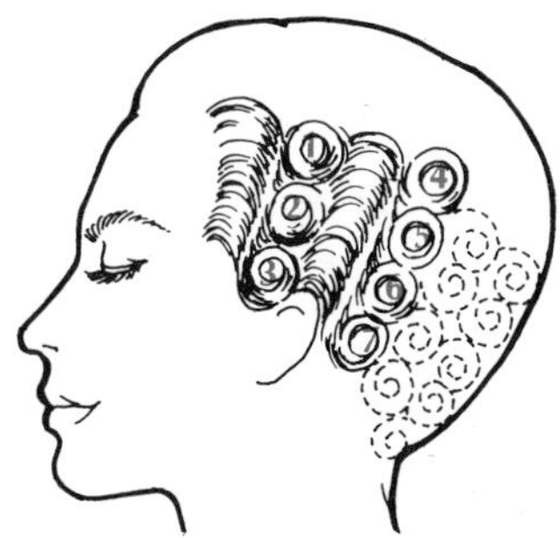

Skip wave pattern for fluff ends

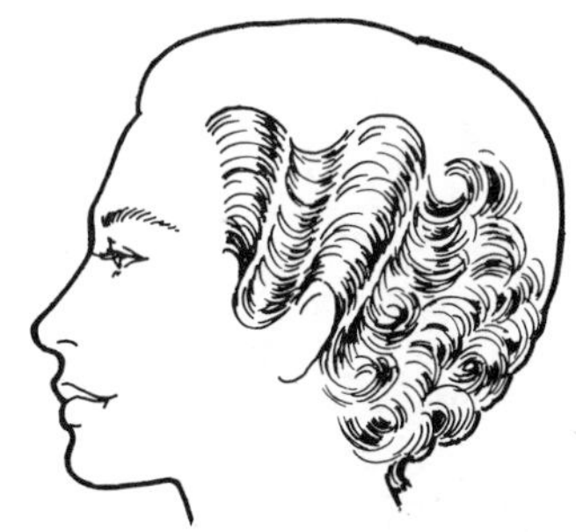

Comb-out with fluff ends

CASCADE OR STAND-UP CURL

The cascade curl, sometimes referred to as a **stand-up curl**, is wound from the hair ends to the scalp. The center opening is made large, and the curl is pinned in a standing position.

The stand-up curl provides a great deal of lift to the hair. It can be used in conjunction with rollers or by itself when volume is desired.

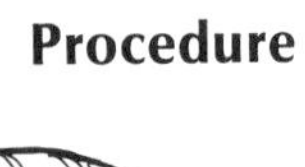

Note To become proficient in hairstyling the student must learn to make stand-up curls with ease and proficiency.

Procedure

Wet the top section with water or setting lotion.

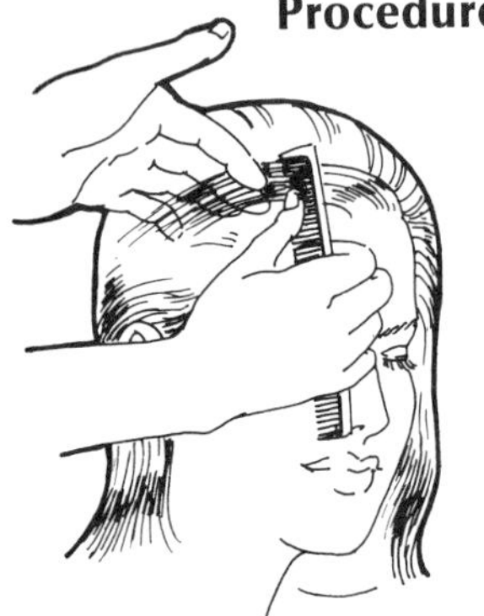

Comb, divide and smooth strand

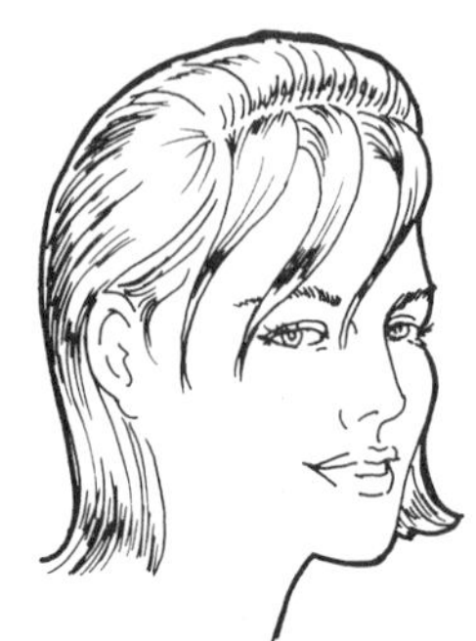

Divide section into strands for easy pick up

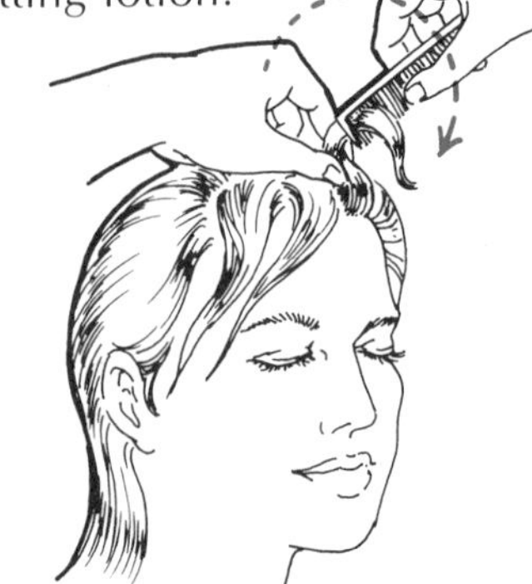

Ribbon the strand

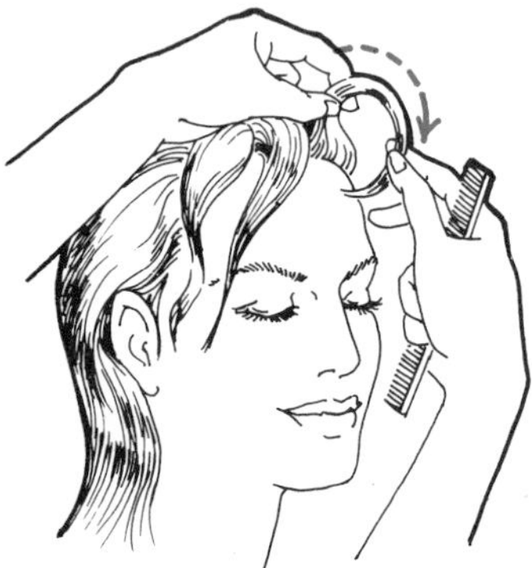

Direct the strand

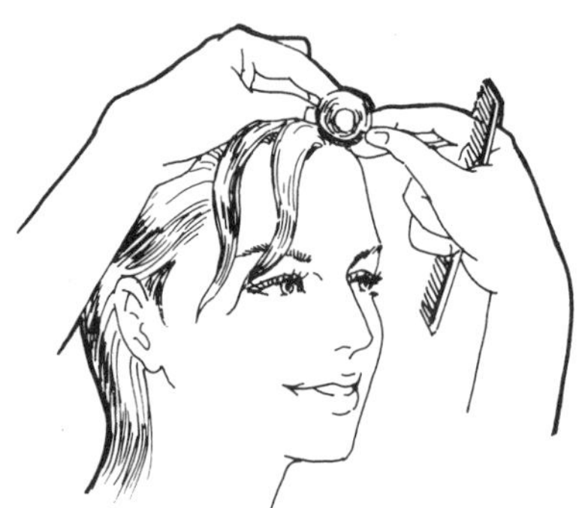

Wind the curl

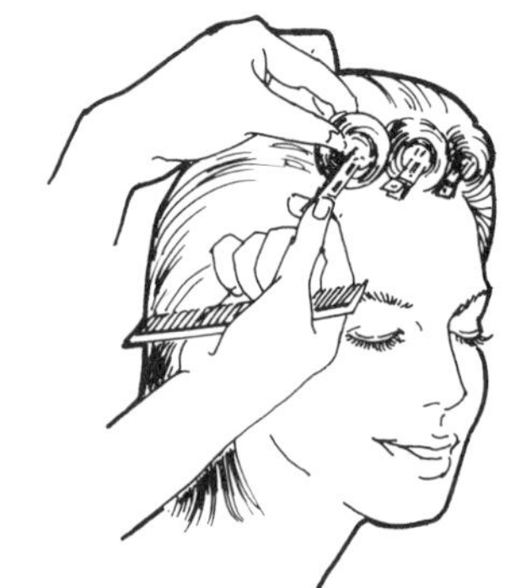

Pin the curl

Effect of Stand-Up Curls

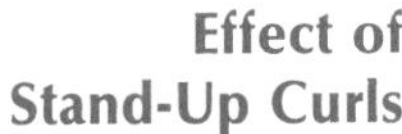

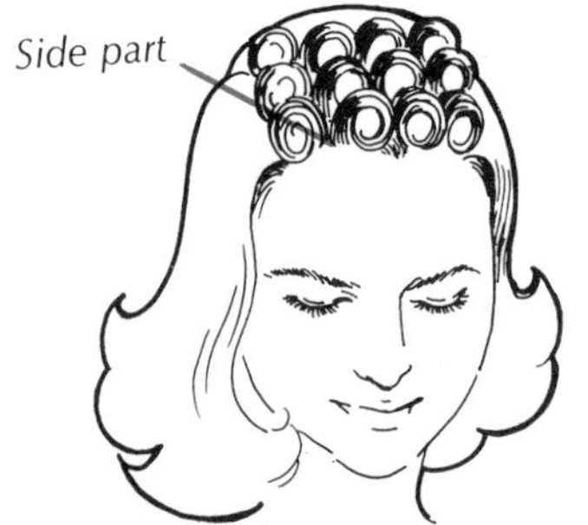

Top of setting

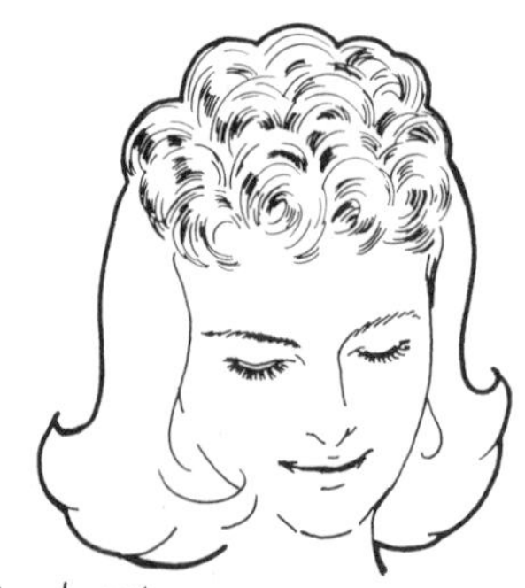

Comb-out

Setting—Stand-up curls for side movement with a side part.

Comb-out—The hair is brushed from the hairline, then sliced off in small sections and flipped over the forehead.

SEMI-STAND-UP CURLS

Semi-stand-up curls are pin curls that have been carved out of a shaping and pinned into a semi-standing position.

Top wave effect can be achieved with stand-up curls by the following procedure:

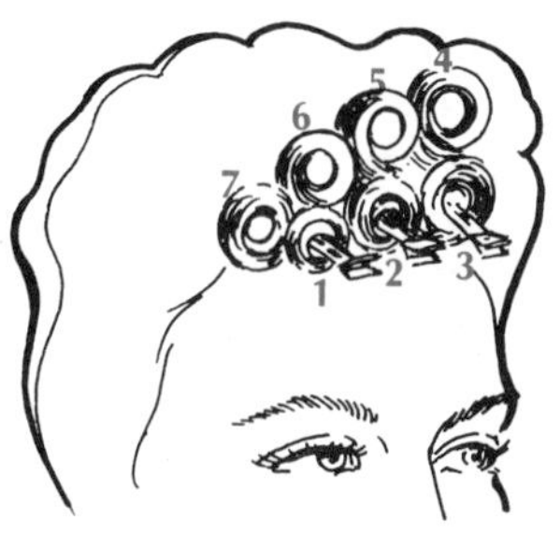

Semi-stand-up curl setting

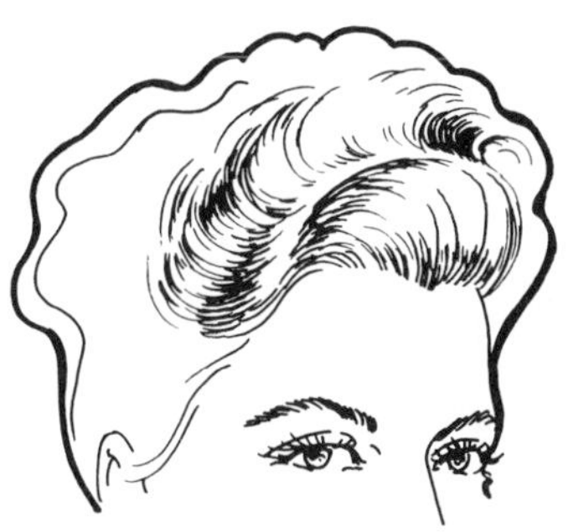
Comb-out

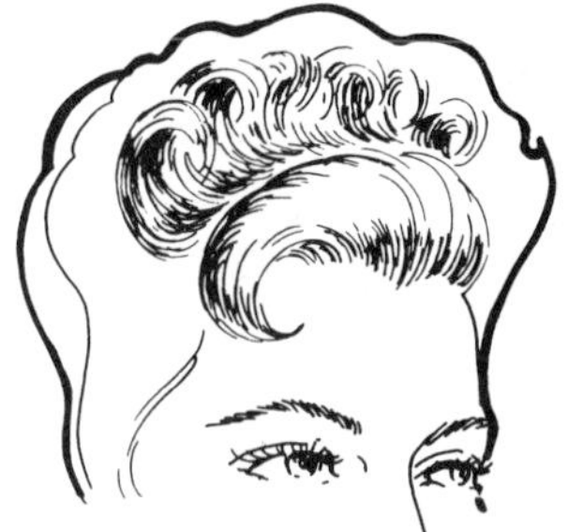
Alternate comb out

1. Shape the top hair.
2. Make three counter clockwise curls.
3. Back up with four clockwise curls.
4. Comb-out. The hair may be combed out as shown in the two illustrations.

ROLLER CURLS

Roller curls are designed to create the same effects as stand-up curls. They are formed over special rollers that come in various sizes to fulfill special needs in a hair design.

The rollers are, in effect, molds around which curls are formed to create added lift or volume. They are especially effective in creating a straight line design with more height and stability than is usually achieved with stand-up curls.

An important difference between roller and stand-up curls is that stand-up curls are formed one at a time and rollers can accommodate the equivalent of from 2 to 4 stand-up curls at one time. In addition, the rollers give far more security to the rolled hair while its wet.

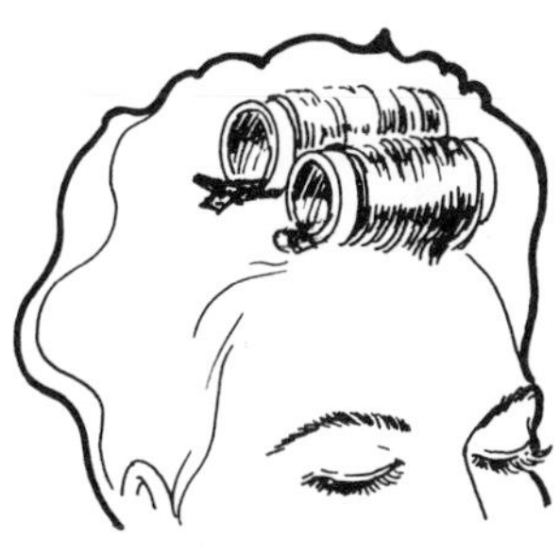
Roller curls

Sectioning the Hair

First, the hair is sectioned into panels, then subdivided into roller bases. The size of the bases should be as near as possible to the length and diameter of the roller.

A good example to follow is if a roller is 3″ (7.5 cm) long and 1″ (2.5 cm) wide in diameter, the base should be 1″ (2.5 cm) wide by 2 3/4″ (6.875 cm) long, about 1/4″ (.625 cm) shorter. If this proportion is followed with the various sizes of rollers, the hair will not be overcrowded nor slip off the sides of the rollers.

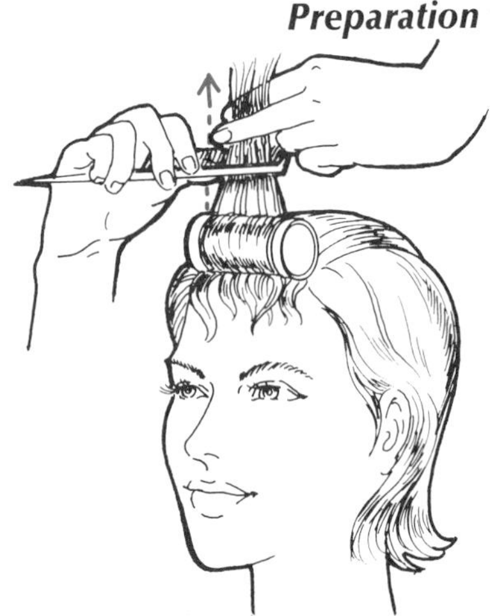

1. Strand preparation

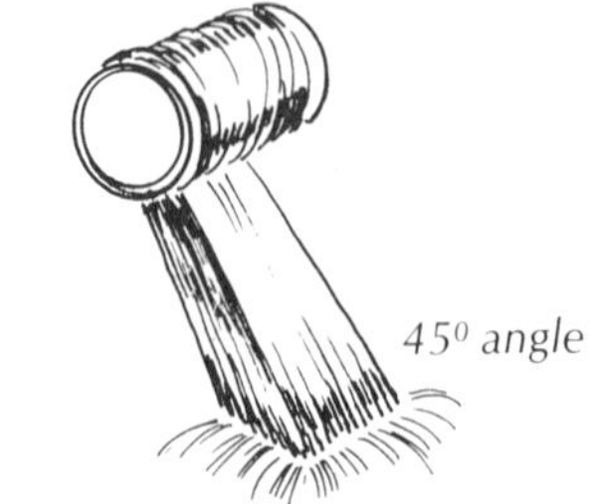

2. Hold the strand at a 45° angle

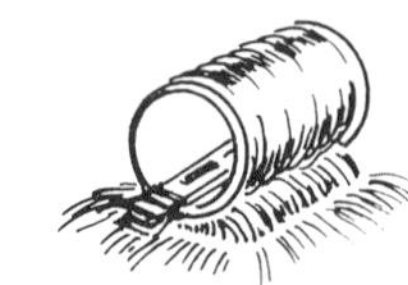

2a. Roll strand on base and anchor with a clip

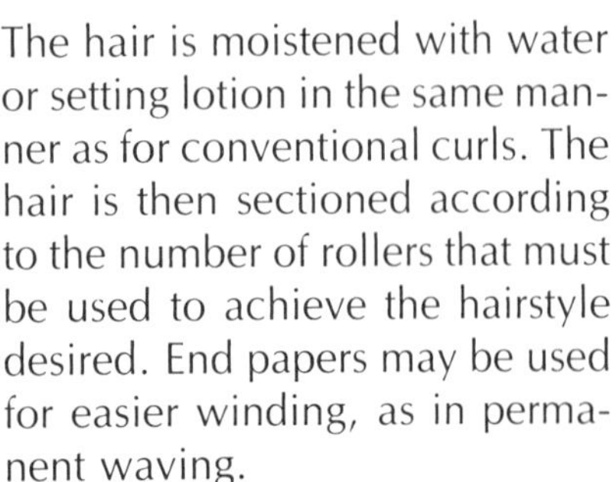

The hair is moistened with water or setting lotion in the same manner as for conventional curls. The hair is then sectioned according to the number of rollers that must be used to achieve the hairstyle desired. End papers may be used for easier winding, as in permanent waving.

Roller setting technique. Hold the strand at a 45° (.785 rad.) angle and roll in the manner shown. The roller will sit directly over the base of the rectangle. The curl will be strong and have maximum volume or body.

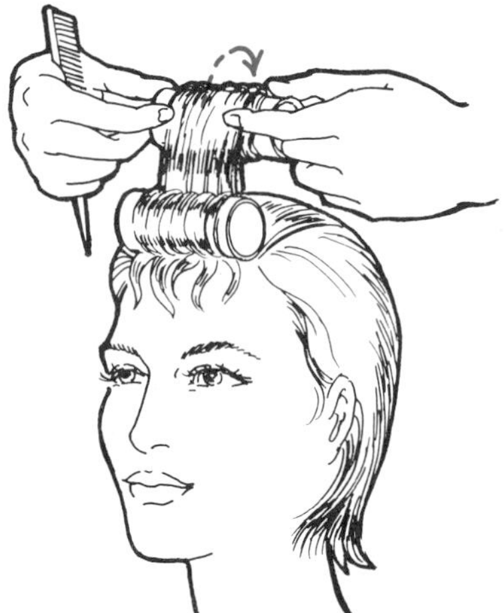

3. Hand position while winding the roller

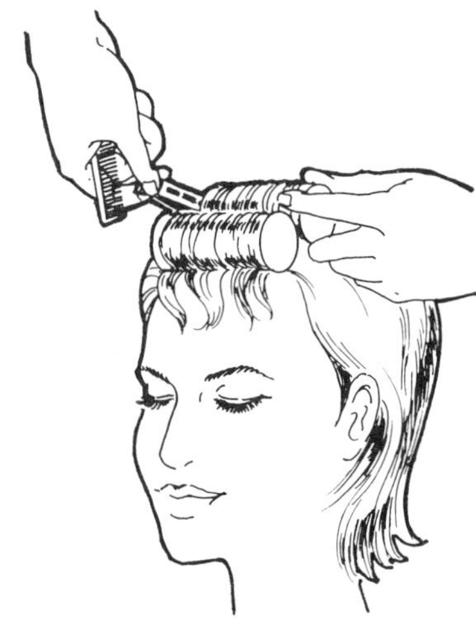

4. Holding roller in position while pinning

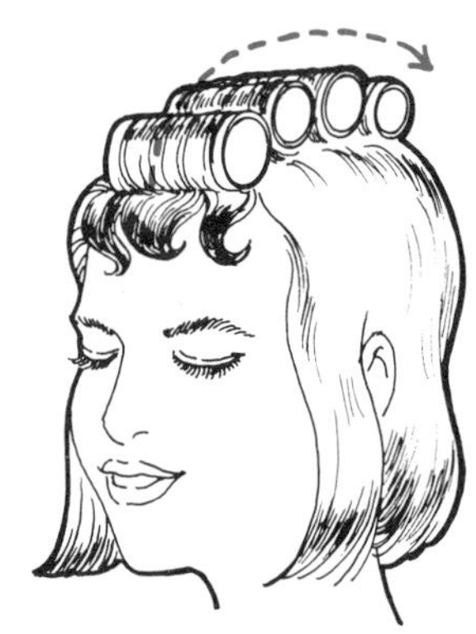

Complete roller curls from hairline to crown with pin curls for bang effect

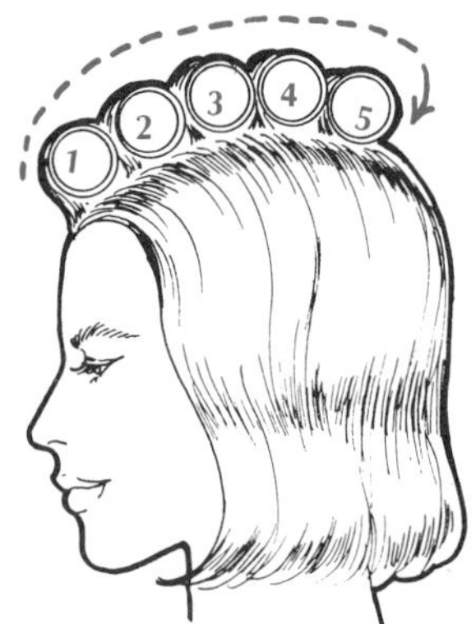

Roller setting for off-the-face effect

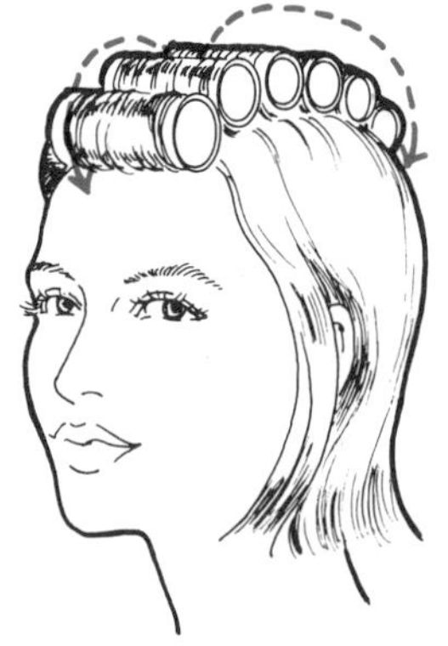

Roller curl pattern for bang effect

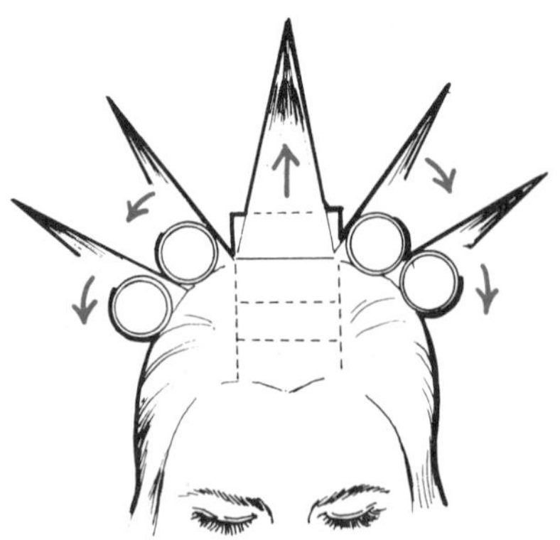

The angle at which the hair is held from the head for roller placement

Effects of Hair Length on Rollers

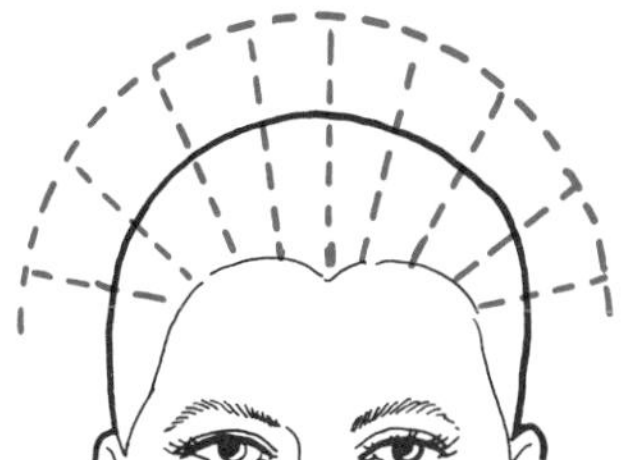

The length of the hair and the size of the rollers affect the finished hairstyle in the top front area in the following manner:

1. When wrapping a 4 1/2" (11.25 cm) strand around a roller 1" (2.5 cm) in diameter, it will go around one full turn. Result: three rollers will produce a soft puff with minimum curl turned in ends.
2. When wrapping a 4 1/2" (11.25 cm) strand around 3/4" (1.85 cm.) roller in diameter, the strand will go around about 1 1/2 times. Result: four rollers will produce a curl fluff with turned in ends.
3. Should the size of each roller be small enough to permit the hair strand to be rolled around it twice, five rollers will be needed to adequately curl the area. The use of these rollers will result in a deep, soft wave because the hair ends are in the opposite direction of the original movement of the hair.

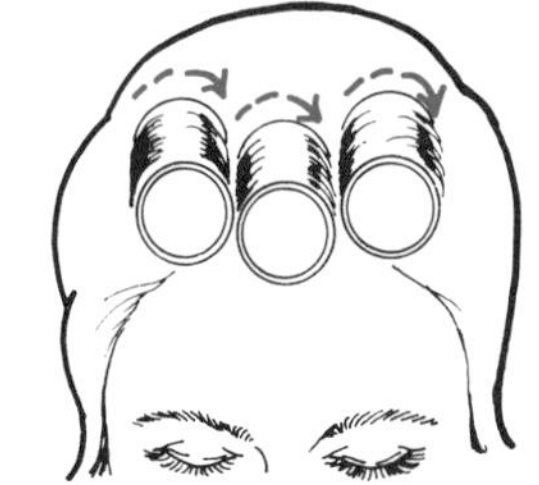

Pattern

Comb-out

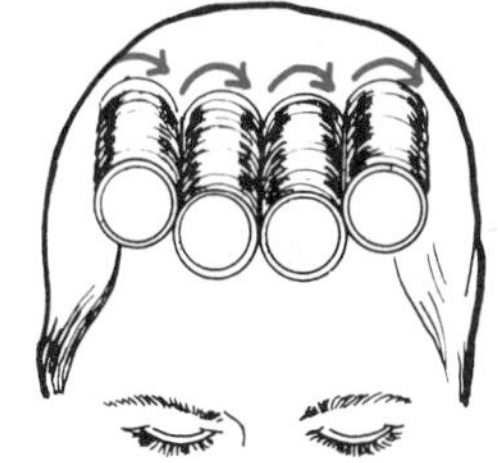

Pattern

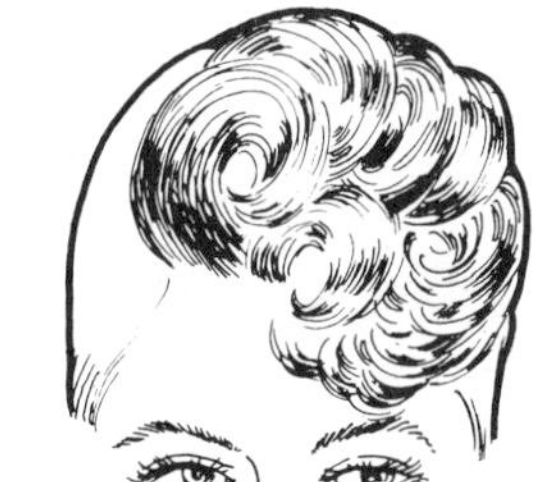

Comb-out

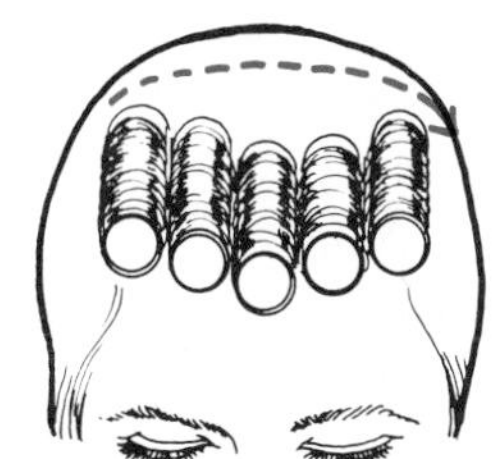

Pattern

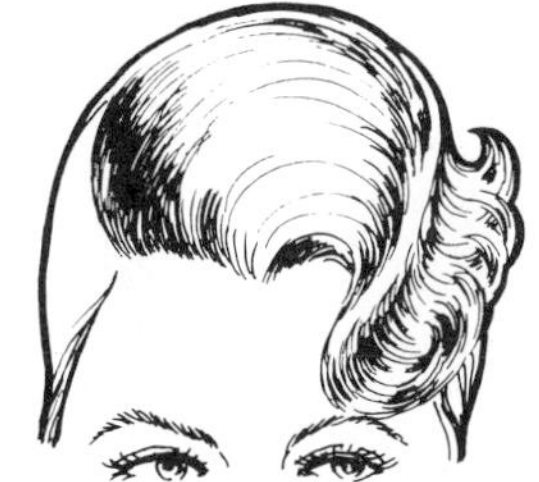

Comb-out

BARREL CURLS

A barrel curl serves as a substitute for a curl formed around a roller and may be used where there is insufficient room to place a roller. However, it does not provide the tension that is present in roller wrapping.

The barrel curl is made in a similar manner as the stand-up curl, with a flat base and containing much more hair.

Barrel curl

VOLUME AND INDENTATION IN ROLLER TECHNIQUE (With Cylinder Rollers)

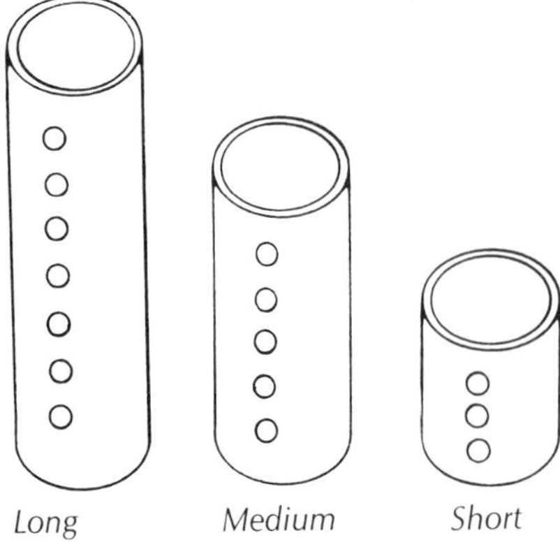

CYLINDER SHAPED ROLLERS (one-half size)

Modern hairstyling incorporates the use of various devices and methods to achieve special designs and effects. One of the most effective devices in this area is the roller which is available in various sizes and lengths. Rollers are especially important in the creation of volume (lift) and indentation (valleys and hollows) in the hairstyle.

Note For the rollers to be used to their maximum efficiency, roll the ends under and then roll the hair down to the scalp on its base.

Volume and Indentation To create indentation, the hair is kept close to the head and rolled over on the rollers.

Angle of strand for full volume

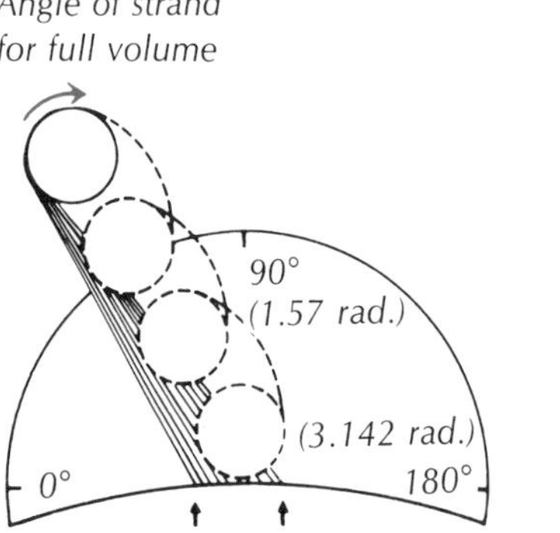

To create full volume, roller rests on its base

Strand kept at scalp level for indentation

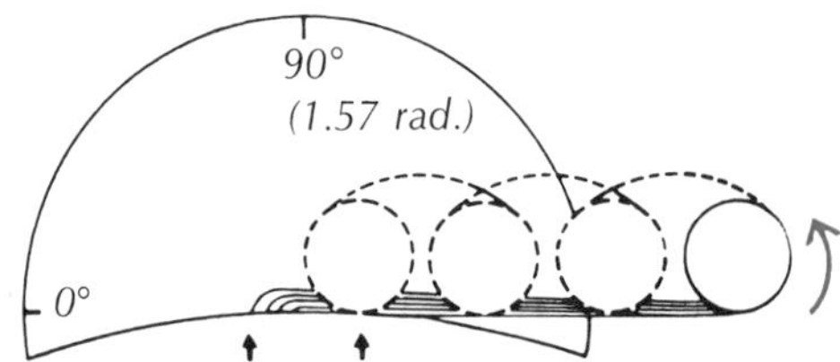

To create indentation or hollowness, keep the hair close to the head and roll to one-half off base

Angle of strand for added volume

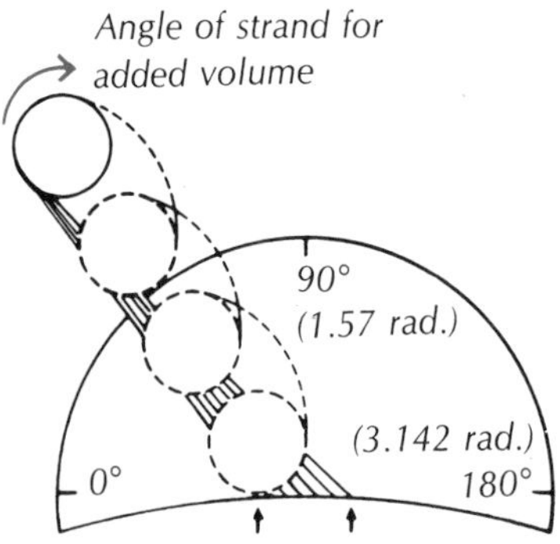

To create maximum volume, roller rests one-half off left side of base

Angle of strand for medium volume

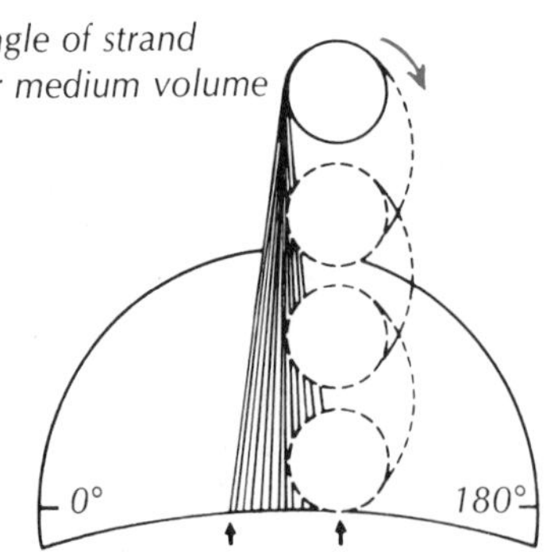

To create a medium amount of volume, roller rests one-half off the right side of base

Angle of strand for less volume

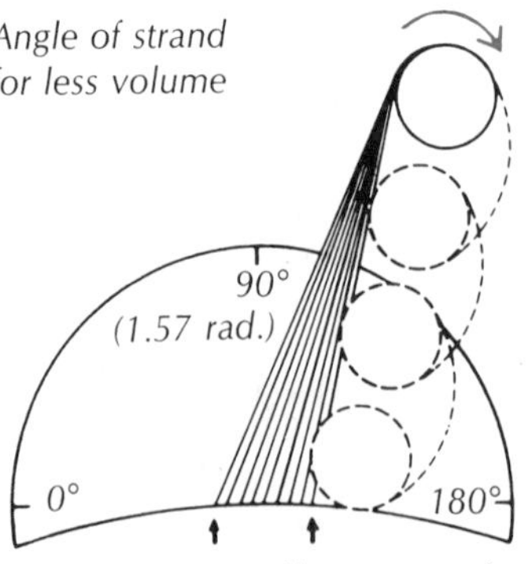

To create a small amount of volume, roller rests off right side of base

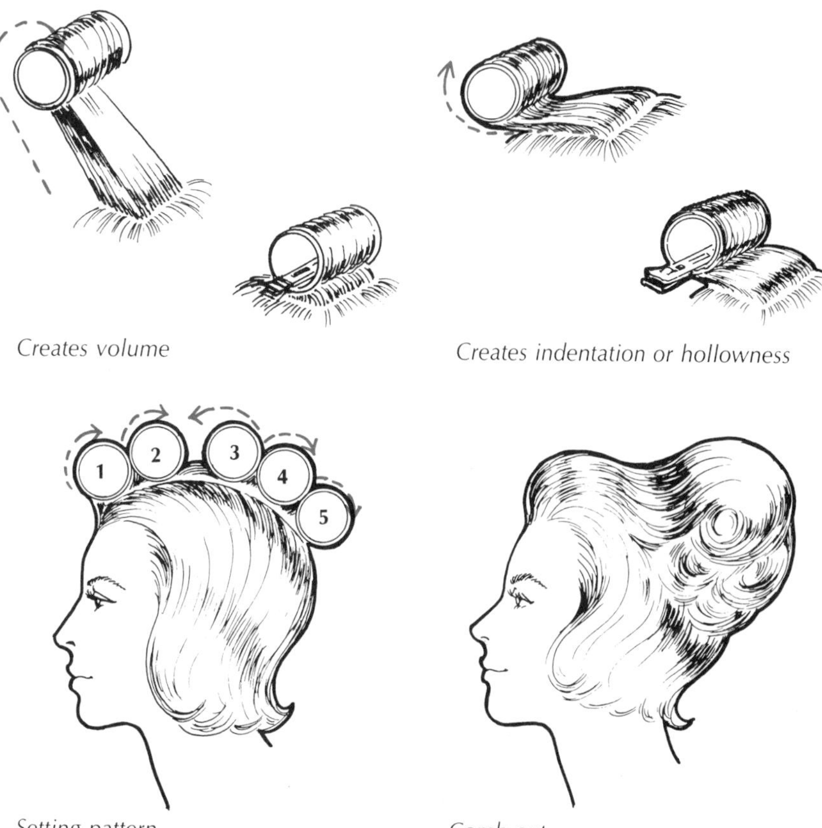

Creates volume

Creates indentation or hollowness

Setting pattern

Comb-out

CYLINDER CIRCULAR ROLLER ACTION

The hair that is directed in a circular manner is referred to by hairstylists in various ways, such as radial motion, circular movement, curvature roller action, rotary motion or movement, spotmatic movement, contour movement and others.

Effects of Hair Lengths on Cylinder Rollers

Short hair (slender rollers)

The point (spot or area) from which the hair is directed to form a circular movement is also referred to by any of the following terms: balance point, swing point, terminal point, pivot point, pendulum point, radial point, fulcrum point, radiation point, rotary point and spotmatic point.

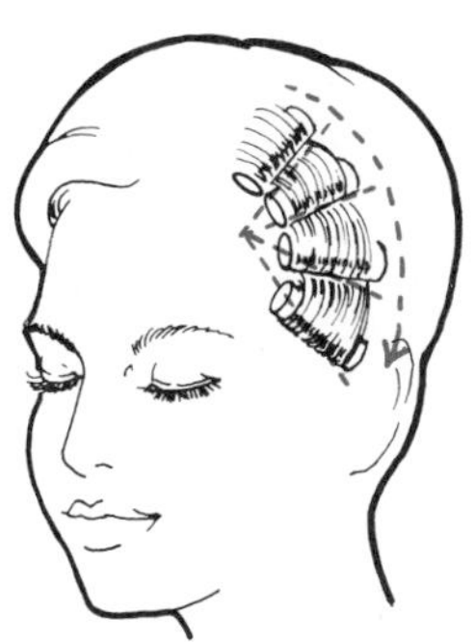

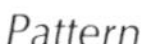

Pattern

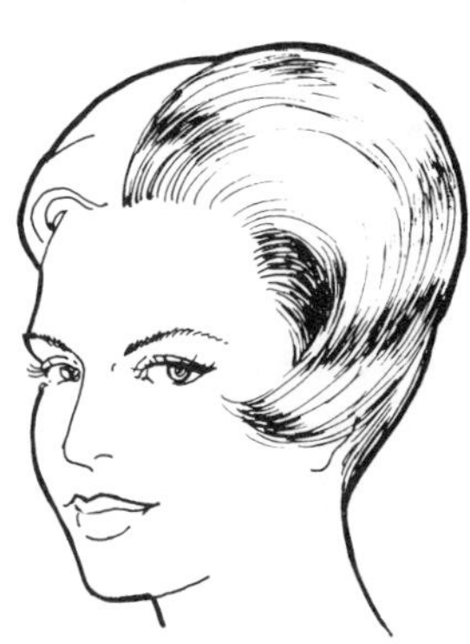

Comb-out

Medium length hair (medium size rollers)

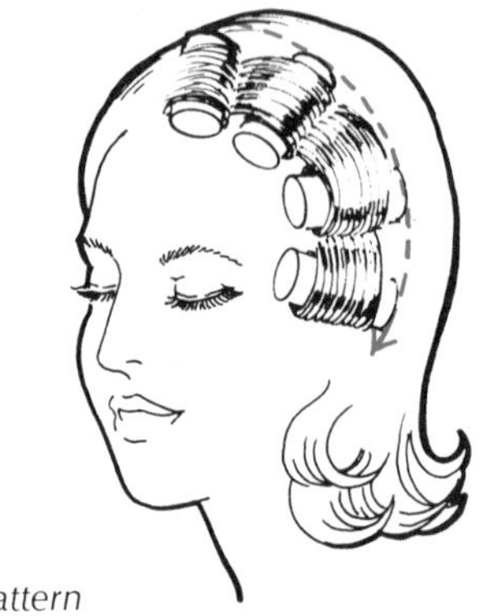

Pattern

Comb-out

Long hair (large rollers)

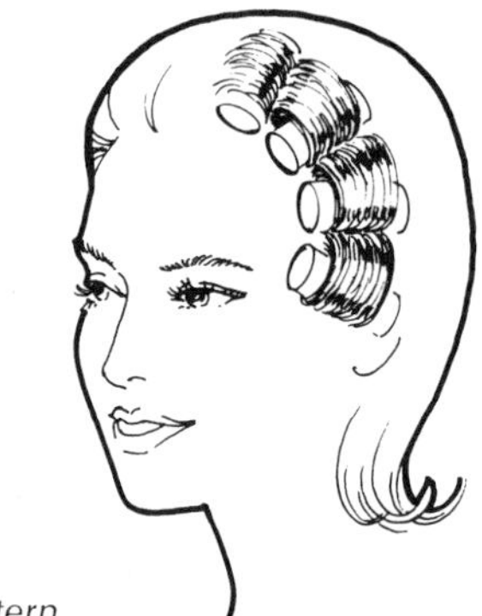

Pattern

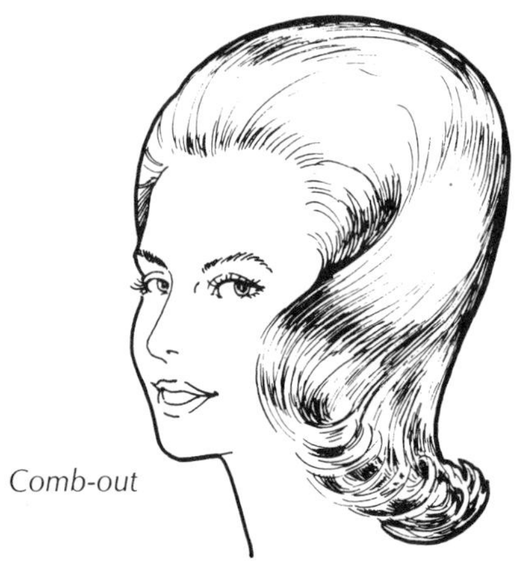

Comb-out

Effects of Same Size Rollers on Different Lengths of Hair
(using the same length and diameter roller)

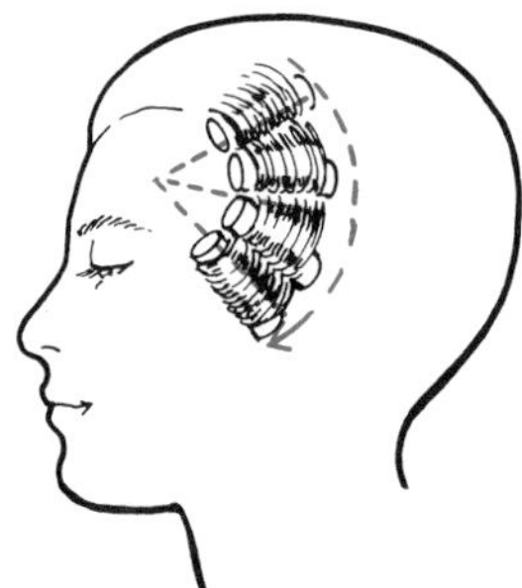

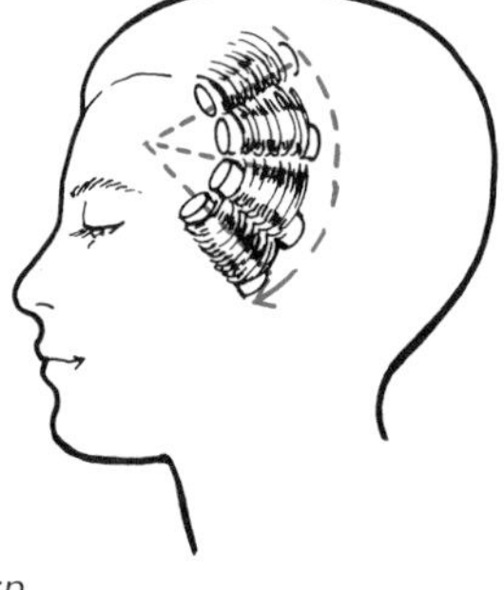

Pattern

Comb-out—short hair

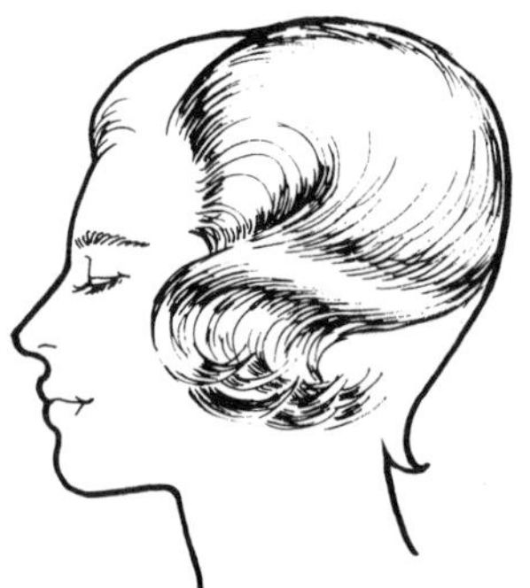

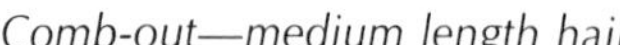

Comb-out—medium length hair

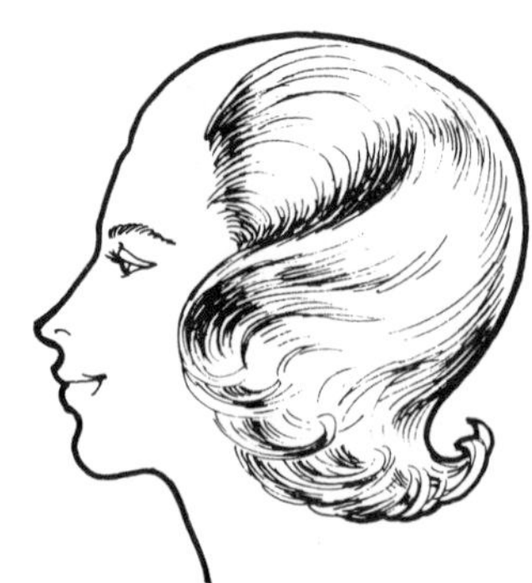

Comb-out—long hair

Effects of Cylinder Rollers—Circular Movement

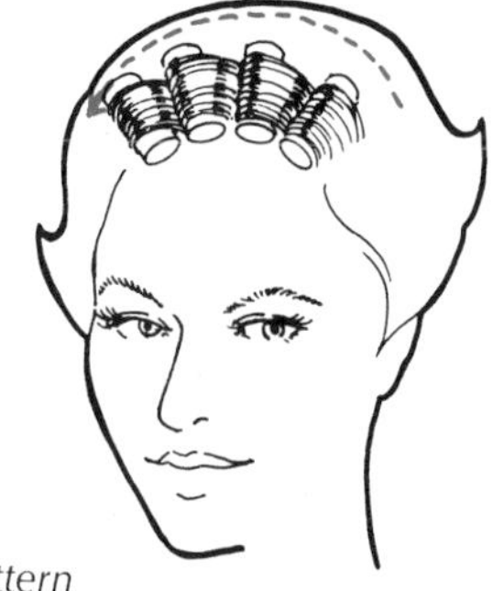
Pattern

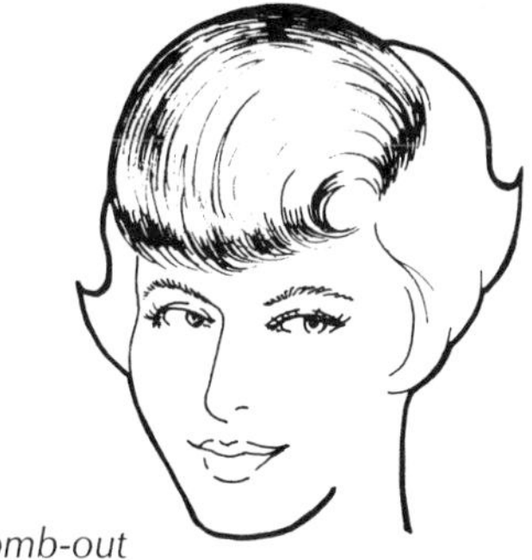
Comb-out

Top—Cylinder rollers set in wedge-shape partings in a circular manner. Comb out in a forward shell effect with bangs.

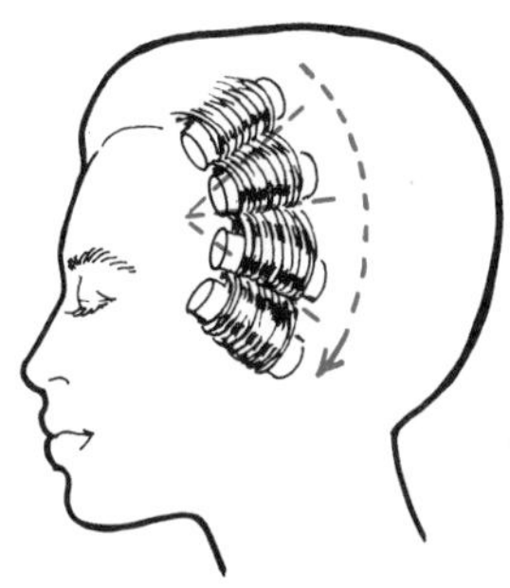
Pattern

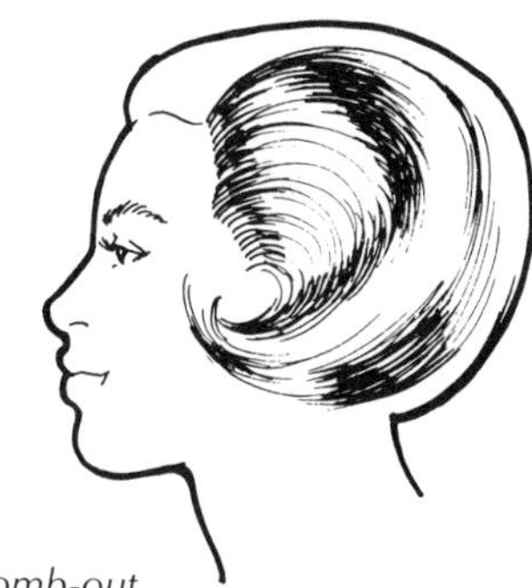
Comb-out

Side—Cylinder rollers set in wedge-shape partings. The comb out gives a circular movement toward the face.

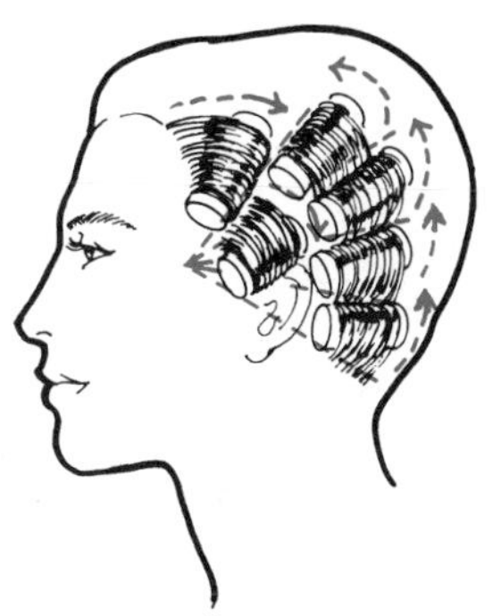
Pattern

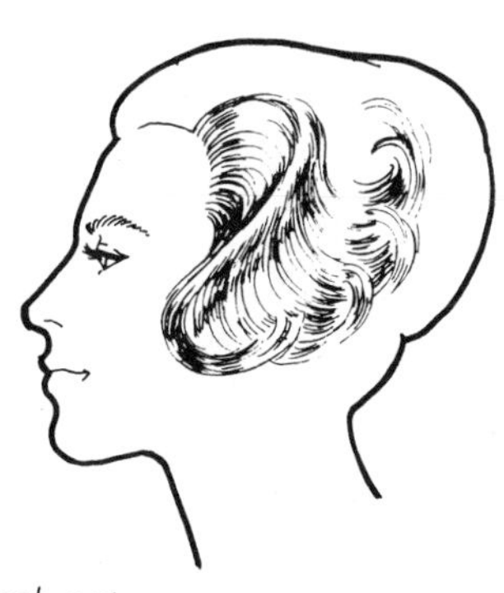
Comb-out

Special side effects—Side roller setting with sculpture curl in front of ear.

The comb-out produces an "S" wave formation effect.

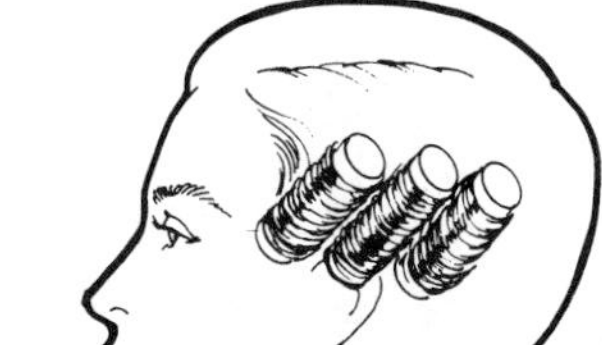
Pattern

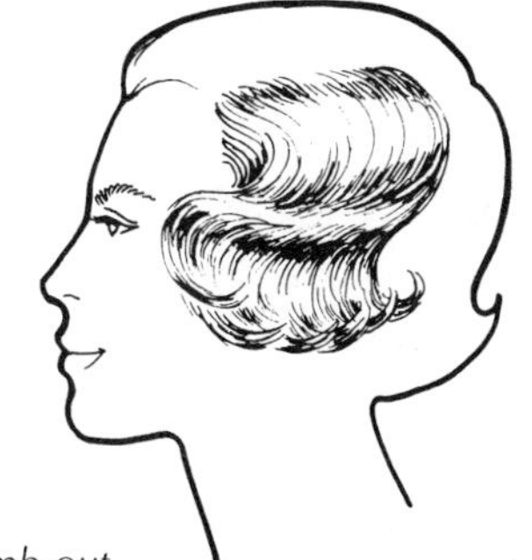
Comb-out

To create a ridge line and indentation (hollowness), set the hair on rollers at an angle as shown in the illustration.

This setting will produce the waved effect shown in the comb-out.

TAPERED ROLLERS

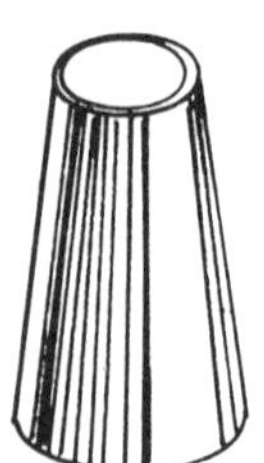

Practically the same styling results can be achieved by using either cylinder or tapered rollers. However, since cylinder rollers must be placed slightly further back from the point of distribution in a pie-shaped parting, the movement of the hair may be weaker. The tapered roller, however, makes it possible to develop a tighter curvature movement.

Size of rollers is governed by the texture of the hair. Fine hair takes smaller rollers; coarse hair takes larger rollers.

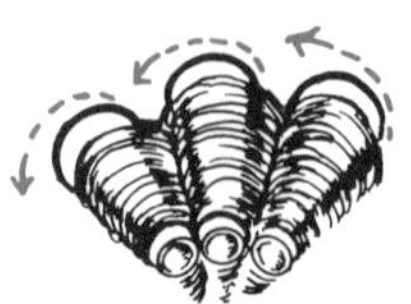

One-quarter circle setting using thinner rollers produces tighter comb-outs

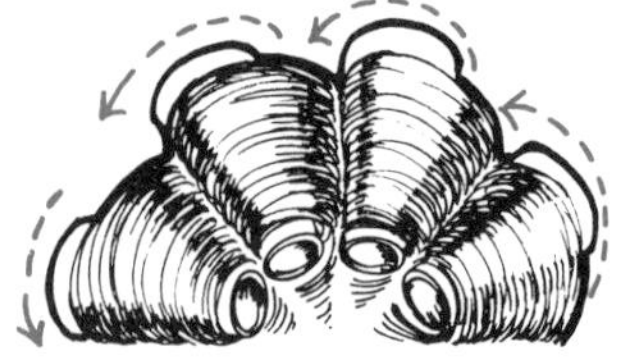

One-half circle setting using larger (thicker) rollers produces looser comb-outs

Effects of Tapered Rollers

Tapered hairline roller setting combs out like a shell shaped front with bangs or curled up ends.

Side tapered roller setting and sculpture ear curls comb out in a forward movement.

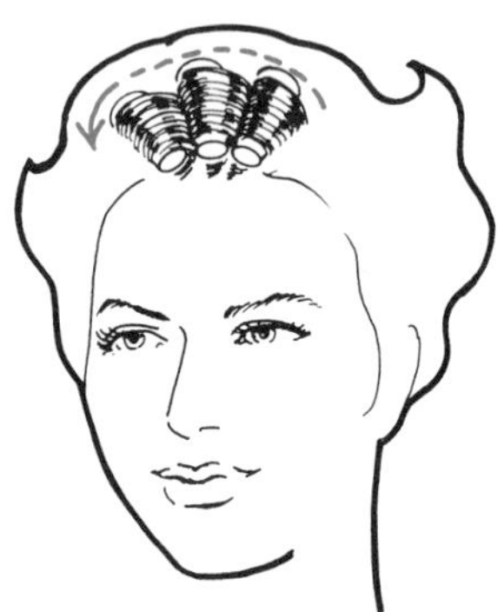

Setting

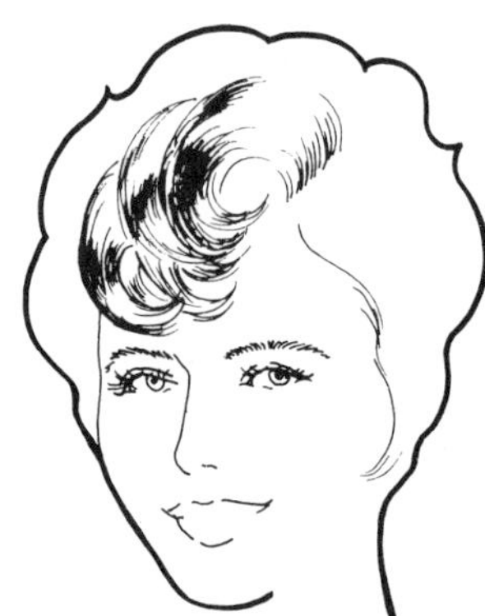

Comb-out

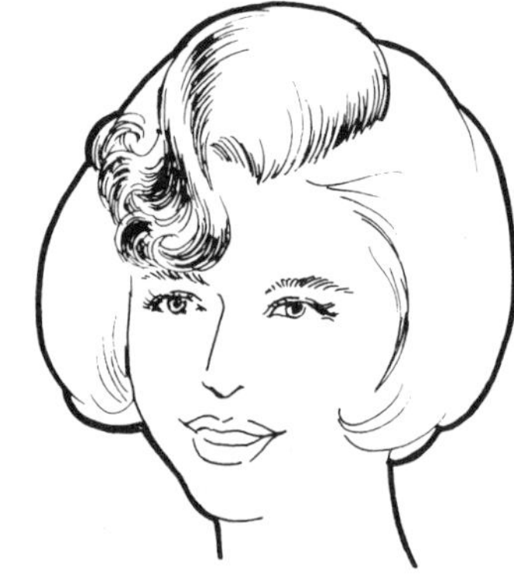

Alternate comb-out

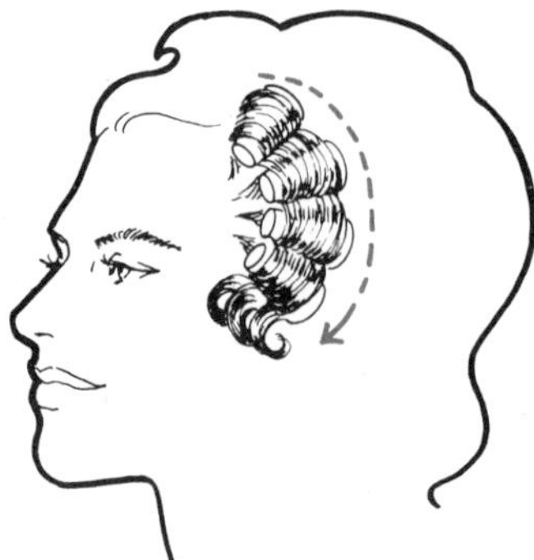

Setting

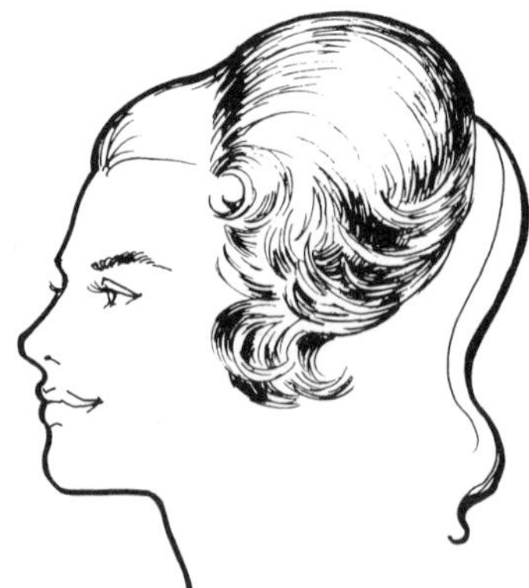

Comb-out

HAIR PARTINGS

The manner of parting the client's hair should be adjusted to the shape of the head, the facial type and desired hairstyle. The cosmetologist also must be guided by the natural parting of the client's hair.

The following are suggested hair partings for various facial types and hairstyles.

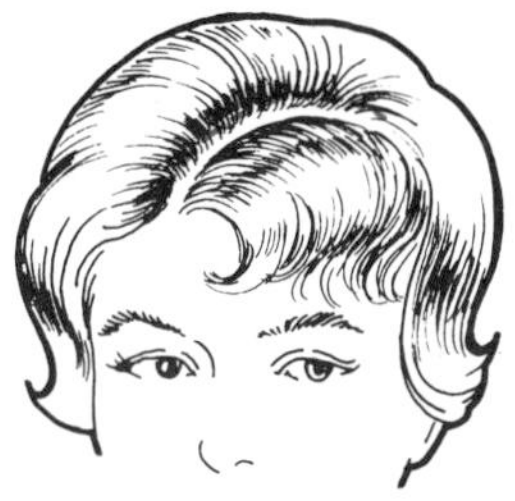

Diagonal part, used to give height to a round or square face

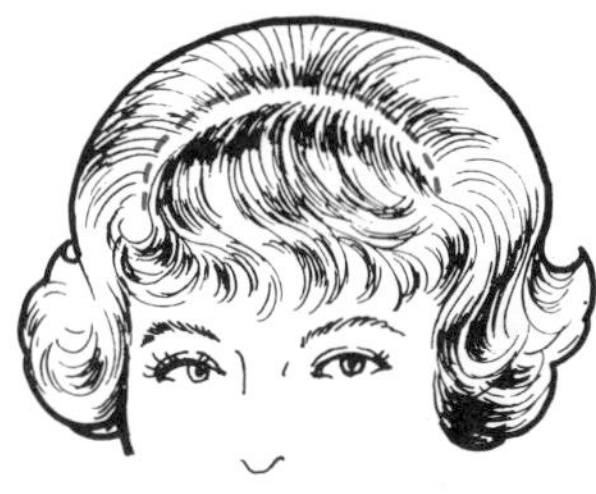

Curved rectangular part, used for receding hairline or high forehead

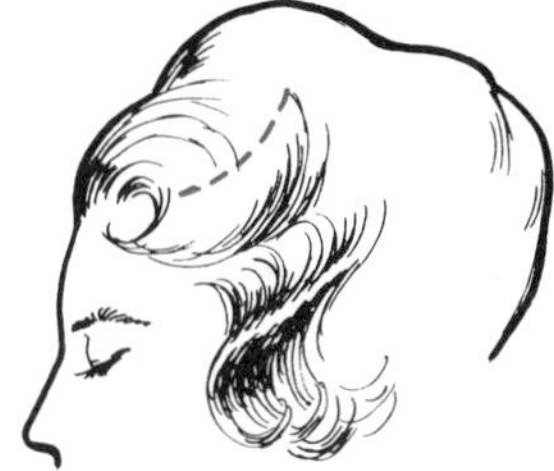

Concealed part, used for height and one-sided style effect

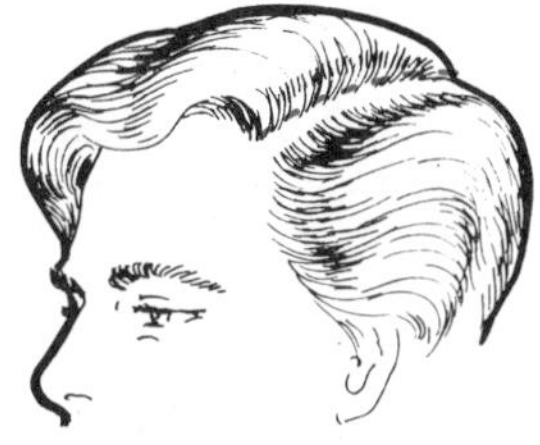

Side part used for styles to be directed to one side. Helps to create the illusion of decreasing width of forehead.

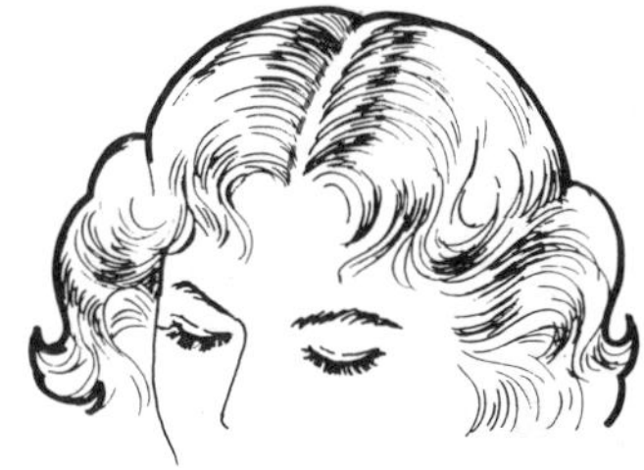

Center part. No rigid rule can be made for a center part style. Always try to create a hairstyle that will give an optical illusion of ovalness to the face.

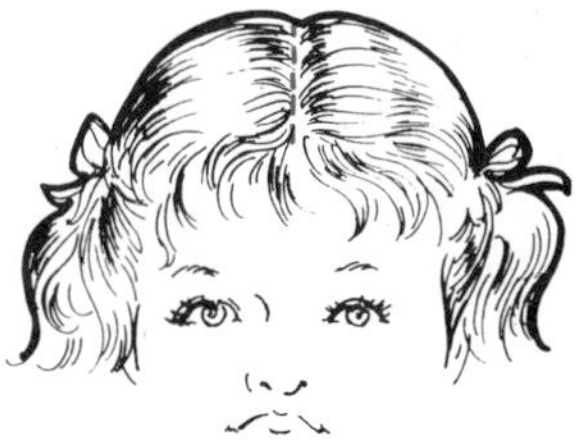

Popular center parting for children's hairstyles with bangs

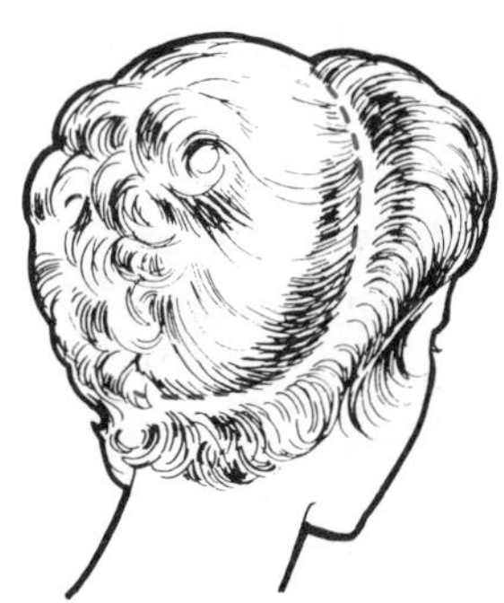

Diagonal back parting, used to create the illusion of width to crown and back of head

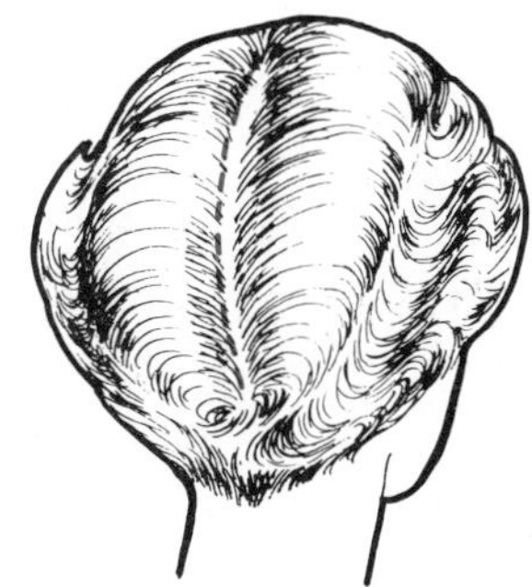

Natural crown parting

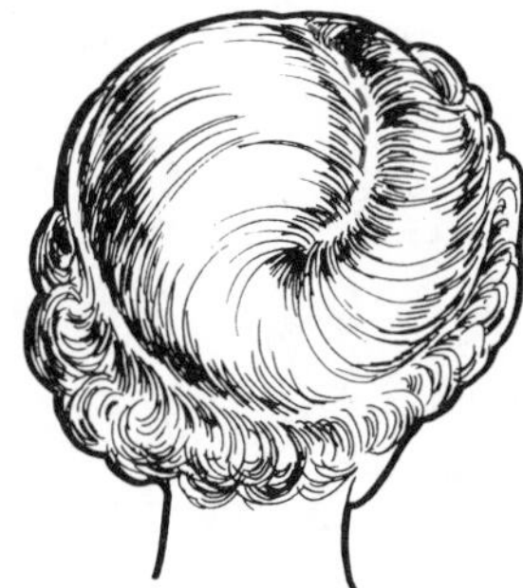

Natural crown parting

It would be extremely difficult to create a hairstyle when working against the natural crown parting. Working against the natural parting would cause problems in getting the hair to fall smoothly or to hold the setting.

BACK COMBING AND BACK BRUSHING TECHNIQUES

Back combing and back brushing are processes of matting the hair by combing or brushing it toward the scalp so that the shorter hair mats to form a cushion or base for the top or covering hair.

Back Combing

Back combing is also called **teasing, ratting, matting** or **French lacing**. After the basic comb-out is completed, it may need back combing or back brushing to achieve the planned hairstyle. When the hair has been brushed and relaxed, analyze the areas that need to be raised.

Procedure

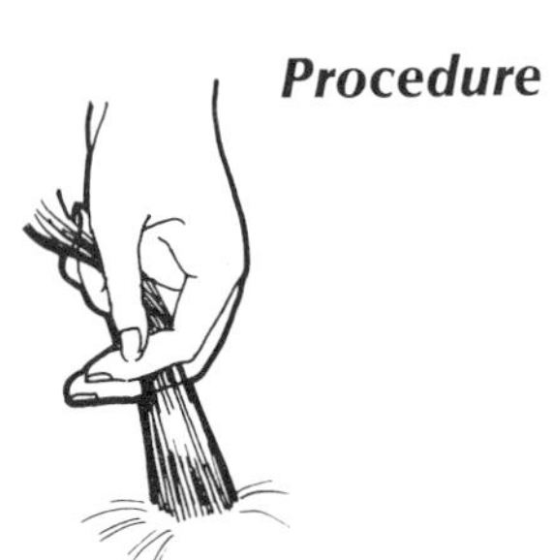

The hair properly held between the index and middle fingers

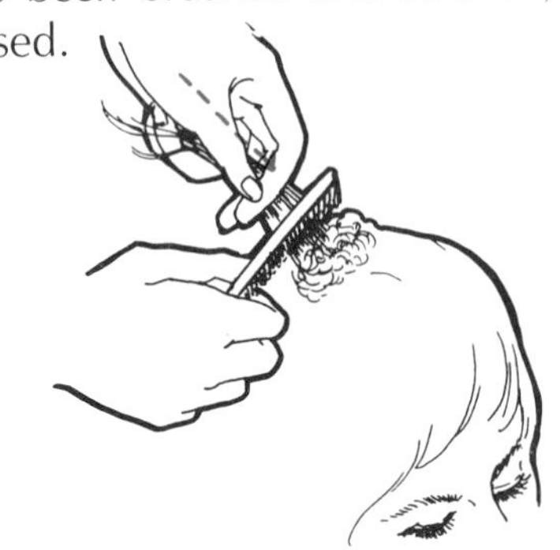

Back combing on top of strand

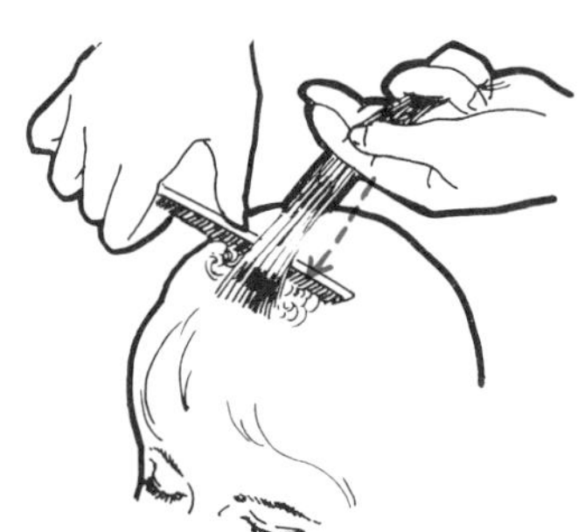

Back combing in back of strand

1. Pick up a section of hair about 3/4" (1.875 cm) wide and hold it up firmly from the scalp.
2. Insert the comb into the strand near its base, press to the scalp and remove.
3. Repeat Step 2 by inserting the comb into the strand a little further away from the scalp, press to the scalp and remove.
4. Repeat Step 3 as many times as necessary, using very small strokes until the desired volume of cushioned hair has been achieved.

Back Brushing

Back brushing, also called **ruffing**, is a technique used to build a cushion to a desired volume at the scalp for the top or covering hair.

Procedure

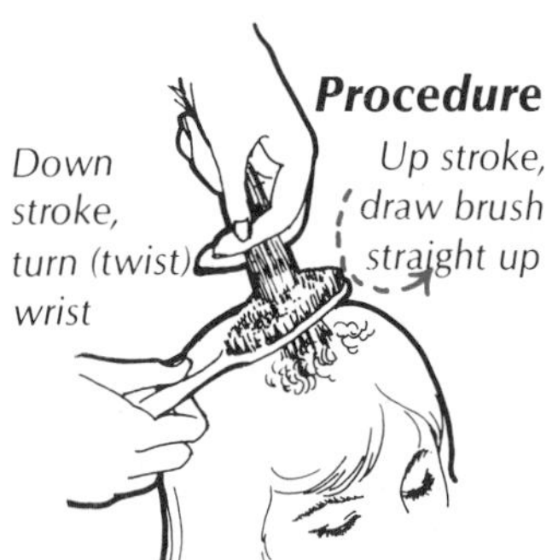

Back brushing

1. Pick up and hold a strand straight out from the scalp.
2. With a slight amount of slack in the strand, place the brush near the base of the strand. Push and roll the brush with the wrist until the brush touches the scalp. Then remove the brush from the hair with a turn of the wrist.
3. Repeat this procedure by moving the brush about 1/2" (1.25 cm) further away from the scalp.
4. Repeat until the desired volume has been achieved.

Note

Only the inner edge of the brush is used. The shorter ends of tapered hair are interlocked to form a cushion at the scalp. For interlocking to occur, the brush must be rolled.

COMB-OUT

To achieve success as a hairstylist, the cosmetologist must first master the art and technique of combing and brushing the hair. The creative skills of the stylist can only be realized when the hair has been properly shaped and molded to produce an attractive and fashionable coiffure.

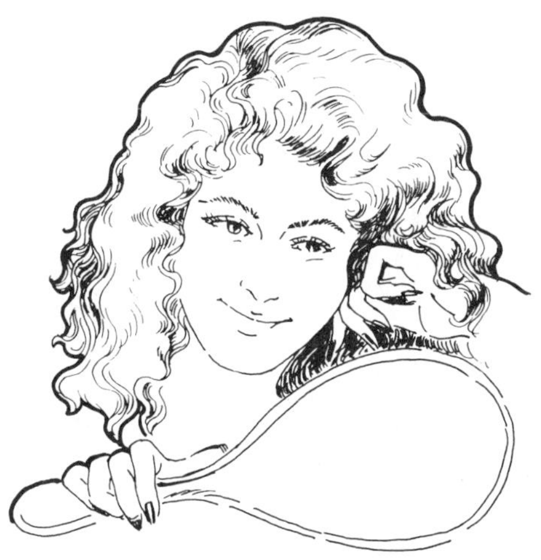

It should be remembered, however, that most comb-out failures are the result of poorly or improperly set hair.

Fast, simple and effective methods for combing and brushing out hair are very important objectives for the creative hairstylist. The real quality of the truly professional hair-style, as developed by the capable hairstylist, is appreciatively recognized by the salon client.

By applying good combing and brushing skill, the imaginative cosmetologist can artistically create almost any hairstyle desired. It is this skill, and the technical ability to handle the comb and brush that forms the foundation for success as a professional hairstylist.

Suggested Procedure

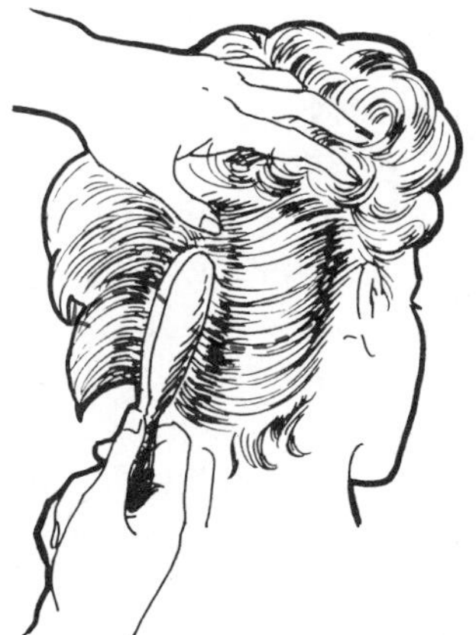

Fig. 14 Brushing back area

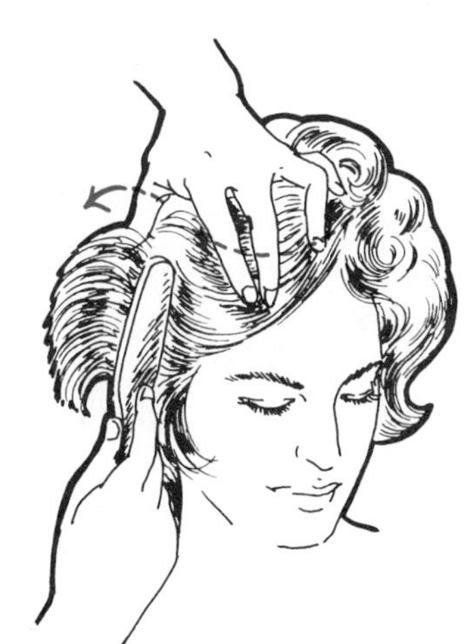

Fig. 15 Brushing sides

A definite system or plan, indicating where to start and the procedure to follow, is required for effectiveness in combing out. Such a planned procedure will help to develop the desired finished coiffure.

A suggested procedure is outlined here.

1. Brush out curls.
2. General wave placement.
3. Accentuate and develop lines and style.
4. Finishing steps.

Brushing Out the Curls

Remove the rollers and clips and relax the set by brushing out the curls with a natural bristle brush. The objective of this technique is to smooth and brush the hair into a semi-flat condition and remove excess curl (figs. 14 and 15). This permits the stylist to position the lines for the planned hairstyle. It is essential that this procedure be correctly executed to achieve a smooth, flowing, finished coiffure.

General Wave Placement

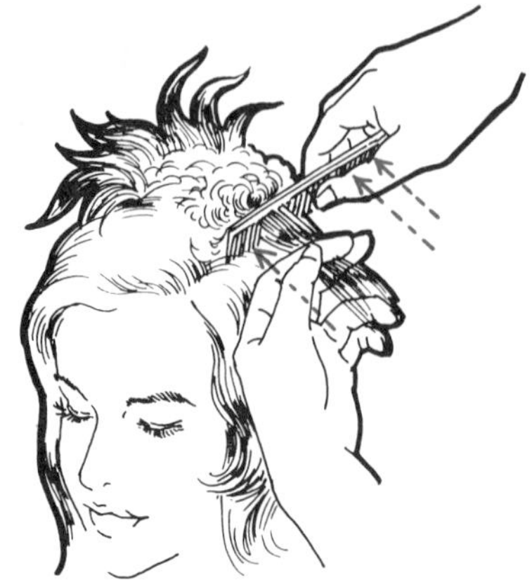

Fig. 16 If desirable, tease from the scalp to about 2″ from the hair ends

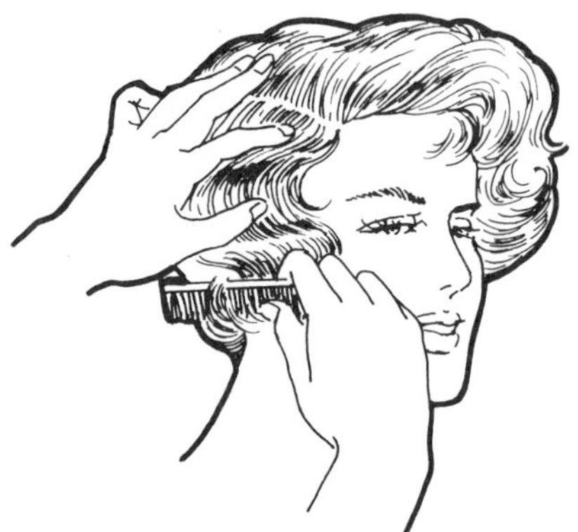

Fig. 17 Molding and combing hair to the desired hairstyle

When brushing is completed, the hair should be combed into the general pattern desired. Lines and direction should be slightly overemphasized to allow for some expected relaxation during the comb-out process. This can be accomplished by placing the hand on the head and gently pushing the hair forward, so that the waves fall into the planned design. Any necessary teasing is performed and volume, indentation and ridges are created as part of the overall arrangement (fig. 16). The entire coiffure is created in exaggerated and over–emphasized lines to provide for the final combing and styling. (fig. 17).

Accentuating and Developing Lines and Style

Taking one section at a time, the proper lines, ridges, volume and indentations are combed and brushed into the finished coiffure. Softness and evenness of flow are created by blending, smoothing and combing. Exaggerations and overemphasis are carefully removed. Finished patterns are created and final evenness and smoothness of line are combed into the final silhouette.

Finishing Steps

After the creation of the style has been completed, it is time for the finishing touches. Lightly spray the hair to hold it in place for the final placement. Using the tips of the teeth of the comb, lightly fit any small hairs or loose ends into place. If necessary, lift and blend disarrayed hair with the tips of the fingers or by carefully lifting with the comb (fig. 31). Even movement and touch during the final stage must be very lightly performed. The objective at this point is to smooth out any visible imperfections.

When the finishing touches have been completed, check the entire set for structural balance, then lightly spray the hair for the desired holding effect.

ARTISTRY IN HAIRSTYLING

The principles of modern hairstyling and makeup are guides to the cosmetologist in selecting what is most appropriate in achieving a beautiful appearance. Best results are obtained when each facial type is analyzed for its own merits and defects.

The face is ideally divided into 3 areas:

Forehead to eyebrows—1/3

Eyebrow to end of nose—1/3

End of nose to bottom of chin—1/3

Each type of face demands a distinctive coiffure that is rightly proportioned, has a balanced line and correctly frames the face. Every accomplished cosmetologist possesses a sense of balance and harmony in visualizing and creating coiffures. The essentials of an artistic and suitable hairstyle must, therefore, be based upon the following general characteristics:

1. Shape of the entire head:
   a) Front view
   b) Profile (side view)
   c) Back view
2. Characteristics in features:
   a) Perfect as well as imperfect features
   b) Defects or blemishes
3. Body structure, posture and poise

Facial Types

The facial type of each client is determined by the position and prominence of the facial bones.

There are seven facial types: oval, round, square, oblong, pear shaped, heart shaped and diamond.

To recognize each facial type and be able to give correct advice, the hairstylist should be acquainted with the outstanding characteristics of each.

Oval Facial Type

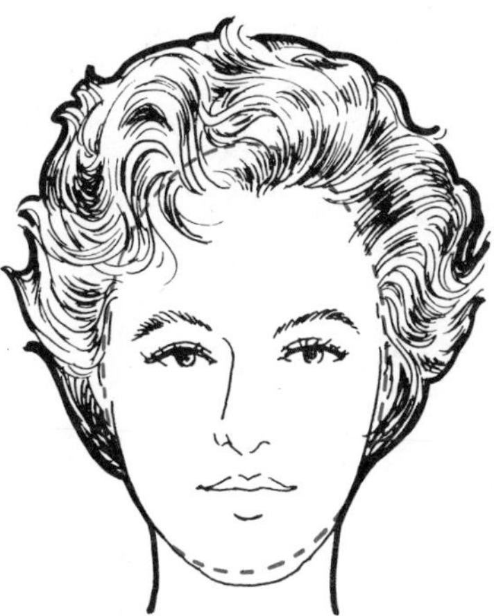

The oval type is generally accepted as the perfect face. The contour and proportions of the oval face form the basis for modifying all other facial types.

Facial Contour: The oval face is about one and a half times longer that its width across the brow; the forehead is slightly wider than the chin.

Any style can be worn because there are no features to minimize.

Round Facial Type

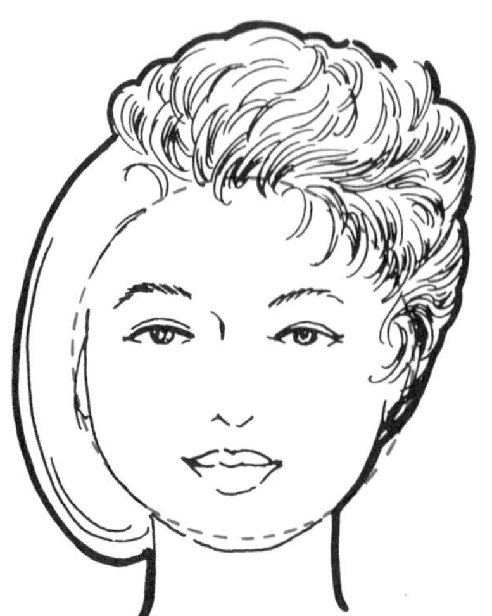

Facial Contour: Round hairline and round chinline

Aim: To create the illusion of length to the face

Arranging the hair on top of the head and dressed over the ears and part of the cheeks, with bangs to one side, will help to minimize the roundness of the face.

Square Facial Type

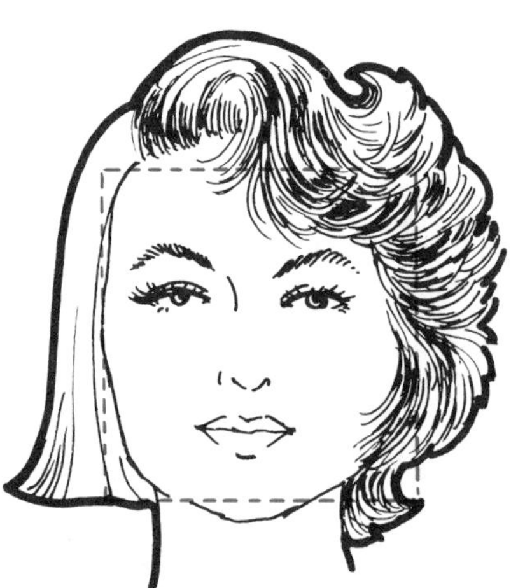

Facial Contour: Straight hairline and square jawline

Aim: To create the illusion of length and offset the squareness of the features

The problems of the square facial type are similar to those of the round. The style should lift off the forehead and come forward at the sides and jaw to create the illusion of narrowness and softness in the face.

Pear-Shaped Facial Type

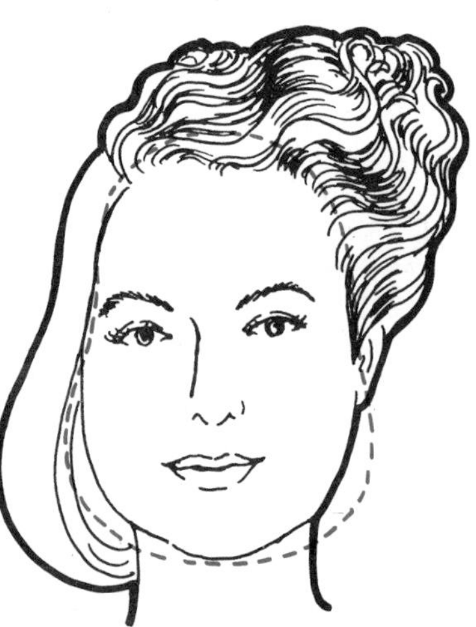

Facial Contour: Narrow forehead, wide jawline and chinline

Aim: To create the illusion of width in the forehead with a fringe of waved hair

The hair should be worn with a semi curl or soft wave effect over the lower jawline. This arrangement will add apparent width to the forehead.

Oblong Facial Type

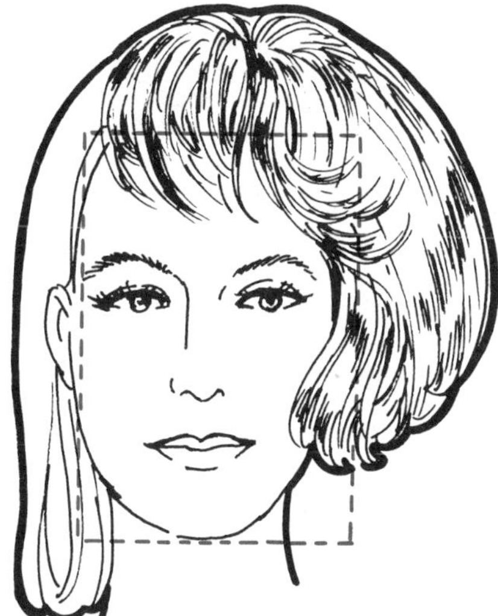

Facial Contour: Long, narrow face with hollow cheeks

Aim: To make the face appear shorter and wider

The hair should be styled fairly close to the top of the head with a fringe of curls or bangs, combined with fullness at the sides. The length of the face will appear to be reduced.

Diamond Facial Type

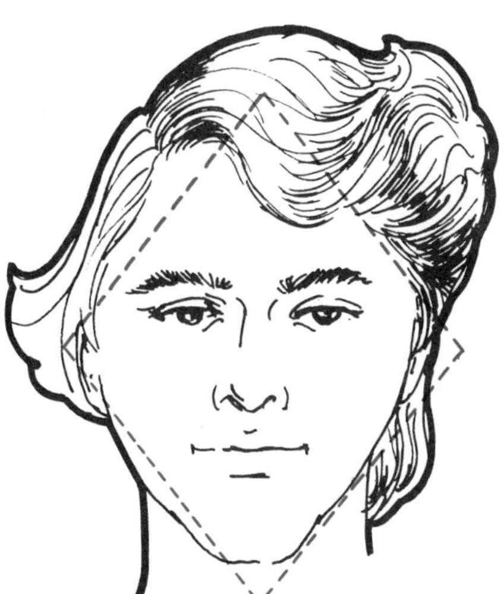

Facial Contour: Narrow forehead, extreme width through the cheekbones and narrow chin

Aim: To reduce the width across the cheekbone line

Increasing the fullness across the forehead and at the jawline, while keeping the hair close to the head at the cheekbone line will help to create the illusion of ovalness in the face.

Heart-Shaped Facial Type

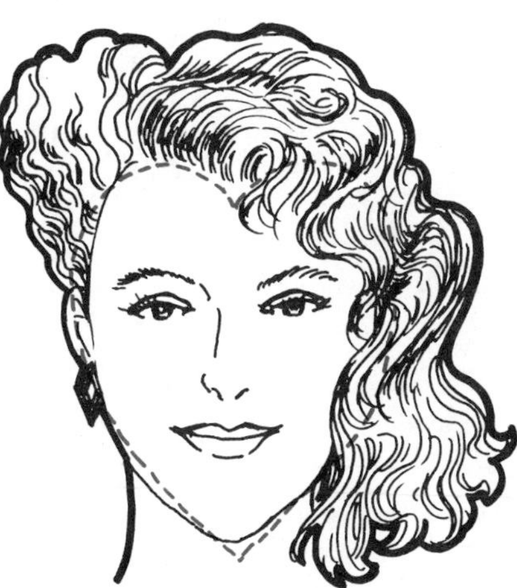

Facial Contour: Wide forehead and narrow chinline

Aim: To decrease the width of the forehead and increase the width in the lower part of the face

To reduce the width of the forehead, a hairstyle with a center part with bangs rolled up or a style slanted to one side is recommended. Add width and softness at the jawline.

Special Considerations

Plump with Short Neck

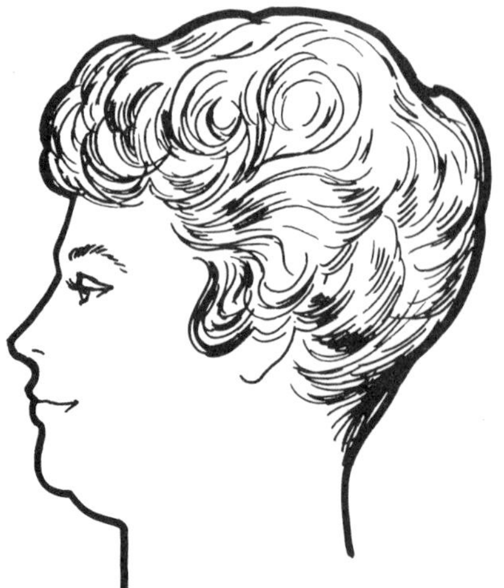

Aim: To create the illusion of length

Corrective Hairstyle: For the forehead, use forward bangs. Style the crown high to lend the illusion of length. Waved-in sides create a slender effect. A smooth head-hugging napeline emphasizes slenderness from the back and side view.

Avoid hairstyles that give fullness to the nape area.

Long, Thin Neck

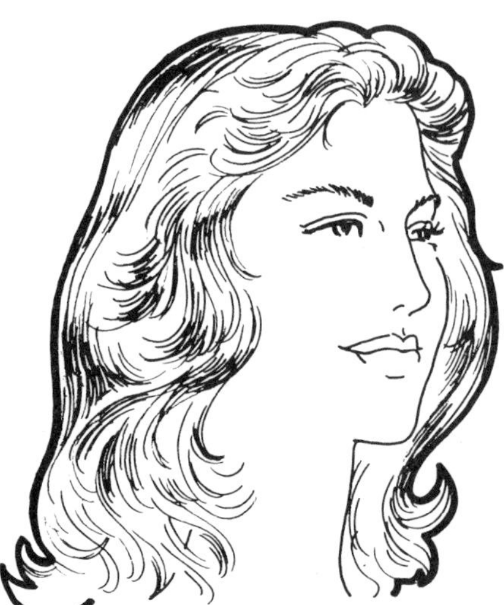

Aim: To minimize the appearance of a long neck

Corrective Hairstyle: Cover the neck with soft waves or curls. Avoid styling the hair up from the back of the neck. Keep the nape hair long.

Thin Features

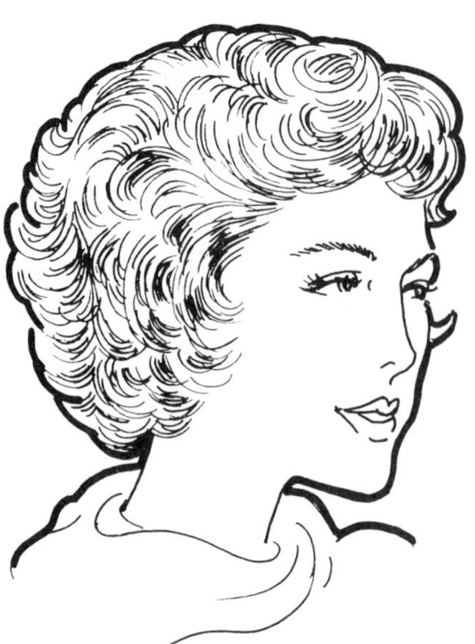

Aim: To minimize thinness of facial features and neck length

Corrective Hairstyle: A high, soft crownline, with the side lifted up and out from the hairline and brushed loosely forward onto the cheeks, will create a softening effect for the face and develop a soft, fluffy effect at the forehead. Keep the nape hair long and full to offset the long, thin neck.

Negroid Features

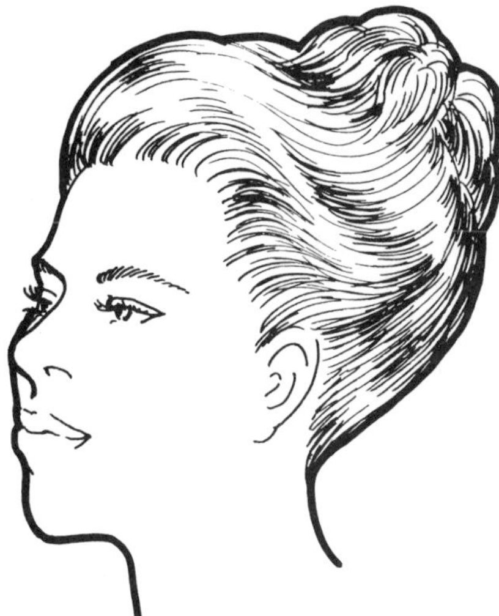

Follow styling rules that relate to each particular facial type.

Styling the hair. It may be accompanied by one of two different methods of hair straightening or relaxing:

Chemically relaxed. The hair should be wet set with rollers and pin curls. It is then dried and combed out in the usual manner.

Thermal straightened (pressed). Use large barrel curls or curl with thermal (marcel) irons. Then comb the hair into a suitable hairstyle.

Uneven Features

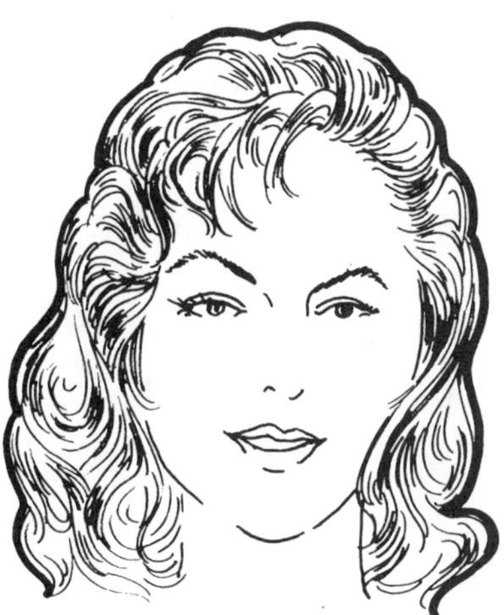

Aim: To minimize the imperfect features

Corrective Hairstyle: Uneven features can be minimized by selection of the proper hairstyle. The suggested hairstyle recommended for this model is a soft effect over protruding features, thereby creating evenness on both sides of the face.

Oriental Features

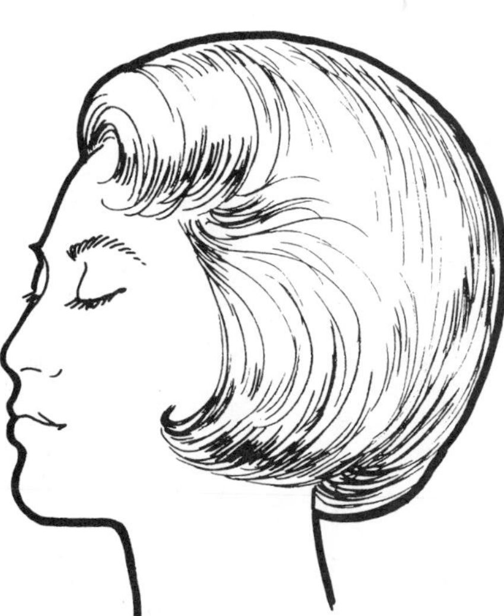

Follow hairstyling rules that relate to the particular facial shape. The oriental hairstyle is very versatile in that it may be combed into a side-upward movement or into a loose, fluffy pageboy style. This is achieved by rolling the hair outward or inward.

Profile

Straight

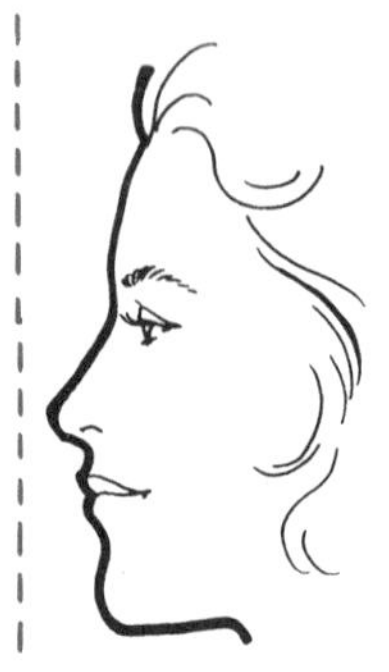

Usually, all hairstyles are becoming to the straight or normal profile.

A normal profile is neither concave nor convex. It contains neither a prominent protrusion nor a receding feature.

Concave (Prominent Chin)

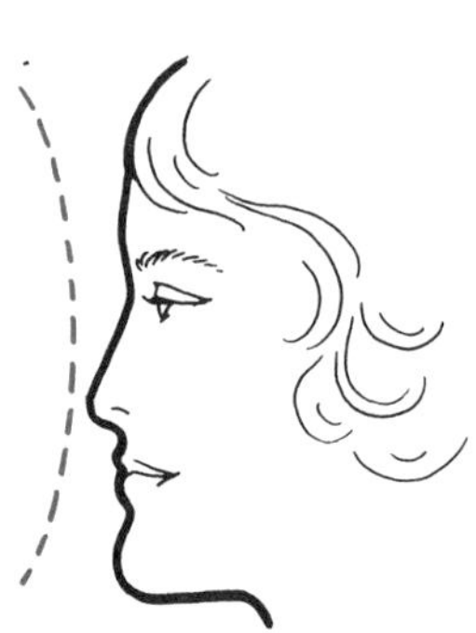

A close hair arrangement or bangs over the forehead minimizes the bulgyness of the forehead. The hair at the sides and nape of the neck should be dressed in small, soft curls or waves to soften the features.

Convex (Receding Forehead, Prominent Nose and Receding Chin)

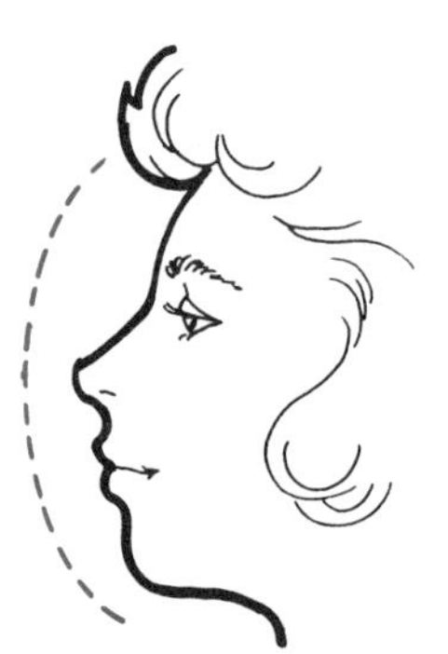

Curls or bangs should be placed forward on the forehead to conceal the receding forehead and irregular hairline. The hair at the sides and nape of the neck should be dressed close to the head to give it perfect balance.

Low Forehead, Protruding Chin

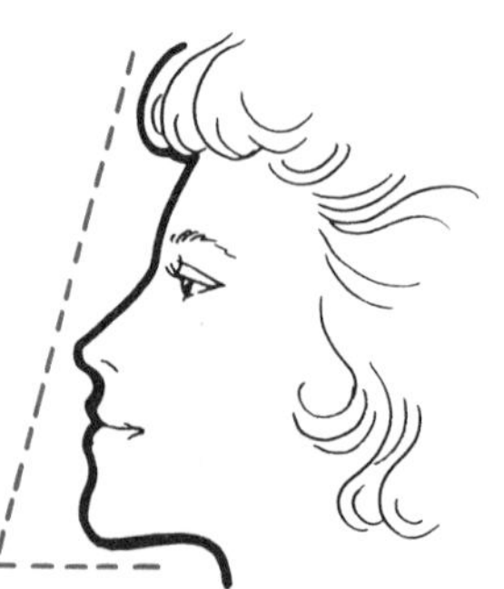

To create the illusion of height to a low forehead and length to the face the hair should be dressed high on the top of the head with curls or bangs on the forehead. An upsweep movement in the temple area with a soft hair arrangement over the jawline will soften the sharpness of the chin.

Nose Shapes

Closely allied to any profile analysis, in fact a very important part of such a study, is the shape of the nose which must be considered both in profile and full face. (Appropriate makeup for nose shapes will be found in chapter 23 on **Facial Makeup**.)

Turned-up Nose

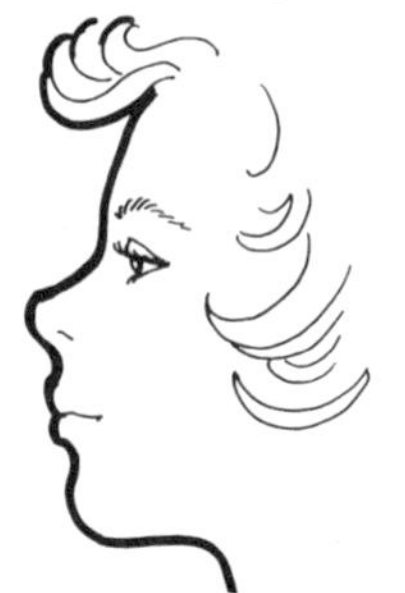

Wrong

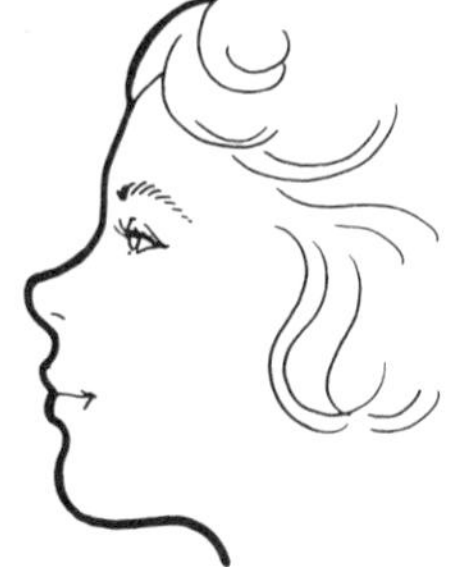

Right

This type of nose is usually small and accompanied by a straight profile. To overcome this, the hair should be swept back off the face at the sides, lengthening the line from the nose to the ear.

Prominent Nose

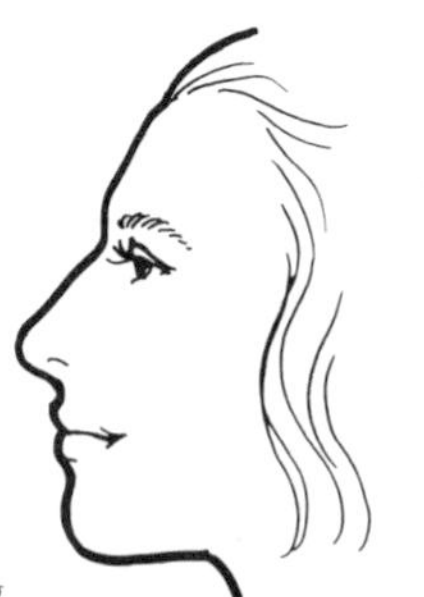

Wrong

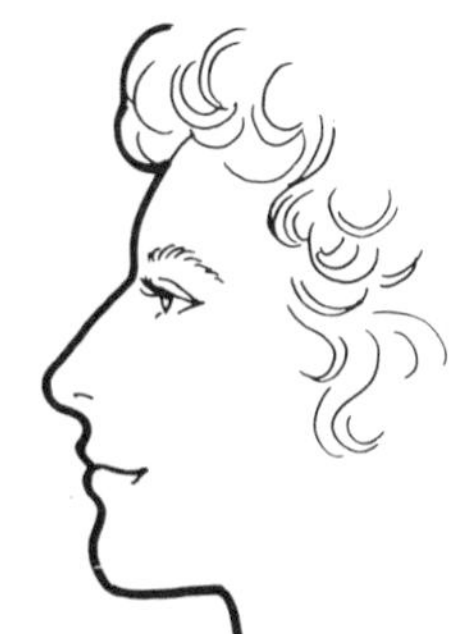

Right

A hooked nose, a large nose, or a pointed nose all come under this classification. The stylist must plan to draw as much attention as possible away from these features.

To minimize the prominence of the nose, bring the hair forward at the forehead with softness around the face.

Crooked Nose

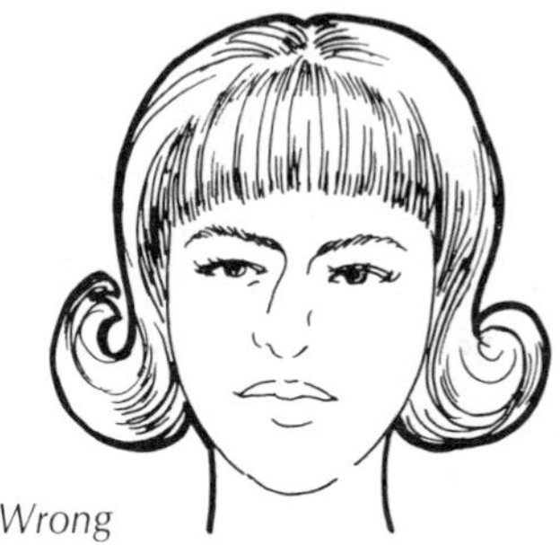

Wrong

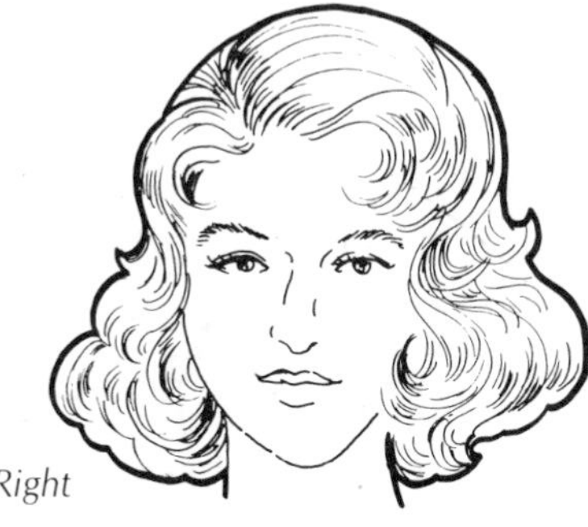

Right

To minimize the conspicuous crooked nose, style the hair in an off center manner, which will attract the eye away from the nose.

Wide, Flat Nose

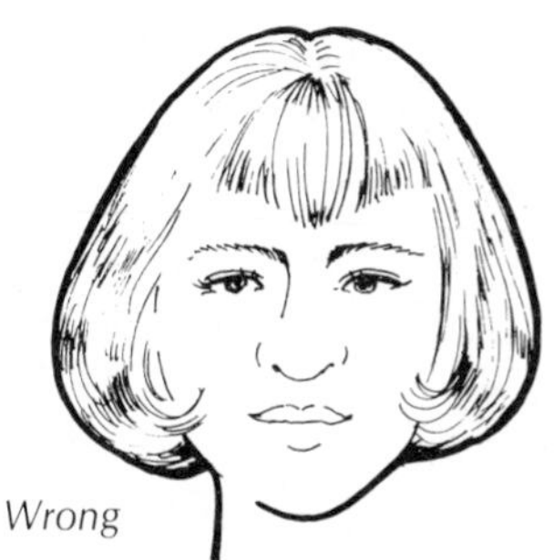

Wrong

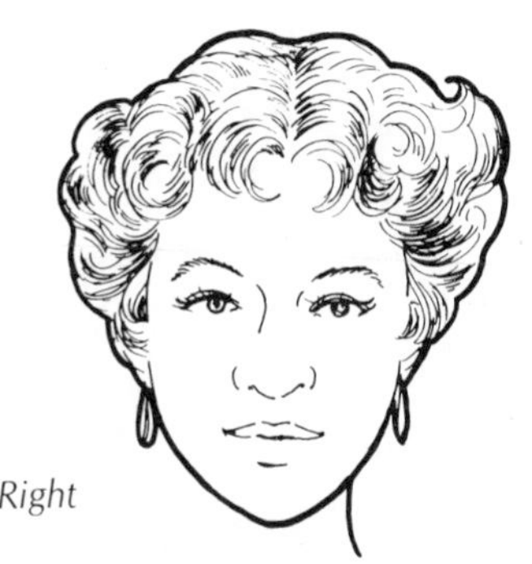

Right

A wide, flat nose tends to broaden the face. To minimize this effect, the hair should be drawn away from the face.

A hairstyle with a middle part and double curled bangs will draw attention away from the nose.

Eyes The eyes are the focal point of all feminine beauty. A professional hairstylist should be qualified to minimize or entirely eliminate any defects in the appearance of the eyes.

Wide-Set Eyes

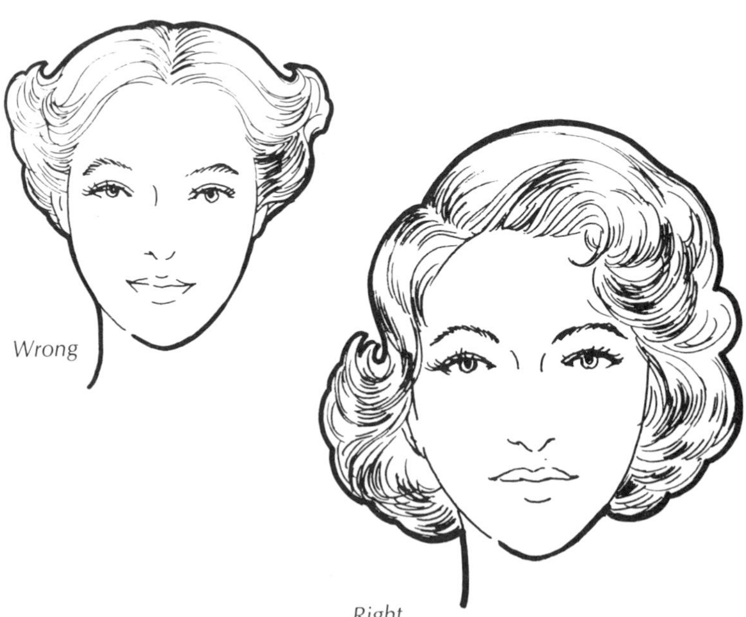

Eyes set far apart are usually found with round, square or strong cheekbone features. The objective of the stylist is to achieve a better balance for the face and minimize the effect of the wide space between the eyes.

To minimize wide-set eyes, lift and fluff the top hair into a side bang. The other side is styled into a dip wave. The rest of the hairstyle is fluff dried and arranged to nestle under, toward the head. The entire hairstyle gives the appearance of minimizing space between the eyes.

Close-Set Eyes

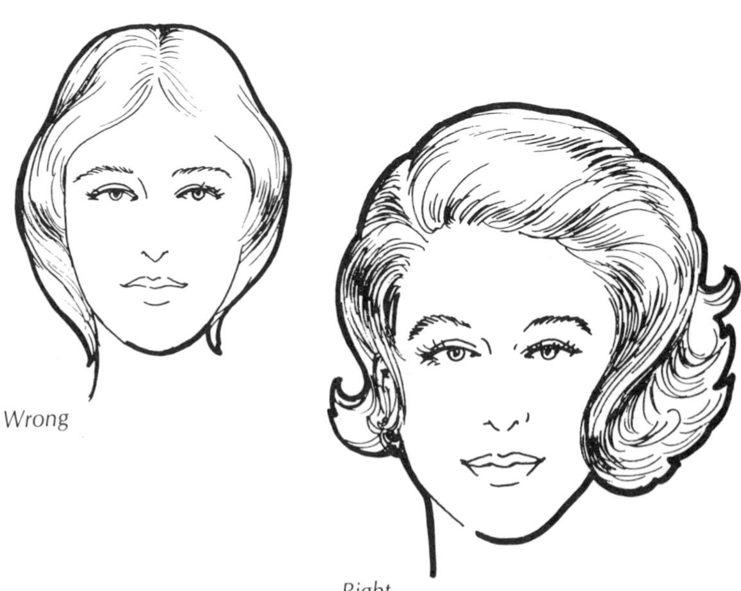

Close-set eyes are usually found in an oval or long, narrow face. The objective of the hairstyle is to open up the appearance of the face and create the illusion of more space between the eyes.

The top crown hair is styled high into a pyramid effect. The side movement may fall over either brow, according to the clients choice, with hair ends turned outward and up. The other side of the hair is styled away from the face, which will give the eyes the appearance of being wider apart.

Styling for Women Who Wear Glasses

Women who wear glasses should be especially careful in their hairstyling and makeup habits. A combination of a becoming hairstyle, the proper makeup and the correct glasses should be blended together to develop and emphasize the wearer's basic feminine beauty. To the beholder, a face wearing glasses can take on an individualistic, special charm if all the elements of good grooming are in proper harmony.

The following are basic good grooming rules that should be followed by all women who wear glasses:

1. Glasses should be modern, with large lenses for good vision.
2. Never wear gaudy, over-jewelled or tricky frames.
3. Do not wear strip false eyelashes. They are too long and function like windshield wipers with every eye movement.
4. Do not use heavy eye makeup. It does not take heavy makeup to bring out the color and best features of your eyes.
5. Hairstyles that fall naturally around the face, making putting on and taking off glasses easy, are most advantageous.
6. Over-styled hair with many tight curls is impractical for women with glasses.

There are numerous **"do's"** and **"don'ts"** in every area of hair and facial grooming. The following are designed to illustrate some of the **"do's"** for those women who must wear glasses.

Round, Oval or Square Face

The natural beauty of the round, oval or square facial types can be further enhanced with proper glasses and grooming.

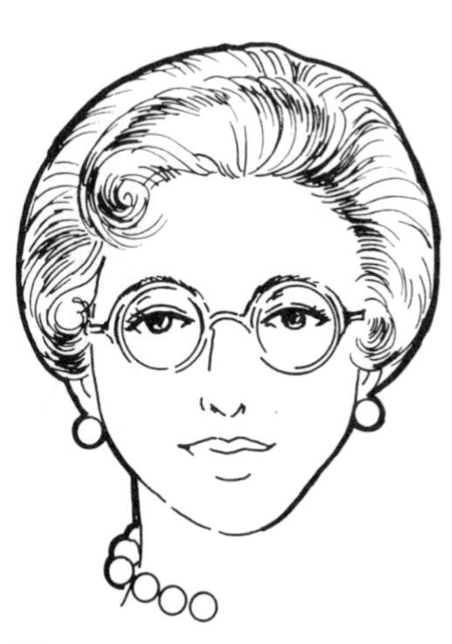

Wrong

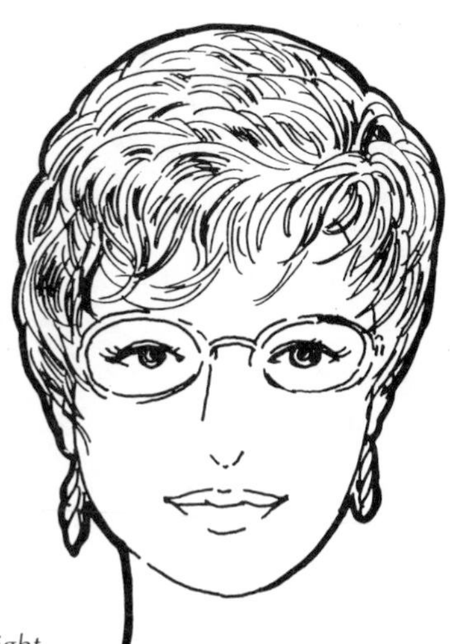

Right

Glasses. A woman with big eyes should wear slender frames with large visual lenses to show off eyes and good eye makeup. (Color of frames should be selected carefully to match her hair.)

Hairstyle. Wear a bouffant hairstyle in natural balance, a simple, uncluttered style, casual but chic.

Bangs. Wear a slashed bang freely touching the eyebrows.

Jewelry. If earrings are worn, they should be long and dangling.

Heart-Shaped or Diamond-Shaped Face

The natural beauty of the heart-shaped or diamond-shaped face can be emphasized, and the glasses can become an integral part of a very pleasing grooming picture.

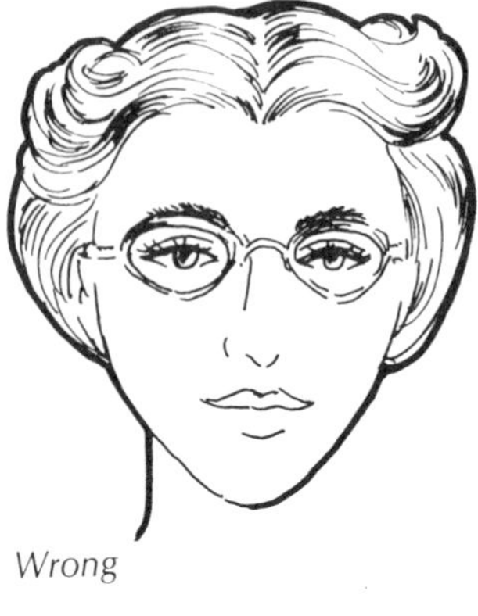
Wrong

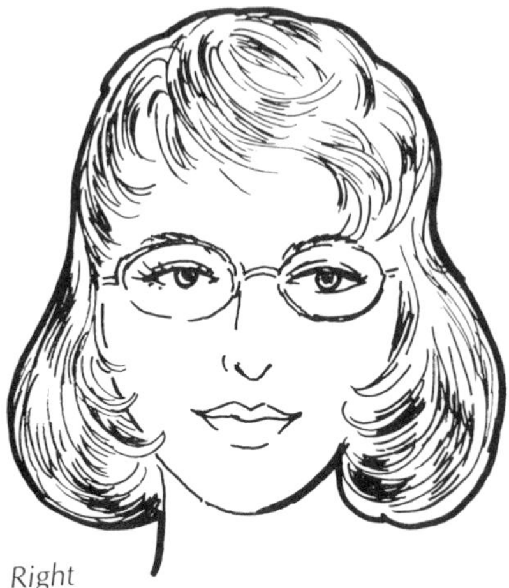
Right

Glasses. Wear smart, slender frames that follow or give a lift to the eyebrows. The frames should be of medium thickness to rest gently against the face.

Makeup. Wear light makeup shades and delicate eye makeup.

Hairstyle. Wear a full pageboy style, or increase the width in the lower part of the face.

Bangs. Wear open, chic bangs which harmonize and balance with the lower part of the face.

Small, Narrow or Oval Face

The small, narrow, or oval face has a special, unique charm that should be emphasized by proper grooming.

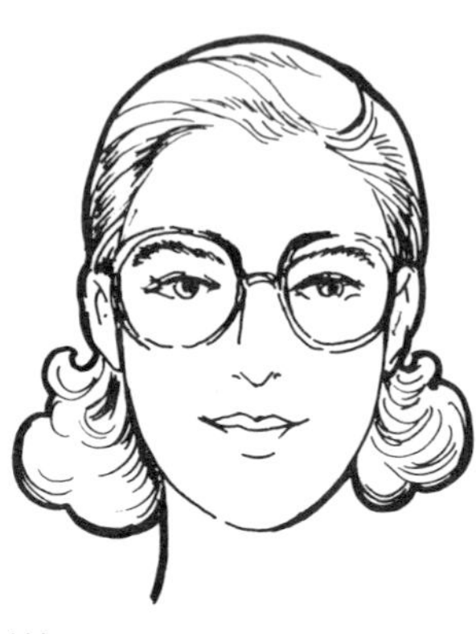
Wrong

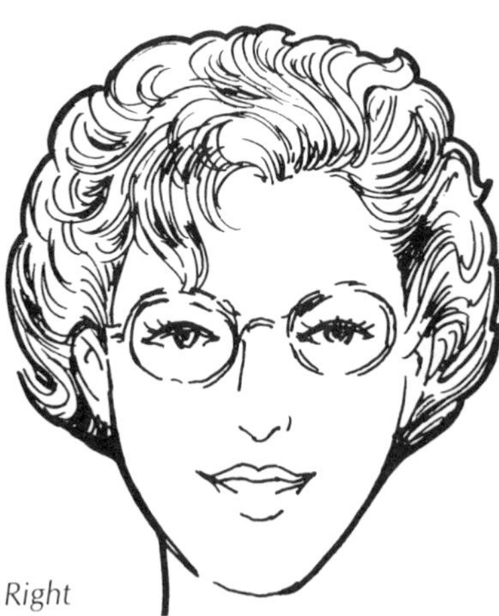
Right

Glasses. Select large, modern frames that are not too exotic or gaudy.

Makeup. Wear only natural tones of makeup. It is essential that eye makeup be applied very carefully. The eyes are seen and magnified through the glasses. Proper eye makeup emphasizes beautiful, sparkling eyes.

Hairstyle. Since the face is delicate in proportion, it is important that the hairstyle have width and height. The hairstyle should be short, with deep wave shapings on the sides, leaving freedom for control of glasses. Use deep waves and flip curls placed well back of the ears and ending lower at the nape.

Bangs. A side wave bang caressing one eyebrow can complement the eyes.

Pear-Shaped Face

The pear-shaped face has attractive features with an attractive hairstyle.

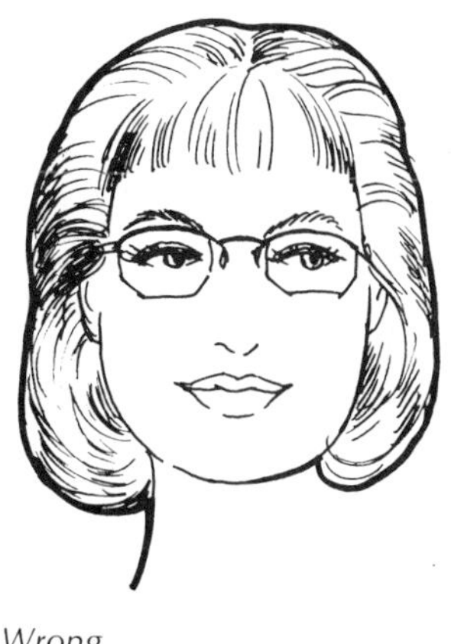
Wrong

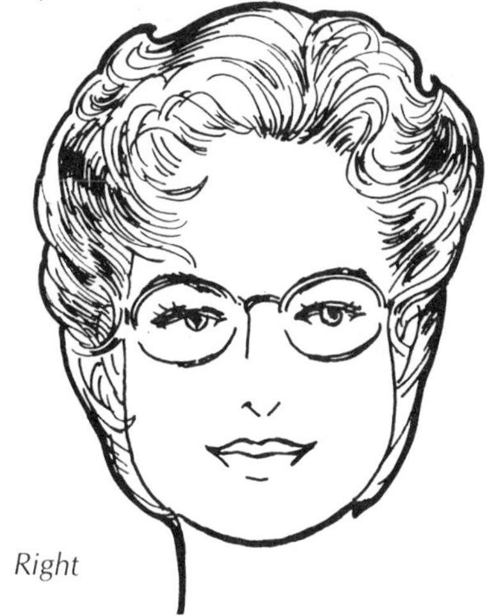
Right

Glasses. Wear large, oval-shaped frames.

Hairstyle. This facial contour requires emphasis on length; therefore, wear the hair up and off the face, high in front and crown. Soft bouffant styling around the face, with softness brushed forward on the cheeks, reduces width and adds beauty.

Bangs. A side wave bang over one eye will add expression and interest.

Proper hairstyling, correct makeup and the selection of suitable and becoming glasses all contribute to making the woman who wears glasses much more attractive.

HEAD SHAPES

The shape of the client's skull (head) has just as many variations as the rest of her physical features. It is the hairstylist's objective to produce this shape by skillfully shaping and arranging the hair. The hairstylist should carefully observe the client's head shape and then mentally impose an oval picture over it. Where there is flatness, the volume of the hair should be adjusted to fill the area.

Types of Head Shapes

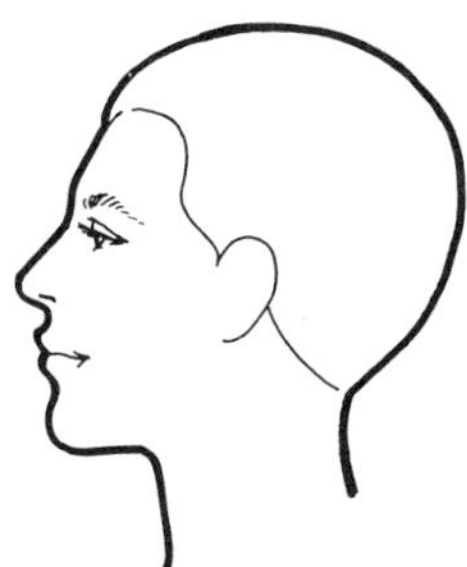
1. Perfect shape

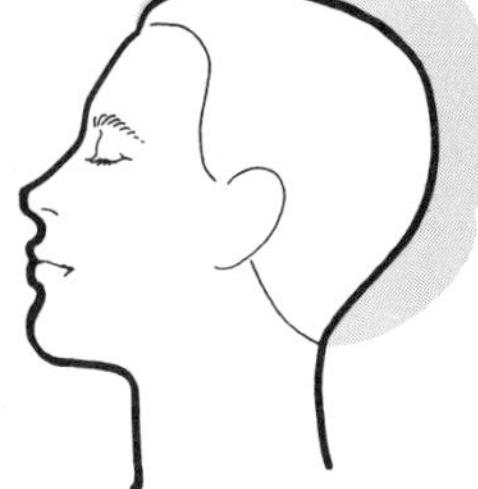
2. Narrow head—flat back

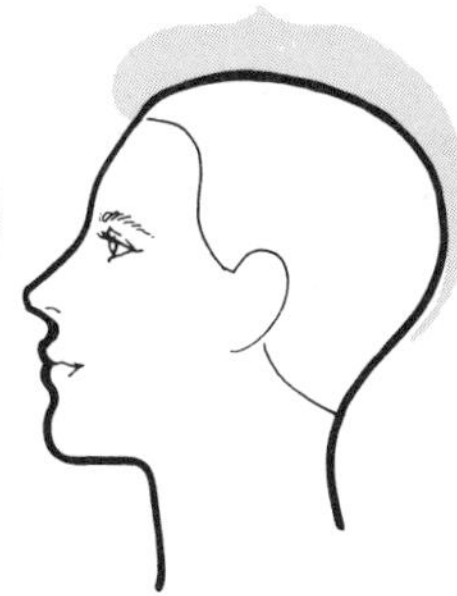
3. Flat crown

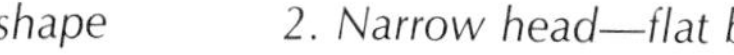

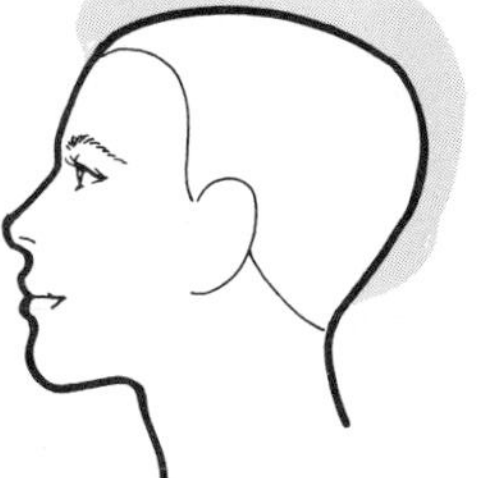
4. Pointed head—hollow nape

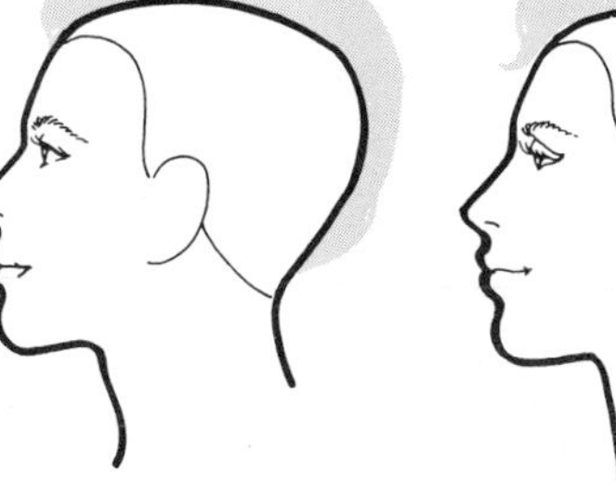
5. Flat top

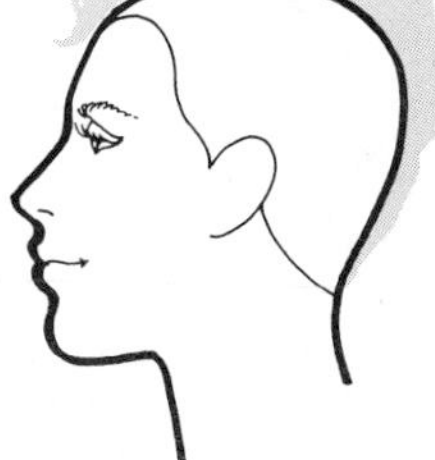
6. Small head

The heavy lines on the diagrams outline the actual shape of the head, and the shaded areas indicate where volume is required. This does not necessarily mean that all heads and all hair designs must be oval. The complete outside shape may be fashioned into many patterns and designs as long as the head shape has been ovalized.

1. Oval (the perfect head shape)
2. Narrow head, flat back
3. Flat crown
4. Pointed head shape, hollow nape
5. Flat top
6. Small head

BRAIDING

Braiding has long been a popular hair grooming technique with both adults and children. Cosmetologists would do well to add the ability to perform this technique to the range of their styling skills. It helps to broaden their professional scope and adds to their versatility as artists.

There are two different types of braiding:

1. French (invisible) braiding—regular braiding
2. French (visible) braiding—inverted braiding

Invisible French Braiding

Invisible French braiding is performed by overlapping the strands on top.

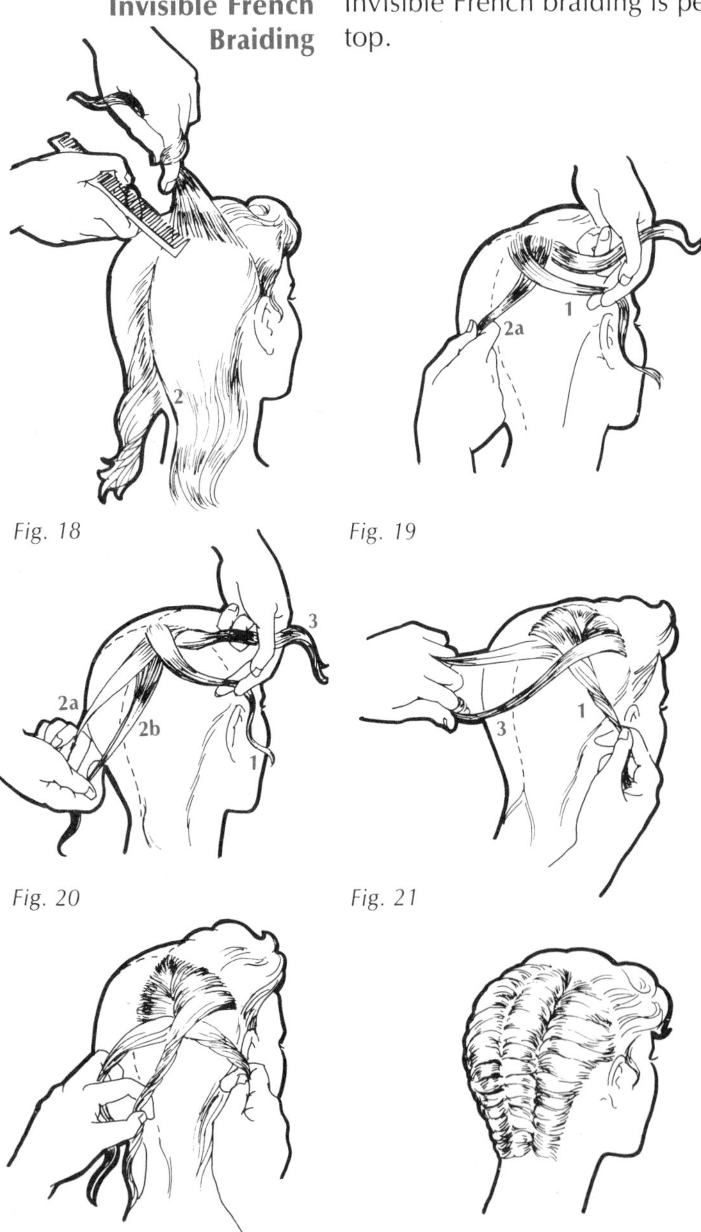

Fig. 18 Fig. 19 Fig. 20 Fig. 21 Fig. 22 Fig. 23

Procedure

1. Part off the crown section and hold out of the way with clips or clamps. Part the back hair from the center of the crown, (fig. 18).
2. Divide the section evenly into three strands. Start to braid by bringing strand 1 (on the left) over strand 2a (in the center) (fig. 19). Draw the strands tightly.
3. Pick up another strand from the left, about 1/2″ (1.25 cm) wide, as indicated by 2b (fig. 20). Join strands 2a and 2b. Tighten the strands.
4. Bring strand 3 over strand 1 and tighten (fig. 21). Pick up another strand on the right, about 1/2″ (1.25 cm) wide and place with strand 1.

Note

Insure neat braids with all short hair ends in place, twist each strand with the thumb and index finger.

5. Continue to pick up strands and braid them (fig. 22), finishing with braiding of the hair ends at the nape. Fasten with a rubber band or string.

Braid the left side of the head, following the same procedure. The final regular French braid is illustrated in fig. 23.

Alternate method: The regular French braid (invisible) also may be started at the nape and braided toward the top of the head. The ends may be finished into rolls or curls.

Fashion

The braids may be crossed and tucked neatly underneath and held in place with hairpins or bobby pins.

When the hair is long enough, braids can be crossed and extended up the back of the head.

Another attractive effect can be obtained by tying the braids with ribbons at the hairline and allowing the ends to fall into clusters of curls.

Visible French Braiding

Inverted French braiding (visible) is done by pleating the strands under thus making the braid visible.

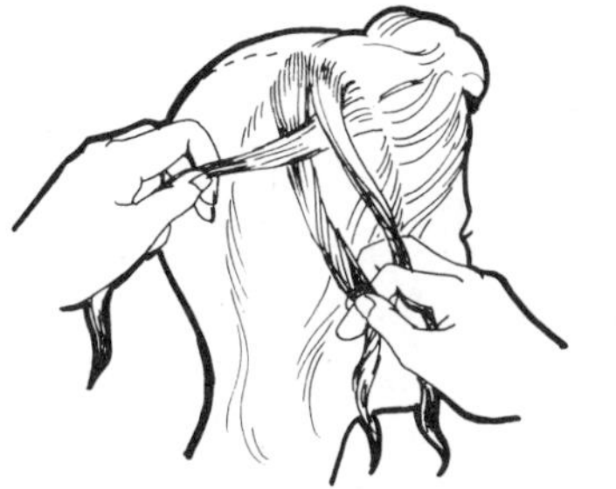

Fig. 24

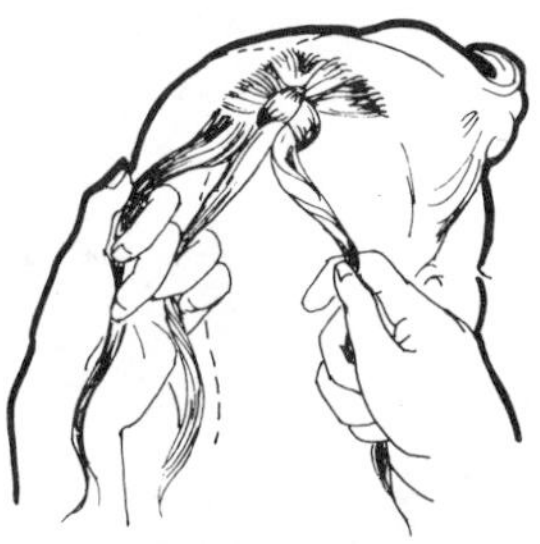

Fig. 25

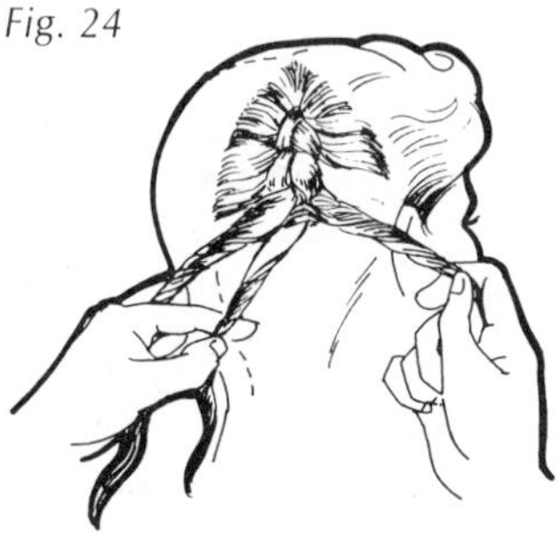

Fig. 26

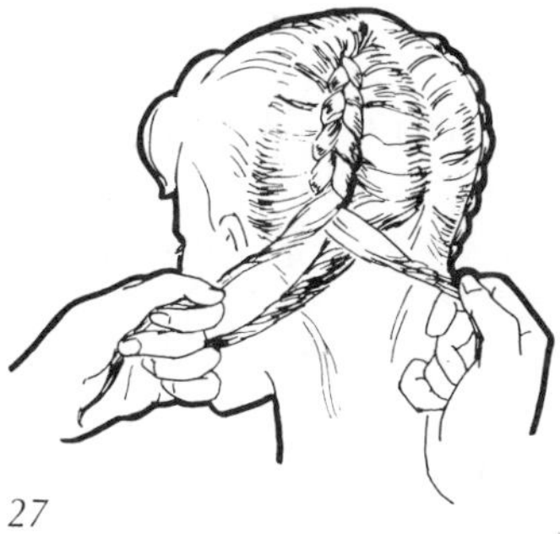

Fig. 27

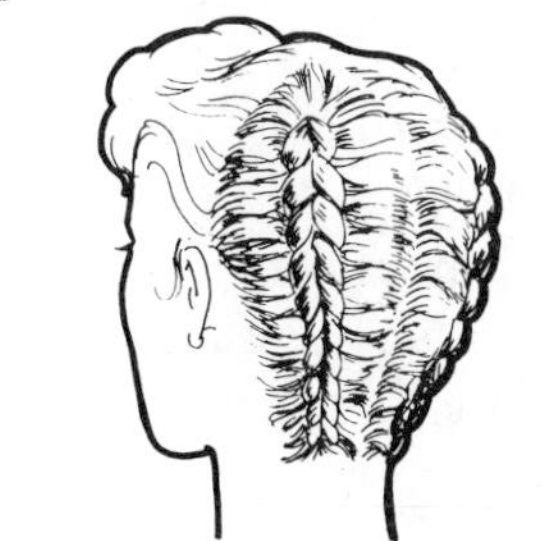

Fig. 28

Fig. 28 Appearance of finished inverted French braid with braids tucked under and held in place with hairpins or bobby pins

Procedure

Part and section the hair in the same manner as for regular French braid.

1. Divide the top right section evenly into three strands. Place the right side strand under the center strand and the left side strand under this one. Draw strands tightly (fig. 24).
2. Pick up 1/2" (1.25 cm) strand on the right side and combine with the right side strand. Place under the center strand. Pick up 1/2" (1.25 cm) strand on the left side and combine with the left side strand. Place under center strand (fig. 25).
3. Continue to pick up the hair and braid as above (fig. 26). Finish braiding at the nape and hold in position with rubber bands.
4. Braid the left side of the head (fig. 27).

Fashion

The same suggestions recommended for the regular (visible) French braiding can be utilized for the inverted (invisible) French braiding.

Cornrowing

Over-curly hair may be fashioned into visible braids with long, narrow sections, sometimes called cornrows, which are popular with children and adults alike.

The technique is similar to the visible method of French braiding with the following exceptions:

1. After a shampoo, apply and distribute conditioner through the hair.
2. Use a hand dryer or blow dryer to dry hair. If a hood dryer is used, apply and spread the conditioner then cover the hair with a hair net. Have the client sit under the dryer.

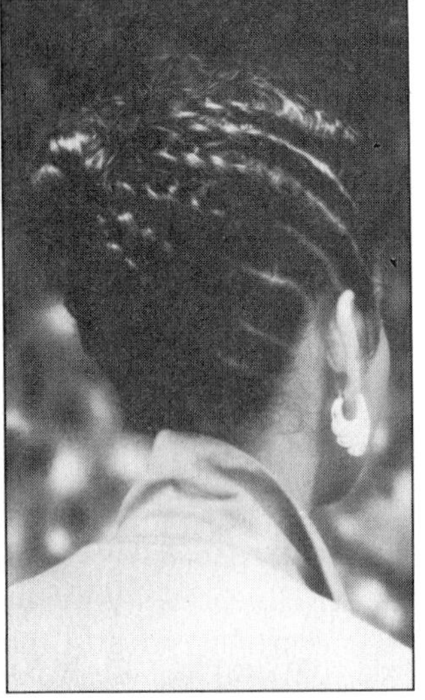

Fig. 29

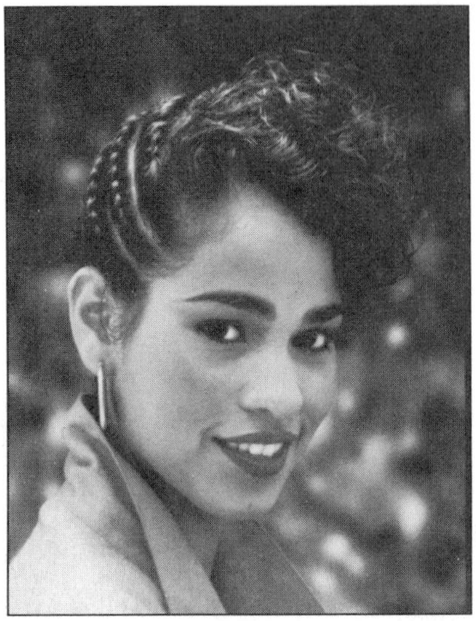

Fig. 30

Procedure

Pre examine the hairstyle to be achieved.

Part a long, narrow section and braid as outlined for **French visible braids.**

Part another section and braid. Continue until the entire head is completed (fig. 29).

Fashion the style to be created so that it will enhance the appearance of the client.

Cornrowing is a hairstyle for young ladies seeking an individualistic effect (fig. 30).

DEFINITIONS PERTAINING TO HAIRSTYLING

Back brushing: The brushing of the hair toward the scalp, so that the shorter hair tangles to form a cushion at the scalp for top covering hair. Another term used for back brushing is **ruffing.**

Back combing: Combing the underside of small sections of hair from the ends toward the scalp, causing the shorter hair to form a cushion at the scalp. Other terms used for back combing are **teasing, ratting** or **matting.**

Barrel curl: A curl that is wound like a roller curl without using a roller.

Base: The stationary or immovable foundation of the curl that is attached to the scalp.

Bouffant: The degree of height and fullness in a finished hairstyle.

Carved curl: A section of hair sliced from a shaping and formed into a curl while holding the strand close to the head.

Circle: That part of the pin curl forming a complete circle.

Clockwise: The movement of hair, in shapings or curls, in the same direction as the movement of the hands of a clock.

Counter clockwise: The movement of hair, in shapings or curls, in the opposite direction to the movement of the hands of a clock.

Curl: A circle or circles within a circle. The size of the curl governs the width of the wave.

Direction: The moving of hair to form a particular pattern or style.

Down-shaping: Directing the hair in a downward movement in preparation for a particular pattern or style.

Extended or **elongated stem:** A space area between two rows of pin curls that permits the first row of curls to unfold without buckling.

Finger wave: A wave formed in wet hair with the use of fingers and comb.

Flat curl (regular pin curl): Gives a flat motion and no lift.

Forward curl: A curl that is directed toward the face.

Forward shaping: Directing the hair toward the face.

Hair shaping pivot: The exact point from which the hair is directed in forming a curvature or shaping.

Indentation: Indicates a curved hollow or valley created in the formation of a hairstyle.

Molded curl: Same as carved curl.

Molding: The forming or directing of the hair to create a desired shape or style.

Movement: Directing and changing the direction of hair.

Over-directed: Excessive direction of the hair in the formation of finger waves, curls or shapings.

Overlapping curl: A pin curl that is placed to partially cover an adjoining curl.

Panel: The area between two partings; also known as **section.**

Pin curl wave: Alternating the direction of rows of pin curls to form a wave pattern.

Reverse (backward) curl: A curl directed away from the face.

Ridge curl: A curl placed behind the ridge of a finger wave.

Sculpture curl (pin curl): A strand of hair that is combed smooth and ribbon like and wound into a circle with the ends on the inside; sometimes called a **flat** curl.

Semi stand-up curl (flair curl): A pin curl carved out of a shaping and pinned into a semi-standing position.

Shaping (in haircutting): The process of shortening and thinning the hair into a particular style or to the contour of the head.

Shaping (in hairstyling): The formation of uniform arcs or curves in wet hair, thus providing a base for finger waves, pin curls or various patterns in hairstyling.

Skip wave: A combination of finger wave and pin curl pattern, the pin curls being placed in alternate finger wave formation.

Slicing: Removing a section of hair from a shaping in preparation for making a curl. (The remainder of the shaping is not disturbed.)

Stand-up curl (cascade curl): A curl with the stem directed straight up or out from the head and pinned in a standing position.

Stem: That part of the pin curl between the base and the first arc of the circle.

No stem: The curl is placed in the center of the base.

Half stem: The curl is placed half off its base.

Full stem: The curl is placed completely off its base.

Stem direction: The direction in which the stem moves from the base to the first arc. (Stem direction may be forward, backward, upward or downward.)

Strand: A section of hair.

Under directed: Insufficiently directing the hair in the formation of finger waves, curls or shapings.

Up-shaping: Directing the hair in an upward movement in preparation for a particular pattern or style.

Volume: The height created in the formation of a hairstyle.

REVIEW QUESTIONS

Hairstyling

1. *Why is styling hair an important part of cosmetology?*
2. *What implements are used in hairstyling?*
3. *What is the procedure for removing tangles from hair?*
4. *What is the correct technique for making a part?*
5. *Describe the procedure used to find the natural part.*
6. *What are the parts of the pin curl and the functions of each?*
7. *What is the difference between "clockwise curls" and "counter clockwise curls"?*
8. *How are shapings important in the formation of pin curls? How is the stem and the circle direction determined by the shaping?*
9. *What are four types of pincurl bases?*
10. *What are the pincurl techniques for the right and left side of the head?*
11. *Why is the anchoring of pin curls an important technique?*
12. *What are six effects of pin curl settings?*
13. *What effect is achieved by a ridge curl? A skip wave?*
14. *What are the effects obtained by stand-up and semi-stand-up curls? Describe the formation of these curls.*
15. *What effect(s) is achieved by the use of rollers in setting? List the steps to correctly using the roller.*
16. *How are barrel curls formed? How are they used?*
17. *How is volume and indentation achieved in setting? For what effects are each of these techniques used?*
18. *What effects are achieved by using cylinder rollers? What effects are achieved by using tapered rollers?*
19. *What hair partings would be suggested for clients with an oval shaped face? Round? Square? Pear? Oblong? Diamond? Heart?*
20. *For what purposes are back combing and back brushing during the comb-out?*
21. *How does hairstyling artistry make it possible for cosmetologists to style hair that will most complement the client?*
22. *How does artistry in hairstyling compensate for facial features? Glasses? Facial types? Head shape?*
23. *In what manner are braids formed?*

Chapter 13

THE ART AND STYLING OF ARTIFICIAL HAIR

LEARNING OBJECTIVES

The student successfully mastering this chapter will be able to:

1. *List some of the reasons wigs are worn.*
2. *Recognize the different types of wigs, extensions and hairpieces.*
3. *Give the procedure for taking wig measurements.*
4. *List the important considerations when ordering a wig.*
5. *Describe the technique in fitting a wig.*
6. *Identify the techniques in wig cleaning and conditioning.*
7. *Shape a wig.*
8. *Set and comb out wigs.*
9. *Color wigs.*
10. *Identify various types of hairpieces and their uses.*
11. *List the safety precautions to be followed in handling wigs.*
12. *Give the definitions pertaining to wigs.*

Throughout history, wigs have served to enhance appearance and beauty. The ancient Egyptians first wore wigs in 4000 B.C., primarily to protect their hair from the sun. From Asia and Europe, wigs spread to America, where their use has become increasingly popular and versatile.

The use of wigs and hairpieces in hairstyling can be an important and exciting part of the beauty industry. The sale, styling and servicing of all hairpieces can be the source of increased salon income.

To offer the best possible services, the hairstylist must be familiar with the following:

1. How wigs and hairpieces can improve the client's appearance.
2. How wigs and hairpieces are made and fitted.
3. How to select and style wigs and hairpieces to the client's best advantage.
4. How to clean and service wigs and hairpieces.

WHY WIGS ARE WORN

Wigs are worn for several reasons:

1. **Necessity**—to cover up baldness and sparse or damaged hair.
2. **Medical**—to cover hair loss from a health problem.
3. **Fashion**—for changes in everyday hairstyles, for decorative purposes and special occasions and to increase length and volume.
4. **Practicality**—for flexibility and ease of style change.

TYPES OF WIGS

Wigs can be made from human hair, synthetic or animal hair or a blend.

A simple match test will tell the difference between human hair and synthetic hair. Cut a small piece of hair from the back area of the wig. With a lighted match, burn this hair and observe these characteristics:

1. Human hair burns slowly and gives off a strong odor.
2. Synthetic hair burns quickly and gives off little or no odor. Small, hard beads can be felt in the burnt ash of synthetic hair.

Modacrylic is the general term used to describe synthetic wig fibers.

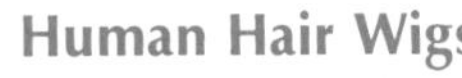

Human Hair Wigs

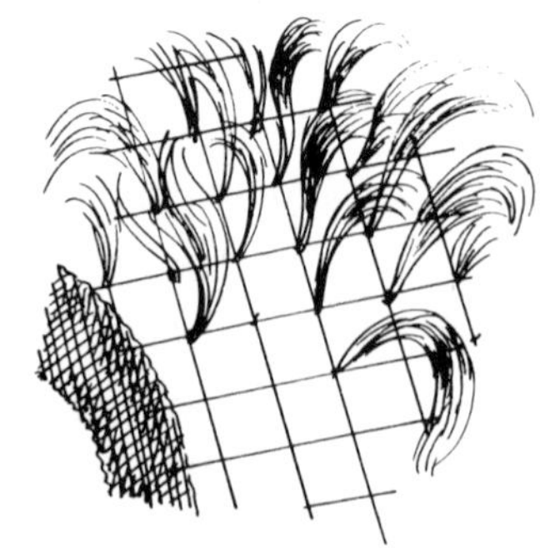

Fig. 2 DETAIL CUTAWAY
Hair is stitched and hand knotted into the mesh foundation.

The quality of a wig depends to a great extent on whether it is constructed by hand or machine. Expensive, custom-made wigs are hand knotted into a fine mesh foundation (figs. 1 and 2). In cheaper weft wigs, hair is sewn by machine into a net cap in circular rows (figs. 3, 4 and 5).

The quality of a wig also varies with the kind of hair it contains, the way it is constructed and how it is fitted to the client's measurements.

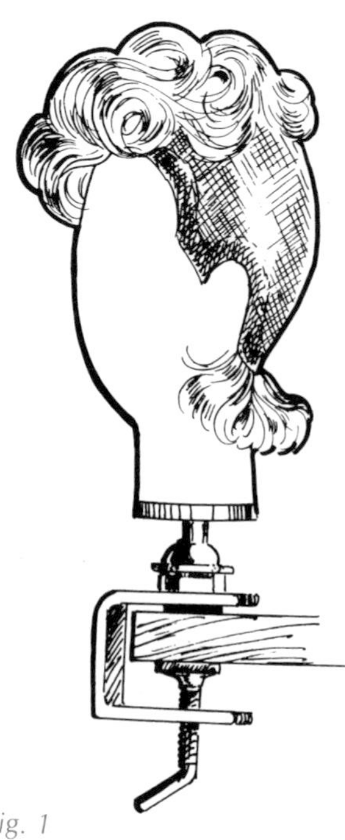

Fig. 1

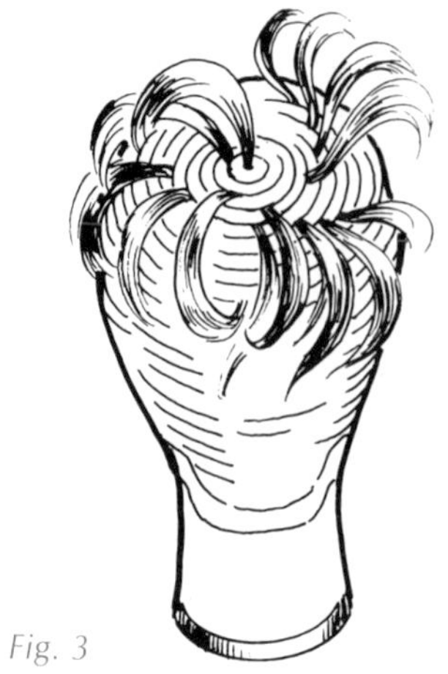
Fig. 3

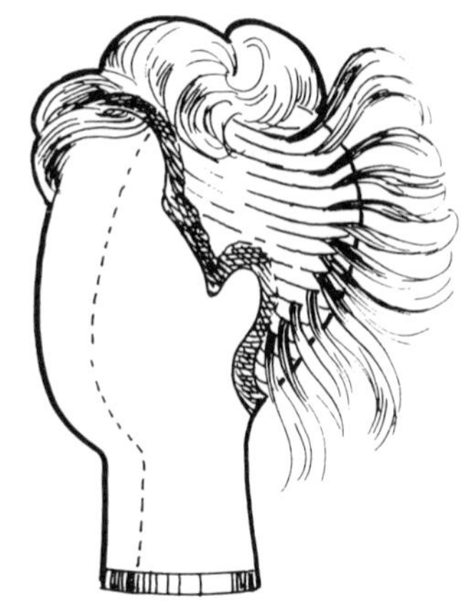
Fig. 4

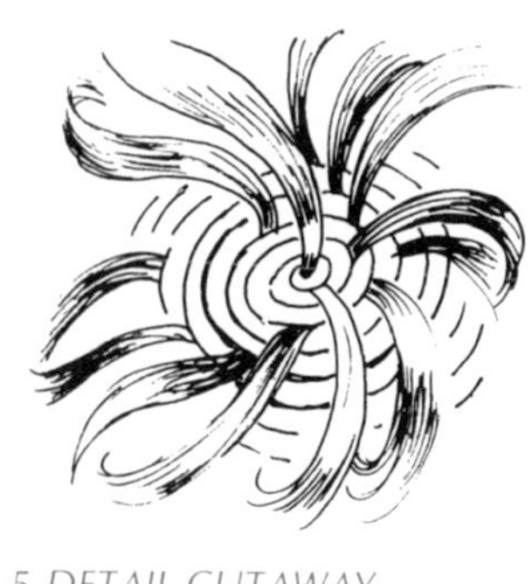
Fig. 5 DETAIL CUTAWAY
Hair is sewn by machine into net cap or weft in circular rows.

Synthetic Wigs and Hairpieces

Great improvements have been made in the manufacture of synthetic fibers. Modacrylic fibers, such as dynel, kanekalon, venicelon and others have eliminated most of the disadvantages of synthetic hairs. Hair fiber research has developed synthetic hair that closely resembles human hair in texture, resiliency, porosity, pliability, durability, sheen and feel. The fibers have good curl retention, are nonflammable and do not oxidize and change color in sunlight. In fact, some synthetic fibers so closely resemble human hair that it is difficult to distinguish between them.

Synthetic hairs have a number of advantages that have contributed to their acceptance for the manufacture of wigs and hairpieces. Since the hair is synthetically produced, it is very economical. The supply is unlimited. The wigs and hairpieces are made from long threads that have been rolled on spools, permitting great efficiency in use. They are made with color fasteners in any color or shade desired.

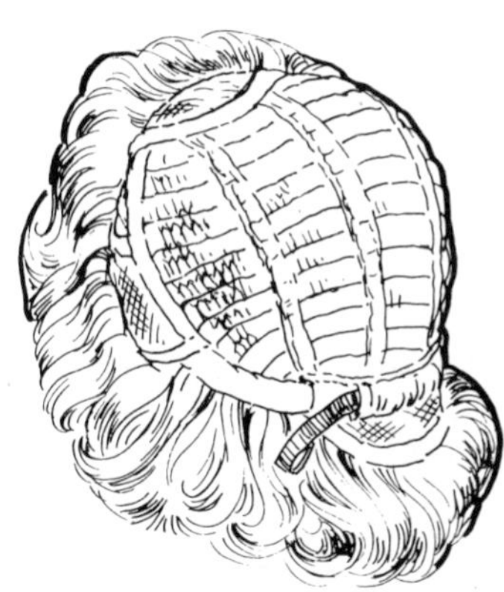
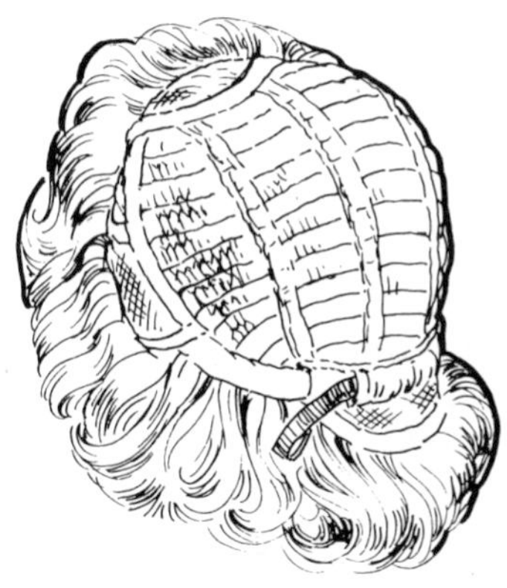
Fig. 6

Synthetic wigs are available as handmade stretch wigs (fig. 6), as machine-made stretch wigs and as handmade fitted wigs. Whatever the type of wig, careful selection of quality, proper fit and good workmanship will give satisfaction in wear, comfort and style.

Also available is the **no-cap wig**, which is composed of rows of wefting sewn to elastic bands. The advantages of no-cap wigs are that they are lighter and cooler than other types of wigs (fig. 7).

Wig caps and hairpieces are made of cotton, a synthetic and cotton all synthetic or reinforced elastic. Hairpieces are generally made with a synthetic bases which do not shrink when shampooed. Synthetic hairpieces are available as wiglets, demi-wigs, braids, chignons, cascades and falls.

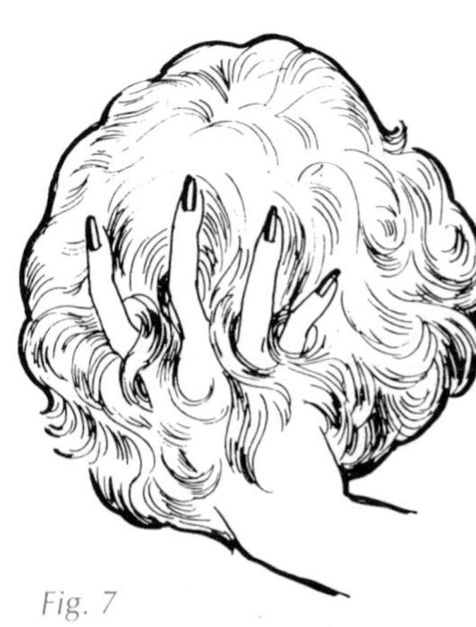
Fig. 7

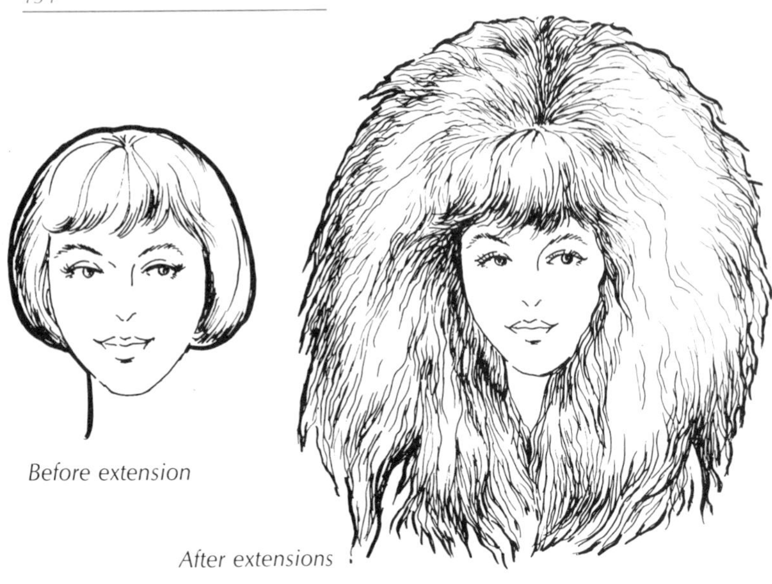

Before extension

After extensions

Hair Extensions

Hair extensions are also available to make hair look longer, to change the already existing hairstyle and to add thickness and volume. Extensions can be made from either human or synthetic hair.

Hair Replacement

Wigs have also become popular for use by those people who have had a hair loss due to illness, heredity or an injury or shock to the nervous system.

Wigs are used by both men and women in this instance to maintain their present hairstyle or to replace the hair that was lost.

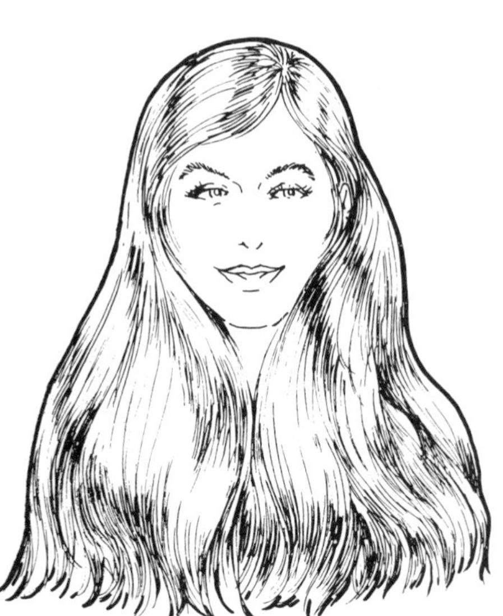

Use of Wigs in Black Hairstyling

Black clients are also increasing their use of wigs for styling flexibility. Many clients may like to wear a straight style without chemically relaxing their hair, and a wig is a styling alternative.

Men's Wigs

An increasing number of men are using wigs or toupees to compensate for hair loss.

Toupees are used with an adhesive applied to the base of the hairpiece so it can remain on the scalp.

To make men's hair appear more full, many clients have begun to have hair extensions added. These extensions are interwoven or braided onto the existing hair, giving the appearance of added thickness to the sparse areas.

Once added, the extensions are then styled to complement the client's hair type and facial features.

TAKING WIG MEASUREMENTS

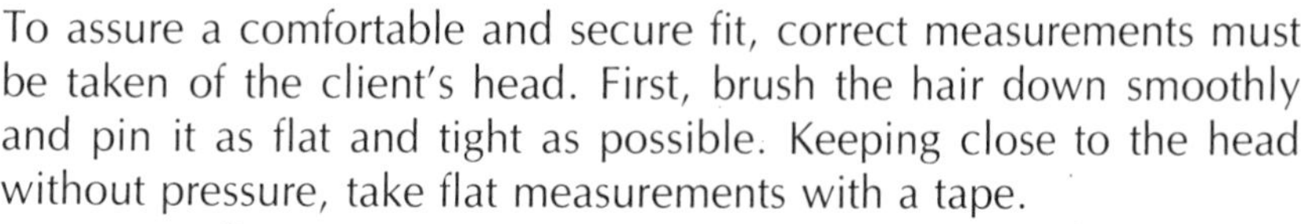

To assure a comfortable and secure fit, correct measurements must be taken of the client's head. First, brush the hair down smoothly and pin it as flat and tight as possible. Keeping close to the head without pressure, take flat measurements with a tape.

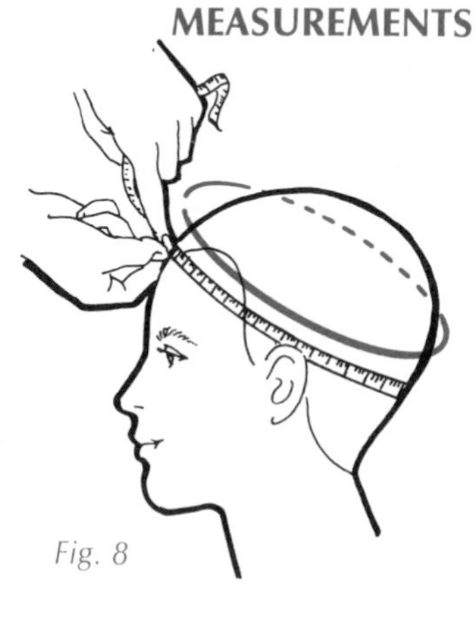

Fig. 8

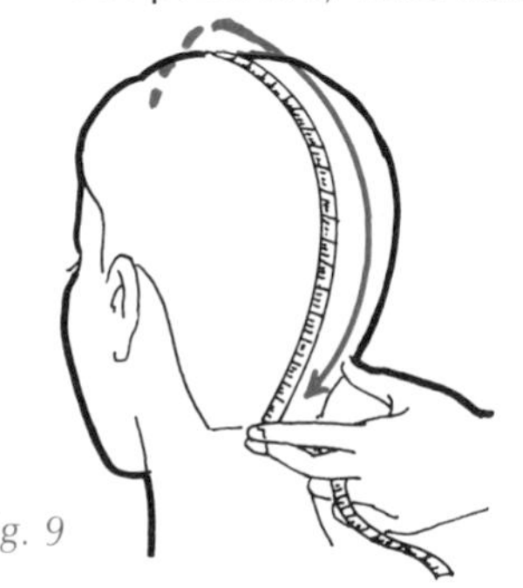

Fig. 9

Procedure

1. Measure the circumference of the head. Starting on the hairline at the middle of the forehead; place tape above the ears, around the back of the head and return to the starting point (fig. 8).
2. Measure from the hairline at the middle of the forehead, over the top, to the nape of the neck. Bend head back and measure to a point where the wig will ride on the base of the skull at the nape (fig. 9).
3. Measure from ear to ear, across the forehead (fig. 10).
4. Measure from ear to ear, over the top of the head (fig. 11).
5. Place the tape across the crown and measure from temple to temple (fig. 12).
6. Measure the width of the napeline, across the nape of the neck (fig. 13).

Fig. 10

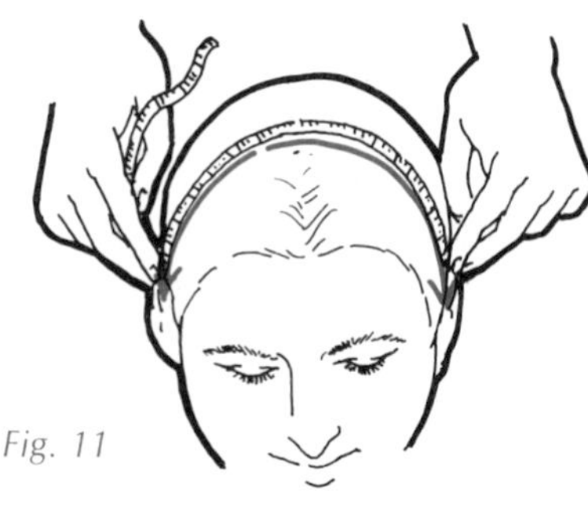

Fig. 11

Fig. 12

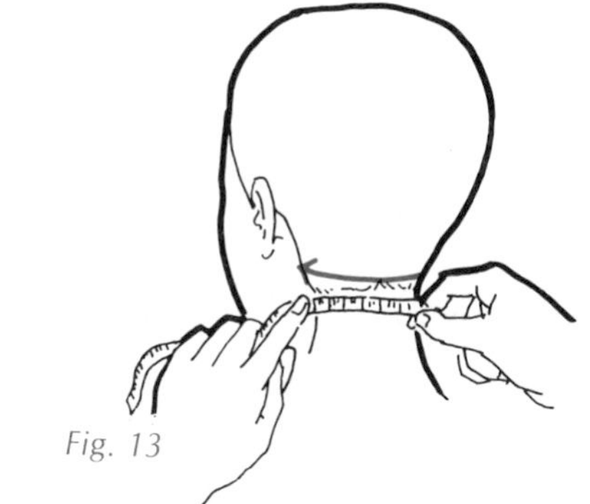

Fig. 13

Note Check to make certain that all measurements are accurate.

ORDERING THE WIG

When ordering the wig, keep a written record of the client's head measurements and forward a copy to the wig dealer or manufacturer. Also specify what is desired as to:

1. Hair shade. If necessary, submit samples of the client's hair to the manufacturer. Hair samples should be of hair that has been freshly shampooed, tinted or rinsed.
2. Quality of hair
3. Length of hair
4. Type of hair part and hair pattern

FITTING THE WIG

After the wig has been made according to specific measurements, it might require some adjustments so it comfortably fits the client's head.

Adjusting the Wig to a Larger Size

If the wig feels too tight, it might require some stretching. Turn the wig inside out and wet it's foundation with hot water. Stretch the wig carefully (without ripping) onto a larger size block and pin securely. Then allow the wig to dry naturally.

Adjusting the Wig to a Smaller Size

If the wig feels too loose, it must be adjusted to fit properly.

Tucking

Tucks are used to improve the fit of a wig that is too big.

1. **Horizontal tucks** shorten the wig from front to nape. They are made across the back of the wig to remove excess bulk (fig. 14).
2. **Vertical tucks** remove width at the back of the wig from ear to ear (fig. 15).

Both earpieces must be checked to be certain they are directly across from each other and do not touch the ears. If the wig touches the ear, make a small horizontal tuck over the ear to raise the wig. If the wig is rubbing or touching the side of the ear, a small vertical tuck behind the ear will pull the wig back and eliminate the problem.

Check the cap fit after each tuck. Excessive tucking will cause the wig to "ride up" and create new fitting problems.

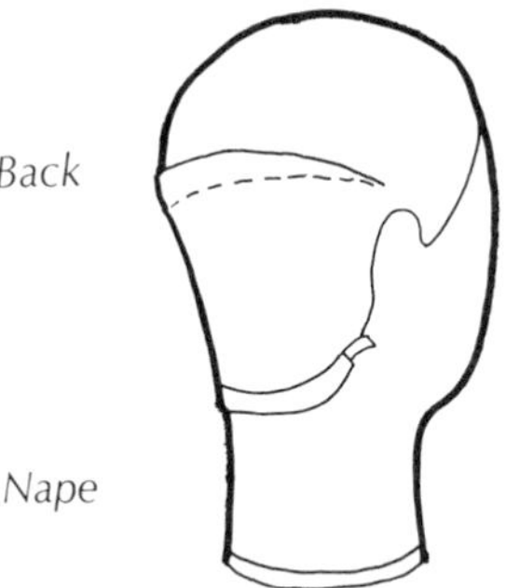

Fig. 14 Horizontal tuck

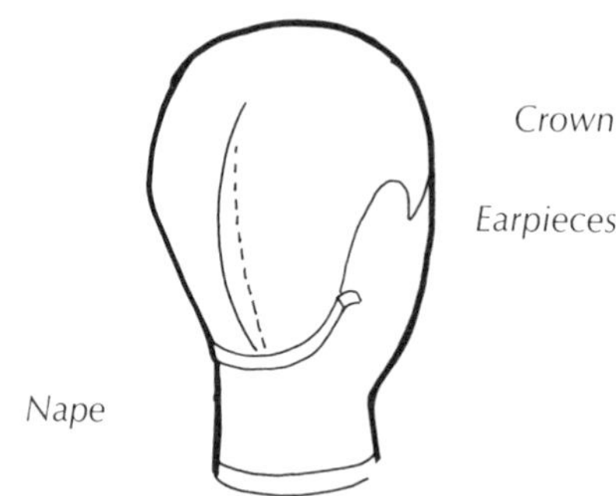

Fig. 15 Vertical tuck

The Elastic Band

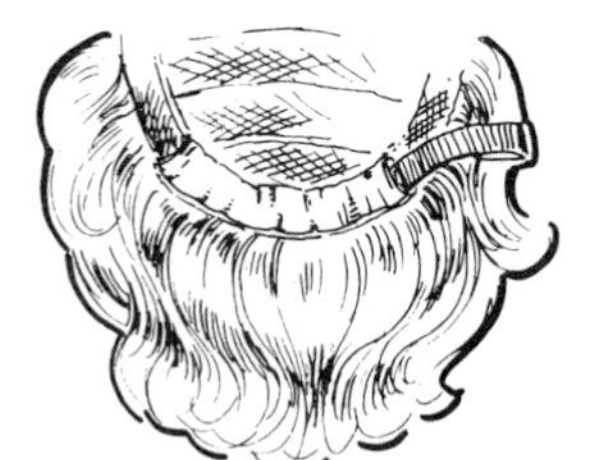

Elastic band

The final step in the wig adjustment process is adjusting the elastic band at the back of the wig. Pull the elastic band to make the wig fit evenly and snugly at the back of the head and then fasten it.

To allow ease when making adjustments, pin the ends of the elastic band in a small safety pin.

The elastic band requires periodic adjustment or replacement because it stretches or deteriorates from its exposure to body heat and cleaning fluids.

CLEANING WIGS

Human Hair Wigs

A human hair wig should be dry-cleaned every 2 to 4 weeks, depending on how often it is worn. Also, when a wig is ready for restyling, it should be dry-cleaned. Refer to the manufacturer's suggestions and cleaning instructions.

Procedure

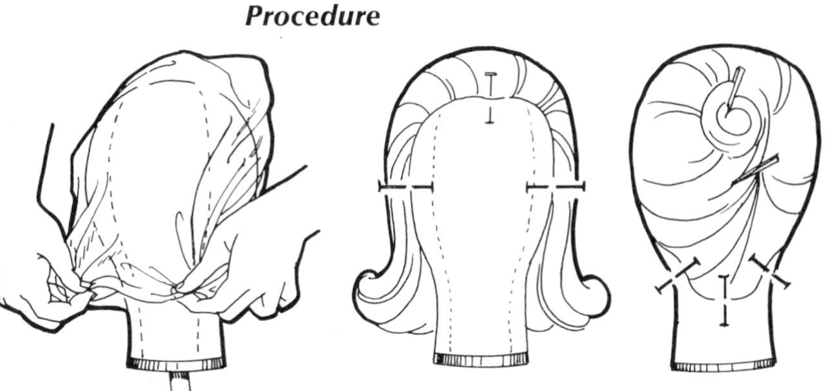

Fig. 16 Covering block *Fig. 17 Front view* *Fig. 18 Back view*

1. Cover the canvas block with plastic to protect the canvas.
2. Clean the edges and inside foundation with a cottom ball or small brush.
3. Block the wig.
4. Saturate the wig in a large glass or plastic bowl containing liquid cleaner.
5. Soak the wig for 3 to 4 minutes.
6. Comb the cleaning solution through the length of the hair with a wide-tooth comb.
7. Work the solution into the entire wig.
8. Carefully towel blot.
9. Allow to dry naturally on the block for about 1/2 hour.
10. Give a conditioning treatment, if necessary.
11. Set and style the wig.

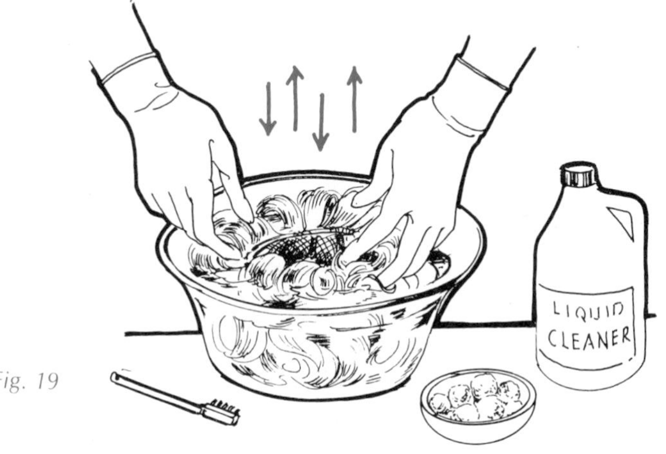

Fig. 19

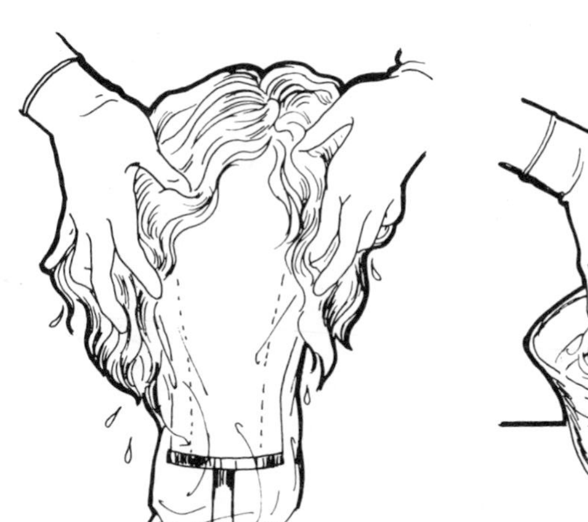

Fig. 20

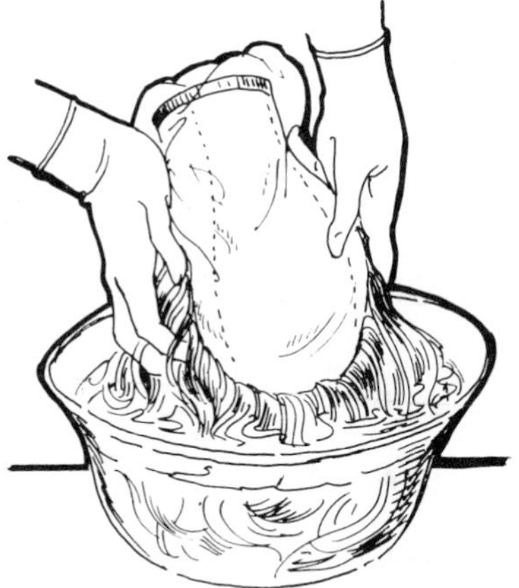

Fig. 21 Saturate wig and work solution through the hair

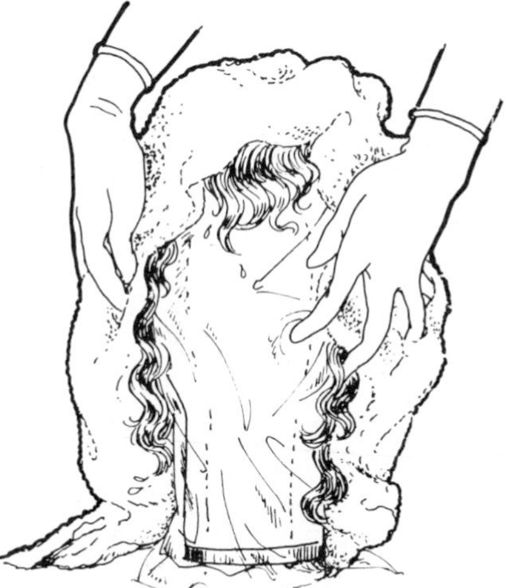

Fig. 22 Towel dry hair

Hand-Tied Wigs

Hand-tied wigs, which are more delicate in structure and far more costly than human hair wigs, should be cleaned on the block.

Synthetic Wigs

Synthetic wigs and hairpieces do not require cleaning as often as human hair wigs. Synthetic fibers are non-absorbent (lack porosity) and do not attract dust and dirt.

Synthetic wigs and hairpieces require cleaning about every three months, depending on the amount of wear and styling. Use tepid or cool water to clean the wig, because hot water will take the curl out of the synthetic wig. Do not comb or brush while wet.

Procedure

1. Cover the appropriate block with plastic to protect the canvas.
2. Mount the wig on the block and outline the size.
3. Brush out tangles and wig spray before cleaning.
4. Fill a container with mild shampoo or a specially formulated cleaner according to manufacturer's directions. Use tepid or cool water.
5. Remove the wig from the block. Swish the wig through cleaning solution for a few minutes. Rinse thoroughly in cool water.
6. Use a small brush or cotton to clean the mesh foundation.
7. Squeeze out excess water and towel blot. (Do not wring or twist wig.)
8. T-pin the wig on the proper size block and let dry naturally.
9. Do not brush a synthetic wig when it is wet; this can remove the curl.
10. Do not expose a synthetic wig to heat.

1.

2.

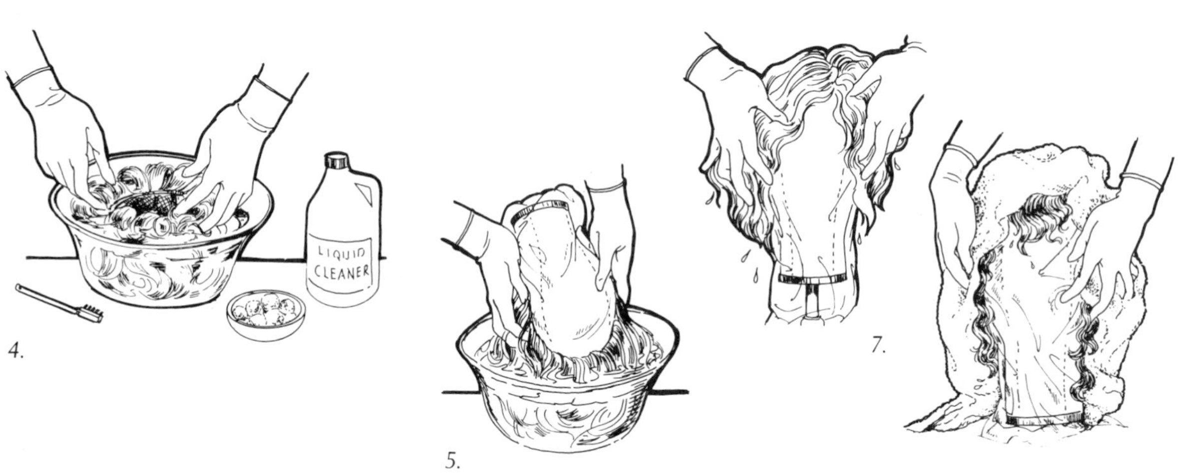

4.

5.

7.

Note

If it becomes necessary to reduce the drying time, the wig may be placed in a cool dryer with only the fan used. Since most synthetic wigs are prestyled, they require no further styling.

Conditioning the Wig

A wig differs from human hair because it does not have its own supply of natural oils for self-lubrication. Since wig cleaners usually are very drying to the hair, it is advisable to use a conditioning treatment after each cleaning to keep the wig hair from drying and looking dull. This will also keep the wig in good condition (fig. 23).

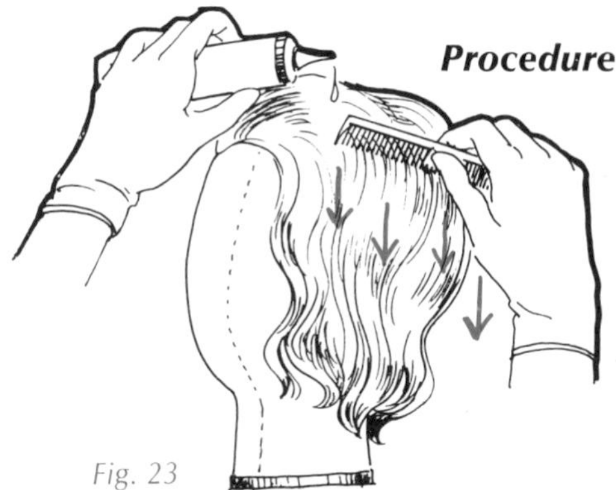

Fig. 23

Procedure

1. Cover the block with plastic and block the wig properly.
2. Apply conditioner. Distribute the conditioner evenly to damp, clean hair with a wide-tooth comb. Keep conditioner in the hair for the length of time indicated in the product's instructions.

SHAPING WIGS

Shaping Human Hair Wig

Basically, a wig may be shaped in the same manner as natural hair is shaped on the head. However, consideration must be given to the fact that a wig has about twice as much hair as a human head. That is why it is important to thin and taper the wig properly or it will look bulky and artificial.

Thinning may be done with either a razor or thinning shears. Because of the excessive amount of hair in the wig, more bulk must be removed in the top section, in back of the ears and around the face.

Most of the thinning should be done as close to the wig foundation as possible, without damage to the cap itself. Thin close to the cap to remove more bulk and to be certain that no hairs are left to stick out after the hair is styled. Special care must be taken so that all knots on the hand-knotted wig are tight. Equal care must be taken not to cut any of the wefts or sewing threads on the wefted wig.

When cutting the wig, remember that the hair will not grow back to cover an error in judgment. Proceed cautiously.

The wig should be cut on the head, to fit in with the natural hair and client's facial features. For convenience, the wig may be cut on a canvas block.

You might prefer to cut a guideline on the client's head and then transfer the wig to the block. This assures that the length of the wig will blend with the natural hair length. By moving the wig to the block, you can secure it firmly for the rest of the shaping process.

Cutting on the block also has the advantage of permitting the wig to be pinned securely, thus avoiding possible slippage during the cutting process.

In placing the wig to be cut on the canvas block, it is important that you carefully set it on the block at the correct hairline distance and continue to cut the remaining hair evenly.

Procedure (Can be done on a block or on the client's head)

Continue the shaping process, section by section, until the entire wig has been shaped.

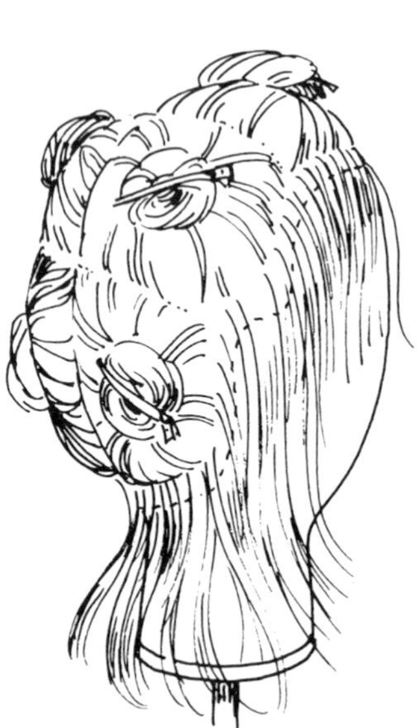

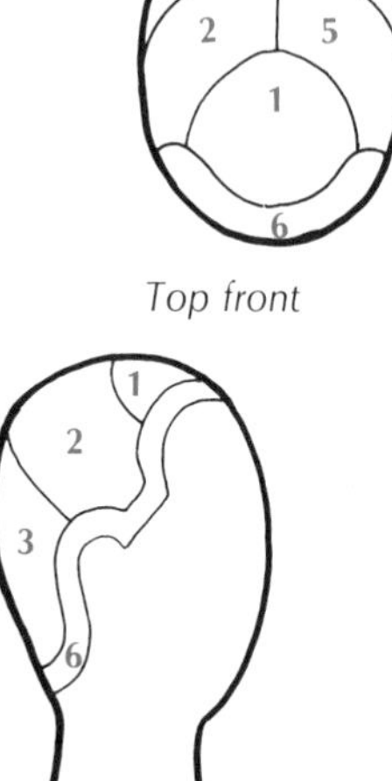

Top front

Right side

RIGHT SIDE OF HEAD. Part off a 2" guideline around the wig. Tie up top hair to keep it out of the way. Cut guideline to the desired length.

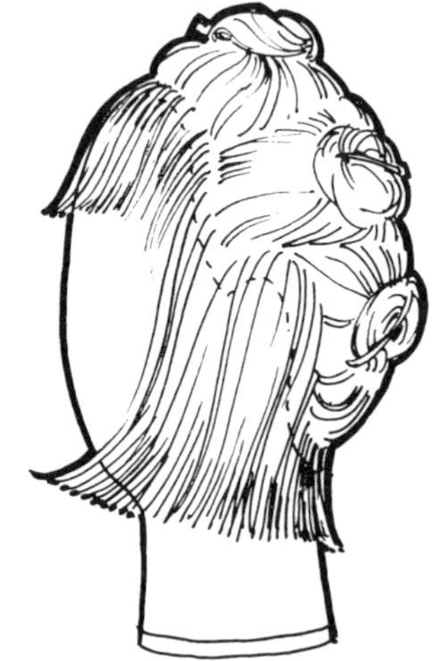

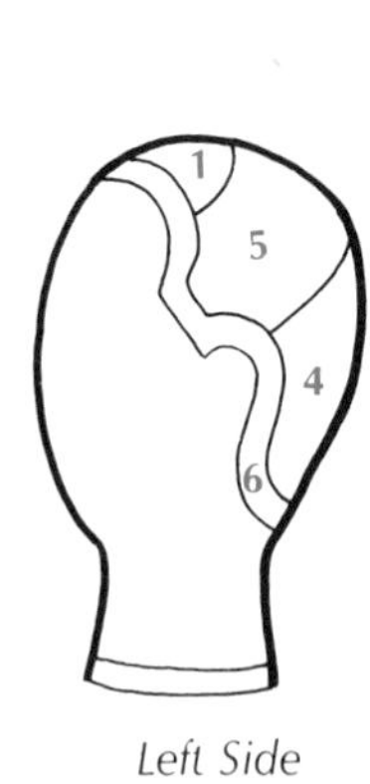

Left Side

LEFT SIDE OF THE HEAD. This illustrates a completely cut guideline.

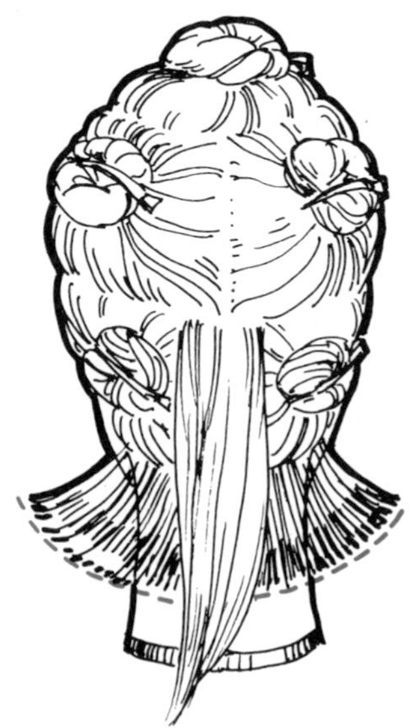

BACK OF HEAD. Let down center back hair. Cut to the same length as guideline.

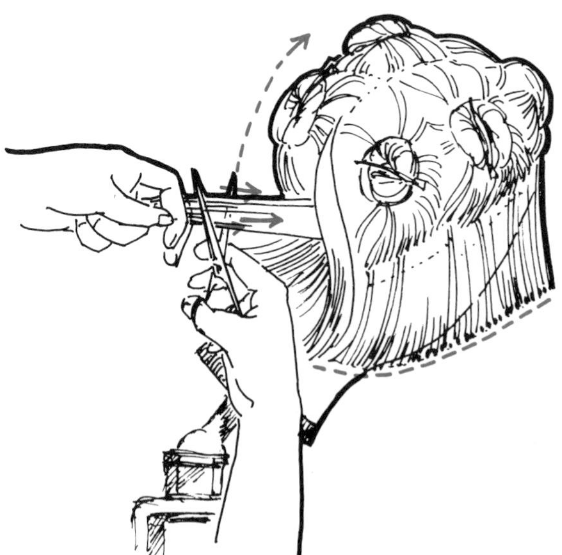

BACK OF HEAD. Pick up a strand of the guideline. With hands arched at a 45° angle, cut into the longer hair. Proceed with a sweeping upward motion.

Shaping Synthetic Hair Wigs

Use only scissors and thinning shears on either synthetic fiber or on a mixture of synthetic and human hair. The durable fiber dulls a razor.

Synthetic wigs always should be cut when dry, because the fibers can stretch when wet.

SETTING AND STYLING WIGS

Setting and Styling Human Hair Wigs

Setting wig hair is similar to setting hair on the human head, except for hairline coverage.

The added fullness of the client's hair, plus the hair and foundation of the wig, are factors to be considered when setting and styling the wig.

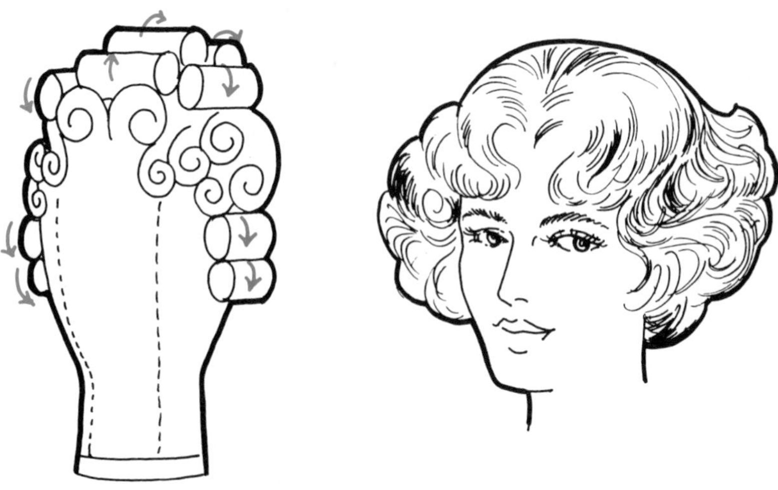

Setting on block *Comb-out*

It is desirable to use T-pins instead of clippies or bobby pins to hold both rollers and curls to insure that they are held securely.

Set, dry and style hair in the usual manner.

Setting and Styling Synthetic Wigs

Cutting and styling synthetic wigs differ from human hair wigs in the following ways:

Teasing or back combing synthetic wigs should be confined solely to the base of the fibers. This is necessary to avoid damage to the fiber, which should be kept perfectly smooth at the wig surface. Damage to the hair shaft (by thinning) will result in a frizzy, fuzzy-looking wig.

Synthetic wigs are precut into definite styles when they are manufactured. If the client desires a change, a good quality synthetic wig can be combed into different styles by a skilled stylist. These comb-out styles are all based on the basic precut factory created style. The synthetic wig never really needs restyling. However, the hairstylist must be guided by the client's wishes.

PUTTING ON AND TAKING OFF A WIG

A simple but very important procedure is the correct way to remove a wig from a block and place it on the client's head. (It is a good policy to show the client the proper way to put on and take off the wig.)

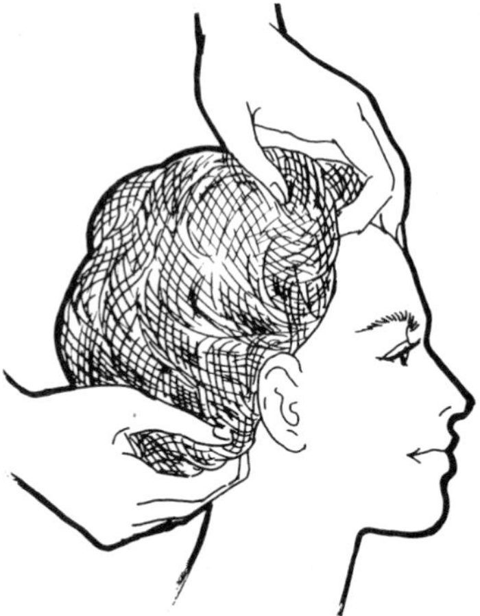

Comb client's hair away from her face. Pile the hair on top. Place long hair in fine net.

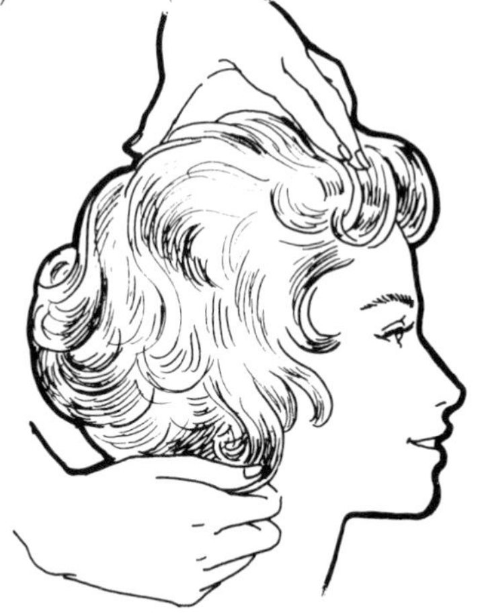

Place wig on front of the client's head. While holding the wig securely on top, glide it back to nape. Pull the wig securely over sides, front and back.

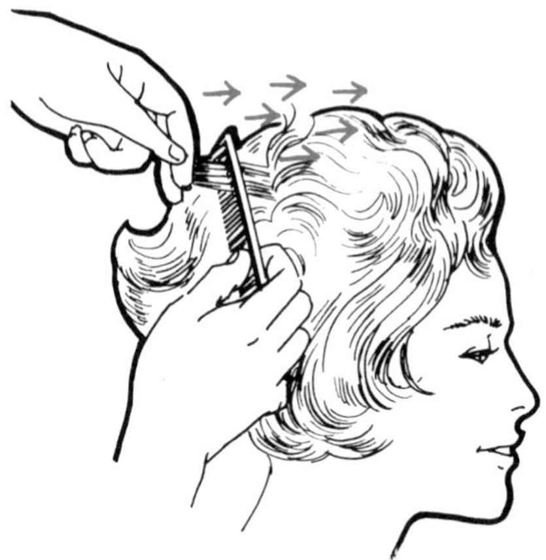

Recomb and adjust the style to suit the client.

Procedure

To remove a wig, place only the thumb under the cap at the nape. **Do not put your fingers into the hair.**

Combing Client's Hair into a Wig

Comb the client's hair away from the face. Bring forward and adjust it to the front hairline.

When the wig is comfortably adjusted, draw out approximately 1″ (2.5 cm) of the client's hair from around the front hairline; then comb and blend the hair into the style of the wig.

WIG COLORING

Color Rinses

Color rinses are used as temporary coloring on human hair wigs and should be reapplied whenever the hair is cleaned. Color rinses can only darken the hair; if a lighter color is desired, a different wig must be worn.

The following method is one way to apply a color rinse. Your instructor's method may be equally correct.

Procedure

1. Pin the wig securely on a plastic covered block.
2. Dampen the clean hair, using a spray applicator bottle.
3. Whenever in doubt of which color to use, strand test the color rinse on the back of the wig.

Note If a color rinse is applied on dry hair, additional rinse is required for complete coverage.

4. Spray the hair with a color rinse. Distribute it evenly with a downward motion, using a small brush and wide-tooth comb (fig. 24).
5. Apply setting lotion in the usual manner (fig. 25).
6. Set, dry (fig. 26) and comb out the hair to the desired style.

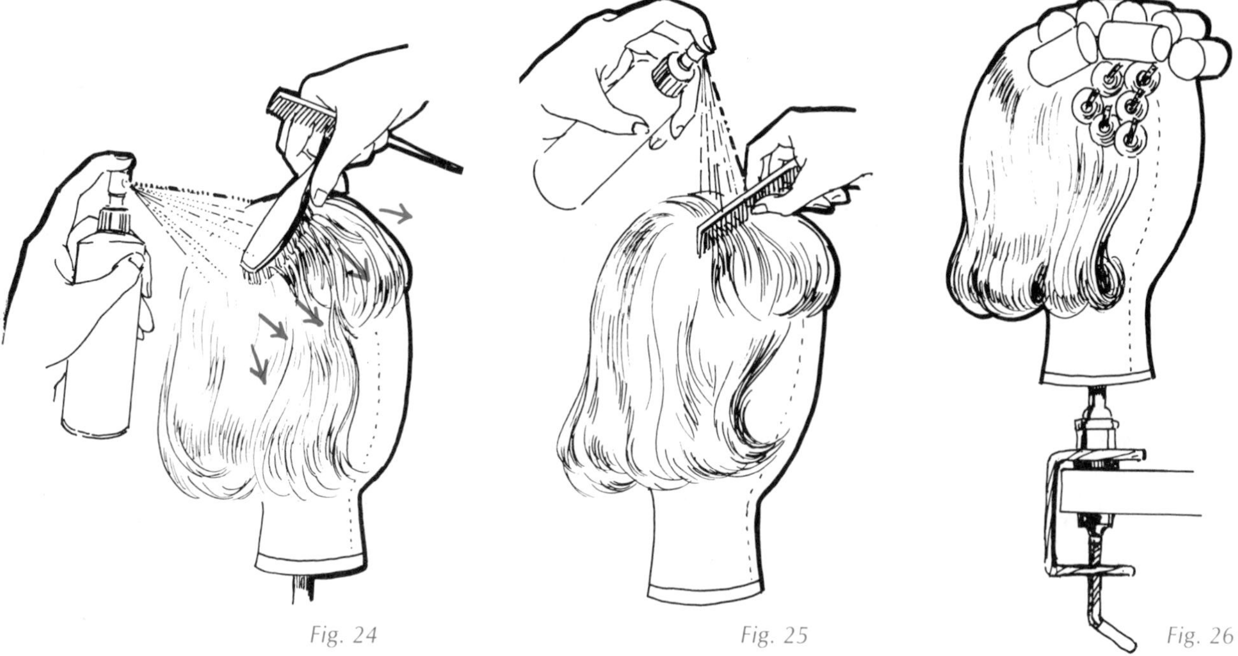

Fig. 24 Fig. 25 Fig. 26

Note In addition to color rinses, human hair wigs may be colored with a semi-permanent tint. However, it is never advisable to attempt to lighten (bleach) any wig or hairpiece.

Semi-Permanent Tints The following is one method of semi-permanent tints to machine-made wigs.

Procedure

1. Mount the wig on the appropriate plastic-covered block and outline the size with T-pins.
2. Remove all teasing, tangles and snarls.
3. Clean the wig and comb the hair smooth.
4. Remove the wig from the block.
5. Immerse the wig in a glass bowl of hot water and semi-permanent tint solution.
6. Leave completely immersed for 10 minutes.
7. Remove and rinse with cold water.
8. Apply conditioner.
9. Block, set, dry and comb out in the usual manner.

Permanent Tints Since 100% human hair wigs and hairpieces have been subjected to extensive processing, it is risky to use permanent tints on such hair because the results may be uneven coloring.

Caution When tinting wigs be sure to follow the manufacturer's directions.

HAIRPIECES AND EXTENSIONS

A variety of hairstyles can be created with hairpieces that can be dressed for either daytime or evening wear. These hairpieces come in various forms, such as:

1. **Switches**—long wefts of hair mounted with a loop at the end. They are constructed with 1 to 2 stems of hair. The better switches are constructed with three stems to provide greater flexibility in styling and braiding. They may be worked into the hair or braided, to create special styling effects (fig. 27).

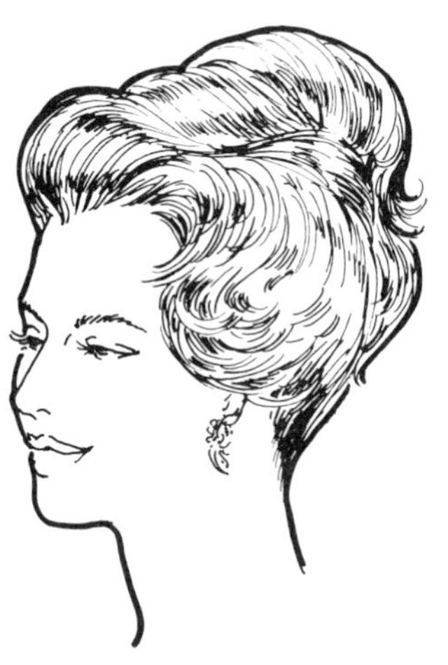

Fig. 27 Switch

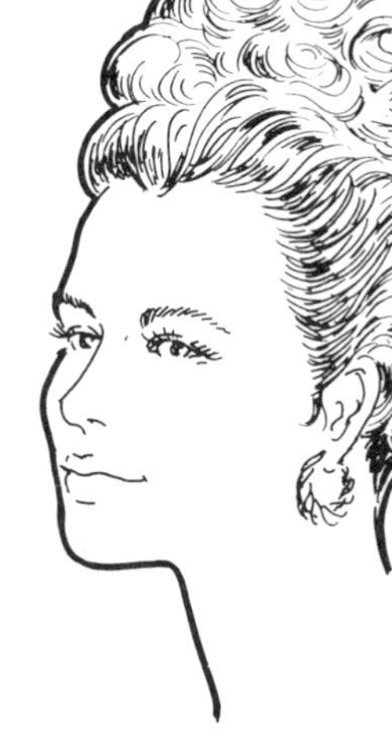

Fig. 28 Wiglet

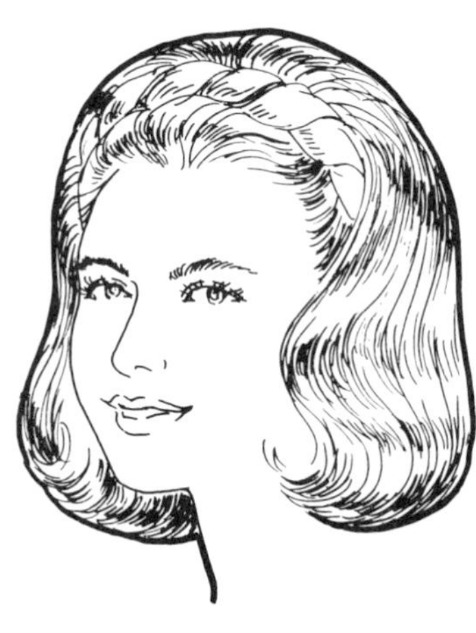

Fig. 29 Bandeau type hairpiece

2. **Wiglets**—hairpieces with a flat base which are used in special areas of the head. They are used primarily to blend with the client's own hair to extend the range of the hair. Wiglets can be worked into the top of the hair in curls or under the hair to give it height and body. They also are used to create special effects (fig. 28).
3. **Bandeau type**—a hairpiece that is sewn to a headband. The bandeau type hairpiece is usually worn over the hair and is dressed casually (fig. 29).
4. **Fall**—a section of hair, machine wefted on a round base, running across the back of the head and available in various lengths. Falls have a thick, full look. Short falls* range from 12″ to 14″ (30 to 35 cm) in length (fig. 30).
   Demi-falls*, 15″ to 20″ (37.5 to 50 cm).
   Long falls*, 18″ to 24″ (45 to 60 cm).
5. **Demi-fall** or **demi-wig**—a large base hairpiece that is designed to fit to the shape of the head and generally ranges in length from 15″ to 20″ (37.5 to 50 cm).

6. **Cascade**—a hairpiece on an oblong base which offers an endless variety of styling possibilities. Cascades can be styled in curls, braids or pageboy or can be used as a filler with the client's own hair (fig. 31).

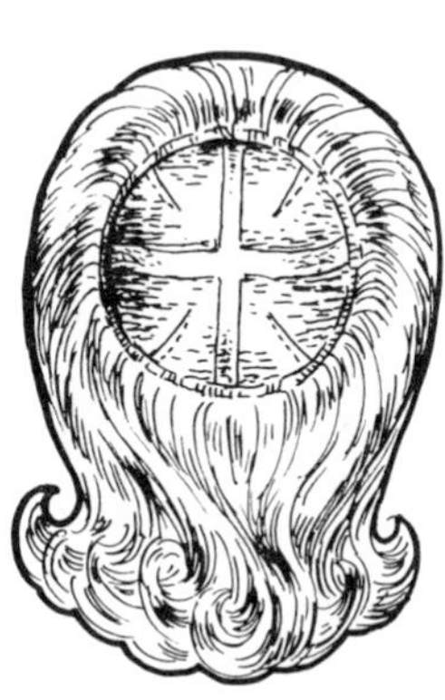
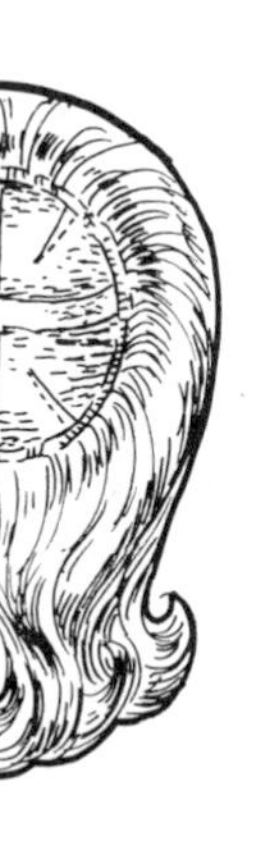

Fig. 30 Short fall

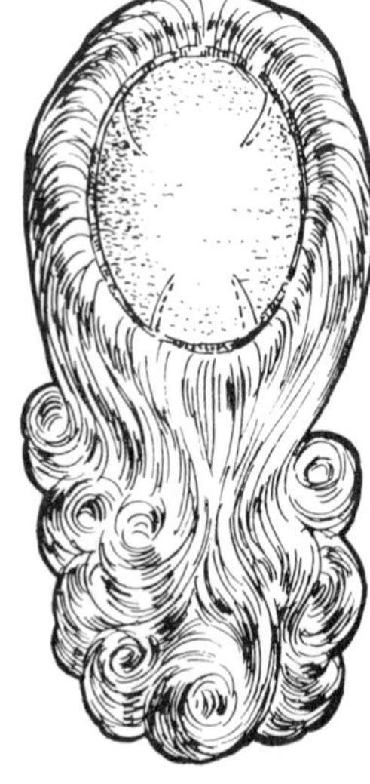

Fig. 31 Cascade

7. **Braid**—a switch whose strands are woven, interlaced or entwined. Some are prepared with a thin wire inside so that they can be formed into various shapes. Others, without wire, are permitted to hang loose on the head.
8. **Extensions**—individual sections of hair that are braided and blended with the natural hair to elongate the style or to make the hair fuller.

SAFETY PRECAUTIONS

1. Great care must be taken when combing or brushing wigs to avoid matting.
2. When dry cleaning a wig or hairpiece, never wring out the cleaning fluid.
3. When shaping a wig or hairpiece, use great care; once the hair has been cut, it cannot grow back.
4. When combing, use a wide-tooth comb to avoid damaging the foundation and to gain greater control.
5. When cleaning or working with a wet wig, always mount it on a block the same head size as the wig to avoid stretching.
6. To assure a comfortable and secure fit, take correct measurements of the client's head.

7. Recondition wigs as often as necessary to prevent dryness or brittleness.
8. If required, dry clean wigs before setting and styling.
9. Brush and comb wigs and hairpieces with a downward movement.
10. Never lighten (bleach) a wig or hairpiece.
11. Never give a permanent to a wig or hairpiece.

DEFINITIONS PERTAINING TO WIGS

The following are the technical words commonly used in wig work:

Angora: Long, silky hair of the Angora goat. It is used primarily in fantasy work.

Band wig: A hairpiece that is sewn to a headband that covers the hairline. The foundation of the hairpiece covers about two-thirds of the head and the overhanging hair covers all of the client's hair. This can be used instead of a full wig.

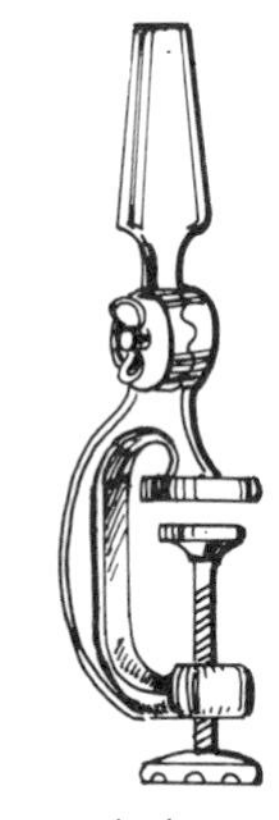
Swivel clamp

Base: The foundation of a hairpiece.

Binding: Ribbon used to protect and reinforce the edges of netting.

Blocking (foundation block): A head-shaped block made to hold a wig upon which work is to be done.

Cap (wig cap): The combined netting and binding of a wig.

Capless wig: Wefts of synthetic hair sewn on a cap made of wide straps; also referred to as **synthetic wig cap.**

Clamp: Device that can be attached to a table and upon which a wig block can be mounted. A **swivel clamp** can be adjusted to hold the block at different angles.

Custom-made wig: Wig that is fitted to the exact measurements of a client's head and styled to suit.

Dart: Tapered seam formed by cutting into a piece of wig net foundation and sewing the cut ends together. A dart is used to reduce the size of a wig cap.

Hairpiece: Small wig used to cover the top or crown of the head.

Hair roll: A sausage-like shape, in various lengths, used to fill under the natural hair to create special effects.

Hem: The bent over edge of a piece of material that has been turned under to avoid fraying. In wig work the netting is so hemmed to place the raw edge between the outside netting and the binding.

Handmade (or **hand ventilated**) **wig:** Wig that is made by hand knotting the hair onto a fine mesh net.

Knotting (or **ventilating**): Process by which hair is attached to the foundation in the creation of a wig or hairpiece. The actual knotting also is referred to as **ventilating.** Two types of knotting are generally used, single and double. **Single knotting** fastens the hair to the net by a single knot. **Double knotting** uses a double knot.

Machine-made (or **wefted**) **wig:** Hair is sewn onto strips of material by machine, then the strips of material are sewn onto a net by machine. The strips of material also are called **wefts**.

Mesh: Open weave foundation used in wig and hairpiece construction.

Refined hair: Oriental hair, which is coarse in texture, is often chemically treated to make it more workable and usable.

Smocking: Length of weft sewn in triangles, diamonds or loops to create the flat, airy base of a hairpiece.

Stretch base wig: Wig cap (foundation) made of elastic material that stretches to fit various size heads.

Styrofoam: Lightweight, plastic foam used for a wig block; recommended for storing wigs.

Switch: Long length of wefted hair mounted with a loop on the end; usually constructed with three stem strands to provide flexibility in styling.

T-pin: Pin resembling the letter "T" used to secure the hairpiece to the block. It is also called a **block** or **wig point**.

Tuck: Reduces the size of the wig cap. Netting is folded into a tuck formation, sewn and folded together.

Ventilate: See **Knotting.**

Ventilating needle: Miniature crocheting needle made of spring steel, which is used to attach hair to a foundation.

Weft: Wig fibers sewn to a ribbon of fabric. Wefts are sewn to a base to form the wig.

Weft: Artificial section of woven (or sewn) hair, used for practice work or as a substitute for natural hair.

Wefted wig (machine-made): Wig made of wefts of hair sewn into a wig base.

Wefting: Art of weaving or sewing hair strands side by side to form a length of hair.

Wig dryers: Cabinet dryers used for drying wigs and hairpieces. They provide regulated heat and can dry many wigs and hairpieces at one time.

Wiglet: Hairpiece with a flat base which is used to extend the area of hair.

REVIEW QUESTIONS The Care and Styling of Wigs

1. *List some of the reasons wigs are worn.*
2. *What are the different types of wigs, extensions and hairpieces?*
3. *Describe the procedure for taking wig measurements.*
4. *What are important considerations when ordering a wig?*
5. *What does "blocking a wig" mean?*
6. *List and describe the techniques in wig cleaning and conditioning.*
7. *What is the procedure for coloring a wig with a semi-permanent tint?*
8. *How should you use a color rinse on a wig?*
9. *List four types of hairpieces and how they are used.*
10. *Describe the safety precautions to be followed in handling wigs.*

Chapter 14

PERMANENT WAVING

LEARNING OBJECTIVES

The student successfully mastering this chapter will be able to:

1. *Give a brief history of permanent waving.*
2. *Explain the purpose of cold waving.*
3. *Explain the use of neutral and acid-balanced solutions.*
4. *Identify the steps in permanent waving.*
5. *List the categories of scalp and hair analysis and demonstrate method(s) for testing each.*
6. *Explain the importance of the pre-permanent shampooing.*
7. *Select the proper size rods to achieve the desired curl effect.*
8. *Describe the chemicals available for modern permanent waving.*
9. *Indicate the importance of sectioning and blocking.*
10. *Demonstrate different patterns for sectioning and blocking.*
11. *Explain the importance of end papers to the wrap and demonstrate three methods of placing the papers when wrapping.*
12. *State the necessity for test curls and demonstrate the correct technique for taking test curls.*
13. *Demonstrate correct lotion application.*

14. *Explain the importance of proper neutralization to the permanent wave.*
15. *Recognize the alternate methods in cold waving.*
16. *List the advantages and disadvantages of heat permanent waving.*
17. *Discuss permanent waving for men.*
18. *List items of importance to be included on the permanent waving record card.*
19. *List at least five safety precautions for the protection of the client during the service.*

HISTORY OF PERMANENT WAVING

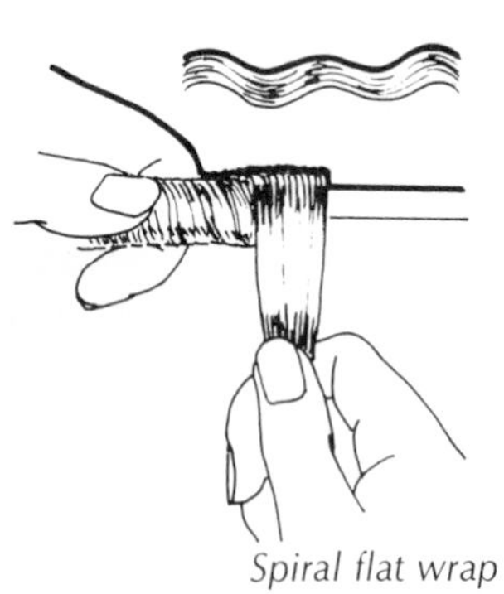

Spiral flat wrap

A crude system of permanent waving was practiced by the early Egyptians and Romans. The first real progress in permanent waving was made in 1905 when Charles Nessler invented the heat permanent waving machine. The machine introduced a method of applying heat to preformed curls through a series of heaters attached by wires to the machine.

The **spiral permanent wave** was the first method used. It involved winding the hair from the scalp to the ends and was suitable for only long hair.

The **croquignole permanent wave** was introduced in 1926 to meet the needs of clients with short hair. The shorter length required that the hair be wound from the hair ends toward the scalp. The hair could then be formed into waves finished with end curls.

A **combination** (spiral and croquignole) **permanent wave** soon came into vogue. The hair in the crown was given a spiral wave to take care of the longer hair and the rest of the hair received a croquignole wave.

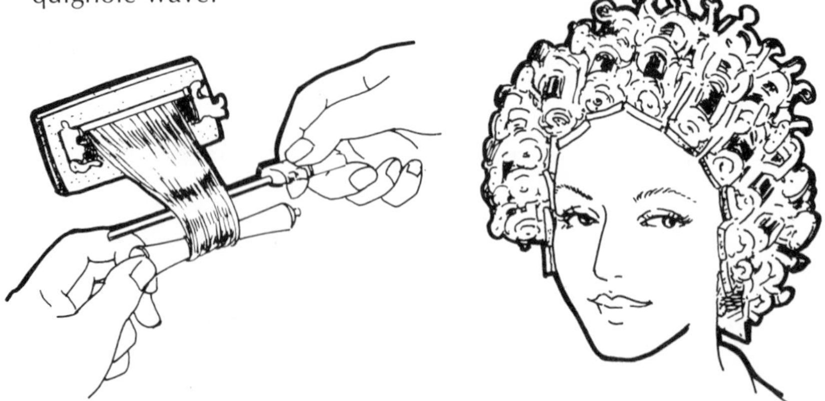

Croquignole wrap *Machineless method (steaming the hair)*

In 1931, the **pre-heat method** of permanent waving was introduced. The procedure was the same as for the croquignole method except for the source of heat. Unlike the machine method, the clamps were first heated by an electrical apparatus and then clamped over the prepared curls.

Another advance in permanent waving was the **machineless method** which was publicly introduced in 1932. This method required no electrical wires or machines. The source of heat was from chemical pads, which were moistened with water.

COLD WAVING

Cold waving (alkaline type) was first introduced in California during 1938–1939. However, in 1940, a nationwide promotion of cold waving got under way.

Why cold waving is so called. Since cold waving does not require heat and is given at room temperature, the manufacturers had to find a suitable name to distinguish this chemical method of permanent waving from the heat method so the name "cold waving" was adopted. As compared to heat permanent waving, cold waving has the following advantages:

1. It is relatively inexpensive since it does not require high-priced equipment.
2. The entire procedure is much faster than the heat method.
3. It is more comfortable for the client.

NEUTRAL AND ACID BALANCED SOLUTIONS

For many years, manufacturers sought to develop a permanent wave solution that did not require the use of excess ammonia. They wanted to minimize the damage caused to hair when permanently waved and to permit hair that had been damaged by lightening or tinting services to receive a permanent. To achieve these goals, they needed a waving solution that was not highly alkaline.

Neutral and acid-balanced permanent wave solutions which did not contain strong alkalines were introduced in 1970 and were less damaging to the hair. These products have a pH of 4.5 to 7.9. Within this range, lotions are slow to penetrate hair and processing time is longer. However, to overcome this problem, **heat** is applied to shorten the processing time.

PERMANENT WAVING

All methods of permanent waving involve two major actions on the hair:

1. Physical action—wrapping.
2. Chemical action—processing and neutralizing.

It is vital to know what takes place when the hair is wrapped around the rods, when the waving lotion is applied to the hair and how the neutralizer re-forms the cross bonds and rehardens the hair in its new position.

Physical Action

Wrapping. The physical action consists of wrapping the hair around the rods without stretching and with minimum tension. It is important that the hair is wrapped so it can expand when completely saturated by the permanent wave solution during processing.

Chemical Action

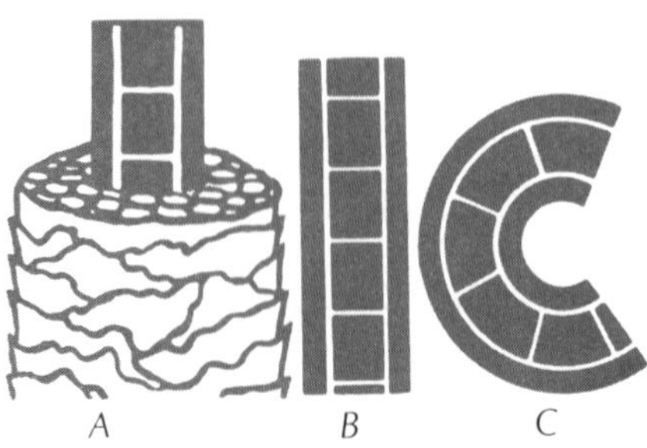

A. Each hair strand is composed of many polypeptide chains. This series of illustrations shows the behavior of one such chain.

B. Hair before processing. Chemical bonds (links) give hair its strength and firmness.

C. Hair wound on rod. The hair bends to the curvature and size of the rod.

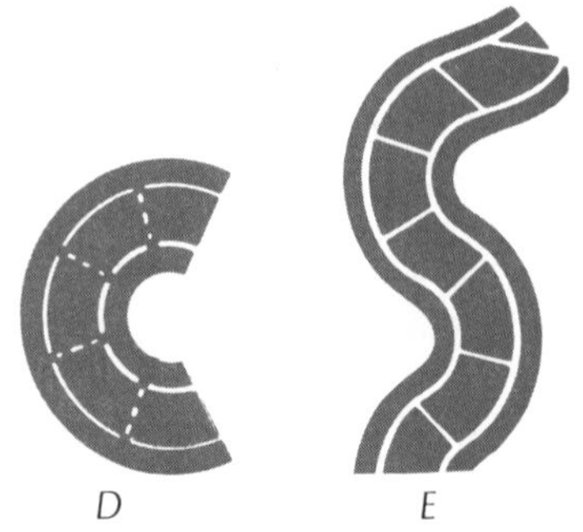

(Permanetly waved hair)

D. During processing waving lotion breaks the chemical cross-bonds (links), permitting the hair to adjust to the curvature of the rod while in this softened condition.

E. The neutralizer re-forms the chemical bonds (links) to conform with the wound position of the hair and rehardens the hair, thus creating the permanent wave.

Hair develops and maintains its natural form by means of hydrogen and sulfur cross bonds in the cortical layer, which hold the hair fibers in position and give the hair its strength. These bonds must be broken before the hair can be changed.

Processing. The bonds are weaker and many are easily broken by the shampooing and rinsing process. However, the chemical action of the permanent waving lotion is required to break the chemical bonds and thus soften the hair. This chemical action permits rearrangement of the inner structure of the hair so that the hair can assume the form of the rods around which it is wound.

Neutralizing. After the hair has assumed the desired shape, it must be neutralized or oxidized to stop the action of the waving lotion and to re-form the cross bonds in the cortical layer. This process rehardens the hair and fixes it into its newly curled form. When the neutralizing action is completed, the hair is unwrapped from the rods and permanently assumes its newly curled formation.

SCALP AND HAIR ANALYSIS

A very important step before giving a permanent wave is to make a careful analysis of the client's scalp and hair condition. The professional approach is to learn all the possible facts, such as:

Scalp condition	Hair texture	Hair density
Hair porosity	Hair elasticity	Hair length

Scalp Condition

The scalp should be examined very carefully. Abrasions of the scalp can make cold waving dangerous to a client. An irritated scalp and badly damaged hair are signs that a permanent wave should be postponed until the conditions are corrected.

Hair Porosity

Porosity (*po-ros-i-tee*) is the ability of the hair to absorb moisture. Since water changes some of the qualities of the hair, this analysis should be made before the shampoo, when the hair is still dry.

The **processing time** for any cold wave depends much more on hair porosity than on any other factor. The more porous the hair, the less processing time it takes, and a milder waving solution is suggested. **The degree at which hair absorbs the cold waving lotion is related to its porosity, regardless of texture.**

Hair porosity is affected by such factors as the client's health, climate, excessive exposure to sun and wind and the use of blow dryers, harsh shampoos, tints and lighteners.

Porosity Classified

Good porosity—hair with the cuticle layer raised from the hair shaft. Hair of this type can absorb moisture or chemicals in average time.

Moderate porosity (normal hair)—hair that is less porous than hair with good porosity.

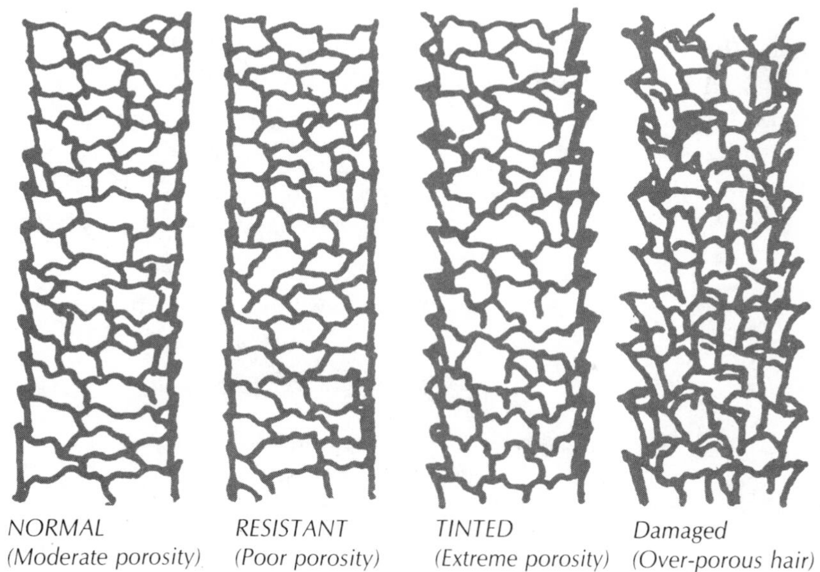

NORMAL (Moderate porosity) — *RESISTANT (Poor porosity)* — *TINTED (Extreme porosity)* — *Damaged (Over-porous hair)*

Poor porosity (resistant hair)—hair with the cuticle layer lying close to the hair shaft. This type of hair absorbs waving lotion more slowly and usually requires a longer processing time.

Extreme porosity (tinted, lightened or damaged hair)—hair that has been made extremely porous by chemical services and abuse. It absorbs the lotion and process very quickly. Either use a mild or a very mild lotion for hair with extreme porosity.

Over-porous hair—hair that is extremely damaged, dry, fragile and brittle. Until the hair is removed by cutting, **it should not receive a regular strength permanent wave.**

Porosity Test To test accurately for porosity, select hair from three different areas: the front hairline, temple and near the crown.

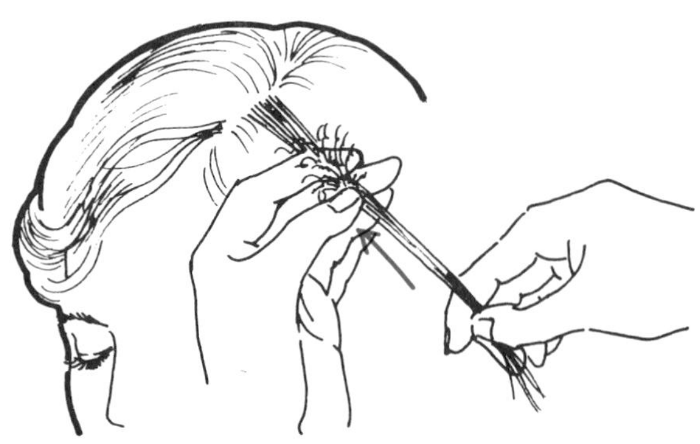
Testing for hair porosity

Grasp a small strand of dry hair and comb smooth. Hold the ends firmly with the thumb and index finger of one hand and slide the fingers of the other hand from the ends toward the scalp. If the fingers do not slide easily, or if the hair ruffles up as your fingers slide down the strand, **the hair is porous.** The more ruffles formed, the more porous the hair; the less ruffles formed, the less porous the hair.

If the fingers slide easily and no ruffles are formed, the cuticle layer lays close to the hair shaft. This type of hair is least porous (most resistant) and will require a longer processing time.

Other ways to test for porosity

1. **Cutting dry hair with scissors.** If the scissors cut through dry hair very easily, meeting little resistance, that hair is porous.
2. **Cupping the hair.** If the hair is squeezed, released in the hand, feels completely soft, showing little or no spring, that hair is porous.
3. **Wetting the hair at the shampoo bowl.** If the hair wets easily and thoroughly with the initial spray of water, that hair is porous.
4. **Placing wet hair under the dryer.** If hair takes longer than usual to dry, it is porous. The faster the hair dries, the less porosity it has.

Hair Texture Hair texture refers to the diameter of the individual hair and its degree of coarseness or fineness. The texture and porosity are judged together in determining the processing time. Although porosity is the more important of the two, texture does play an major part in estimating the processing time. Fine hair, having a small diameter, will become saturated with waving lotion more quickly than hair with a large diameter, if both are equal in porosity. However, when coarse hair is very porous, it will process faster than fine hair that is not porous.

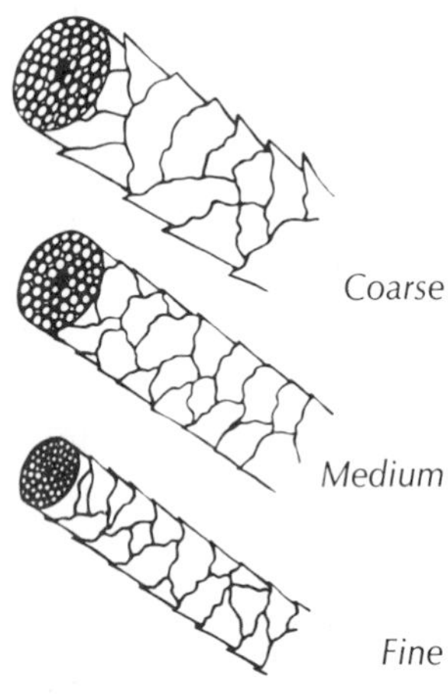

Hair texture also should be considered in deciding the size of the wave pattern. The texture and density of the client's hair must be taken into consideration when planning a hairstyle.

Variations in hair texture are due to:

1. **Diameter of the hair shaft:** coarse, medium, fine or very fine.
2. **Feel of the hair:** harsh, soft or wiry.

Hair Elasticity

Hair elasticity is a very important factor to consider when giving a permanent wave. Elasticity is the ability of the hair to stretch and contract. All hair is elastic, but its elasticity ranges from very good to poor. Without elasticity, there will be no curl in the hair. The greater the degree of elasticity, the longer the wave will remain in the hair, because less relaxation of the curl occurs.

Testing for Elasticity

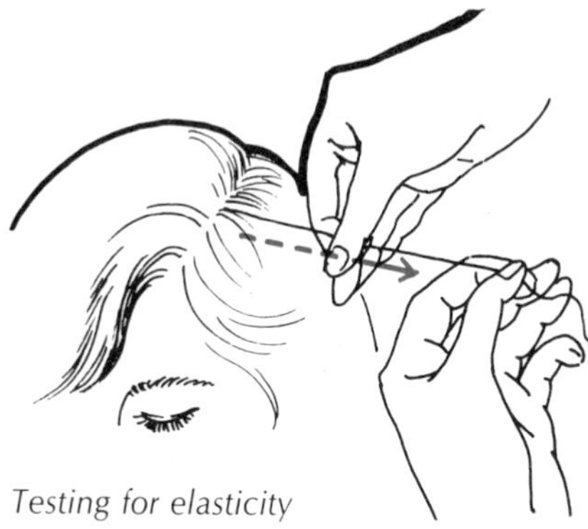
Testing for elasticity

Take a single dry hair and hold it between the thumb and forefinger of each hand. Stretch the hair slowly. The further it can stretch and return without breaking, the more elastic it is. If the elasticity is good, the hair slowly contracts after stretching. Hair with poor elasticity will break quickly and easily when stretched.

Normal hair is capable of being stretched about one-fifth its length and will spring back when released. However, wet hair can be stretched 40 to 50% of its length. Porous hair will stretch more than hair with poor porosity, but it will not completely return to its original state.

Limp hair will not develop a firm, strong cold wave. However, there are special waving lotions available for this type of hair. Limp hair requires a smaller diameter rod than hair having good elasticity.

Hair Density

Hair density is the amount of hairs per square inch (6.452 sq. cm) on the scalp. Density has nothing to do with hair texture. Smaller blockings (subsections) and larger rods are often required for thickly growing hair. However, if the hair is thin, smaller blockings and smaller (thinner) rods are required to form a good wave pattern close to the head.

Avoid blockings that are too large on a thin hair growth, because the strain may cause breakage.

Hair Length

Hair length is another important factor that must be considered. Waving hair of average length presents no real problem. However, if the client wears her hair 6″ (15 cm) or longer, follow **Piggyback, Double Rod Wrap** or other long hair techniques.

PRE-PERMANENT SHAPING AND SHAMPOOING

Shampooing for a Permanent Wave

It is advisable to use an acid-balanced or mild shampoo with a pH between 4.5 and 5.5, as suggested by the manufacturer. Avoid brushing or massaging, which may cause the scalp to become sensitive to the waving lotion.

Use **extreme care in rinsing** to make certain that all the shampoo is removed. Proper rinsing equalizes the porosity of the hair.

While the hair is still wet, carefully examine it for signs of a previous perm. Any hair that indicates it has recently received a wave could be in a weakened condition and should be treated with extreme caution to avoid hair damage. The hair should be treated gently and not wound with tension to avoid pulling and possibly causing breakage.

Shaping Suggestions for Permanent Wave

Shaping the hair may be done before or after a shampoo with a razor or scissors.

1. A **razor** may be used to blunt cut damp hair after a shampoo.
2. **Scissors** may be used on dry hair before a shampoo or on damp hair after the shampoo.
3. If the finished style is very short, your instructor may advise you to perform the cut after the permanent wave.

Shaping Precautions

The texture of the hair must be considered carefully in planning the shaping procedure.

Coarse or **medium hair.** Taper the hair ends sufficiently to form strong, resilient curls. Excessive tapering may make it difficult to wrap the hair or may cause the hair ends to frizz.

Fine, thin or **damaged limp hair** should be shaped with the scissors. Use a blunt cut or short taper. Excessive thinning or tapering will result in frizzy hair ends.

Length of hair. The hair should be long enough to wind around the rods at least two full half turns. Otherwise, there will be no wave pattern. If the desired hairstyle requires short hair, use small diameter rods. If necessary, trim the ends of the hair strands after the permanent is completed.

Slithering the hair prior to the permanent wave may cause some damage to the cuticle, resulting in a poor permanent wave.

To avoid a distorted wave formation, any thinning necessary should be done after the permanent wave is given.

CURLING RODS

Proper selection of curling rods is essential for successful permanent waving.

The size of the rods controls the curl of the hair during the waving process. There are several types of rods available. Most are made of wood or plastic and they each vary in diameter, length and design.

1. Diameter is the distance through the center of the rod.
2. Circumference is the distance around a rod. The circumference determines the size of the wave or curl formation.

Rods are available in various lengths: full, 3/4, 1/2 and short (3 1/2″ to 1 3/4″ [8.75 to 4.375 cm] in length).

They also come in varying thicknesses. These range in diameter size from large to very thin (3/4″ to 1/8″ [1.875 to .3125 cm]).

All rods must have some means of securing the hair on them in the desired position to prevent the curl from unwinding.

Types of Rods

There are two types of rods in general use: concave and straight.

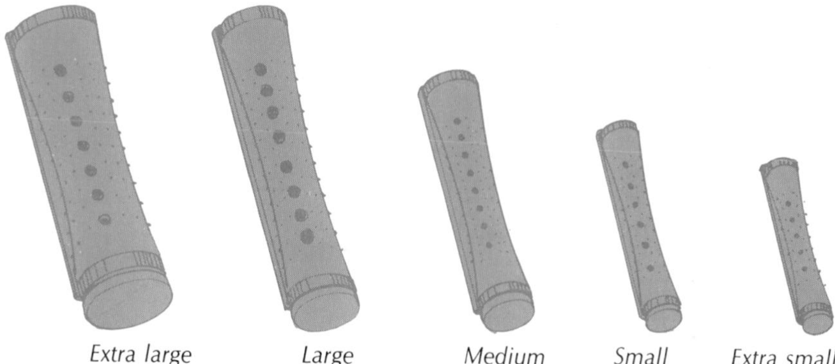

Concave rod

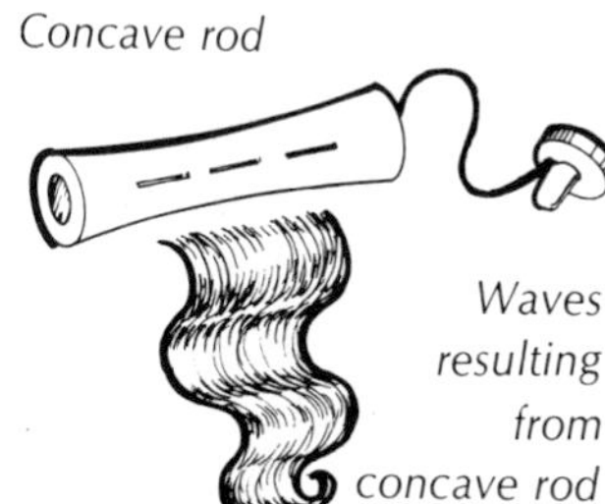

Straight rod

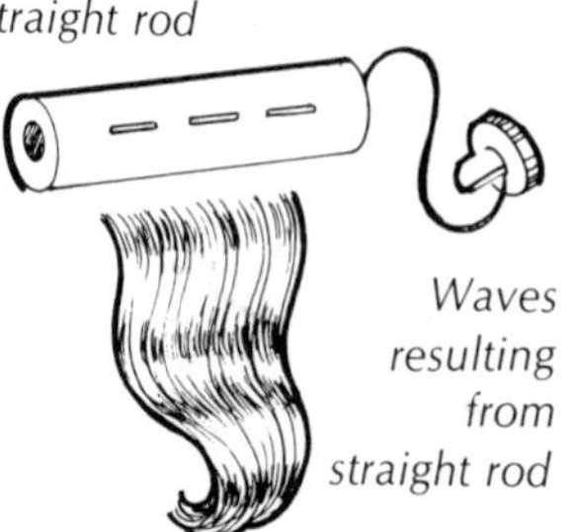

Concave rods are usually thinner in diameter than the straight rods. They have a smaller circumference in the center area, which gradually increases to a larger circumference at both ends. When hair is wound on a rod, the outside hair of the winding forms a larger curl or wave than the hair next to the rod. This creates a tighter curl or ringlet at the hair ends, which gradually becomes slightly wider as it nears the scalp. Because the end of each rod is larger in circumference the curl will be looser at the ends of each rod than in the center.

Straight rods are made so that their circumference and diameter are the same throughout their entire length.

This type of rod usually creates the same size curl throughout the entire hair strand and is used to imitate a natural curl.

Large, straight rods are usually used to give a body wave or style wave. They permit the formation of a permanent with a large enough wave to be dressed into any desired hairstyle.

CHEMICALS

For successful permanent waving, it is essential that the curling rods and lotion be selected properly.

Waving Lotions

Alkaline waving lotions have as their basic ingredient ammonium thioglycolate, commonly referred to as "thio," which permanently changes the structure of the hair. This compound is prepared by combining ammonia and thioglycolic acid. Other ingredients of the waving lotion may be lanolin or its derivatives, wetting agents, protein or other conditioners. Ammonia is added to make the solution alkaline.

Acid waving lotions also contain a thioglycolate base. However, their pH range is much lower, 4.5 to 6.5.

Pre-conditioning. Over-porous or damaged hair might require a preconditioning treatment before the application of waving lotion. Conditioners containing hydrolized protein that condition the hair and equalize its porosity are now available. Some fillers contain oils and moisturizers, which may help to protect the hair against the harshness of the cold waving lotion.

Conditioners. The alkaline cold waving lotion has a tendency to remove natural oils from the hair, causing it to dry out rapidly through loss of moisture. Essential oils, lanolin or lanolin derivatives are added to the waving lotion or can be used in a separate application to replace natural oils. By the conditioner remaining in the hair after the lotion has been rinsed out, the moisture content is somewhat preserved, and the feel and appearance of the hair are improved.

The **strength of the waving lotion** can be adjusted by either increasing its pH (alkalinity) or by increasing the amount of active ingredient (ammonium thioglycolate). To adjust the pH of the lotion, the ammonia content is either increased or decreased by the manufacturer, not to exceed pH 9.6, which is a strong solution.

Most manufacturers of cold waving products provide three or more strengths, such as:

1. **Damaged hair**—weak or mild strength.
2. **Normal hair** (having good porosity)—average strength.
3. **Resistant hair** (less porosity)—stronger strength.
4. **Over-lightened** or **tinted hair** (over-porous)—extra mild strength.

Note Manufacturers of cold waving products are constantly improving their formulas. It is advisable to follow their directions carefully.

Neutralizers

Neutralizers contain either hydrogen peroxide or sodium bromate. Lanolin, vitamins, oils, protein and other special ingredients can be added. They come in various forms, such as liquids, powders and crystals. Depending on the method of application, they may have a thick consistency and have to be diluted. Conditioners are often incorporated in the prepared liquid neutralizer to give some protection to the hair.

SECTIONING AND BLOCKING

Sectioning is dividing the head into uniform working panels.

Blocking, also known as **subsectioning,** is the subdividing of panels into uniform individual rectangular rod sections. Uniform wave patterns depend on:

1. Uniformly arranged sections.
2. Equally subdivided sections (blockings).
3. Clean and uniform parting (length and width).

The size of the blockings is determined by the diameter and length of the rods.

Depending on the pattern used in hair sectioning, the number of hair blockings can vary with each client.

The **average blocking** for a standard wave should match the diameter (size) of the rod being used. The length of the blocking can be the same as or a little shorter, but not longer, than the length of the rod.

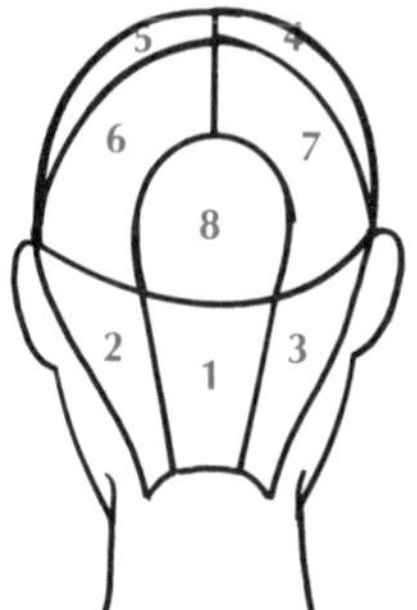

Sectioning

Blocking (sub-sections)

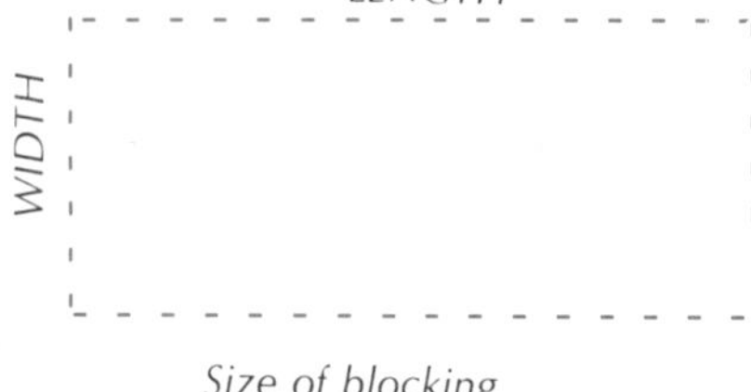

Size of blocking

LENGTH denotes span of blocking WIDTH refers to the depth of the blocking. Small or large blockings usually refer to its width.

Suggested Hair Blockings and Rod Sizes

Although hair elasticity and texture must both be considered in the choice of rods, the texture should be the determining factor.

Coarse hair—good elasticity. Thickly growing hair requires smaller (narrower) blockings and larger rods to permit better arrangements for a definite wave pattern.

Medium hair—average elasticity. Medium or average textured hair requires average blockings and medium size rods.

Fine hair—poor elasticity. Thin hair requires smaller blockings and smaller (thinner) rods to prevent strain or breakage and to form a good wave pattern close to the head.

Lightened or **tinted hair**—very poor elasticity. Use smaller hair subsections and larger rods. If the lightened or tinted hair is fine in texture, use smaller hair sub-sections and medium rods.

Hair in nape area. Use smaller subsections and smaller rods.

Long hair. To permanently wave hair longer than 6″ (15 cm), wrap it smooth and close to the scalp in smaller blockings. The use of smaller blockings permits the waving lotion and neutralizer to penetrate more easily and thoroughly.

If the hair is more than seven inches long use alternate methods of wrapping if an even wave pattern is desired.

PATTERNS FOR SECTIONING AND BLOCKING

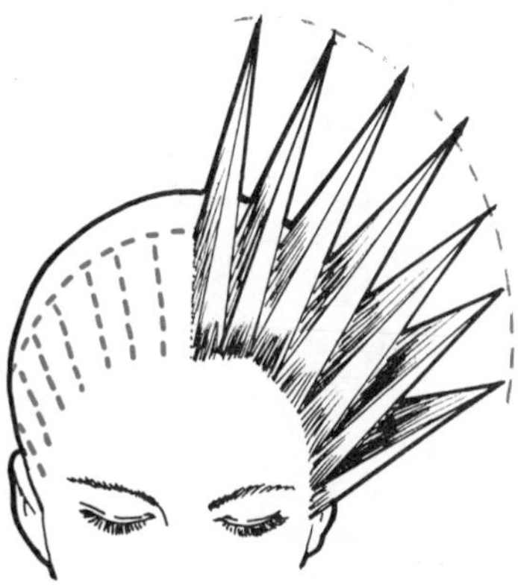

By knowing the texture, elasticity, porosity and condition of the client's hair, the cosmetologist is better able to judge how the hair is to be sectioned, blocked, which rods to use and at what part of the head the application of waving lotion should begin.

(Be guided by your instructor.)

The size of the rods and blockings determines the size of the curl or wave pattern. Processing time has no bearing on the size of the wave pattern.

Five popular blocking (subsectioning) patterns:

1. Single halo
2. Double halo (Double Horseshoe)
3. Straight back
4. Dropped crown
5. Natural hair movement wrap

These are known by other names in various areas of the country.

The following patterns are suggested blockings. However, your instructor might suggest different patterns, which are equally correct.

Single Halo The **single halo** wrap is commonly used for average size heads.

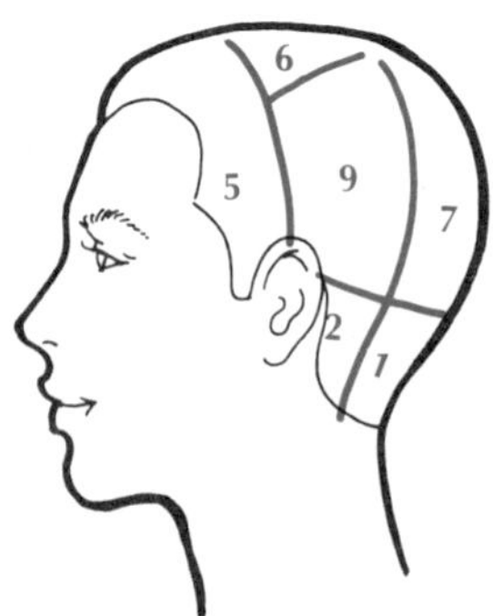

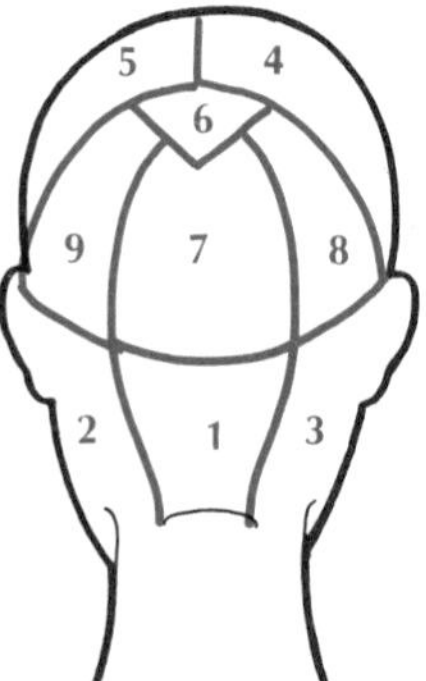

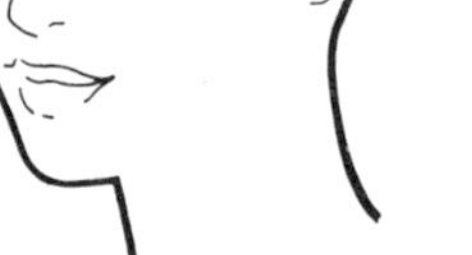

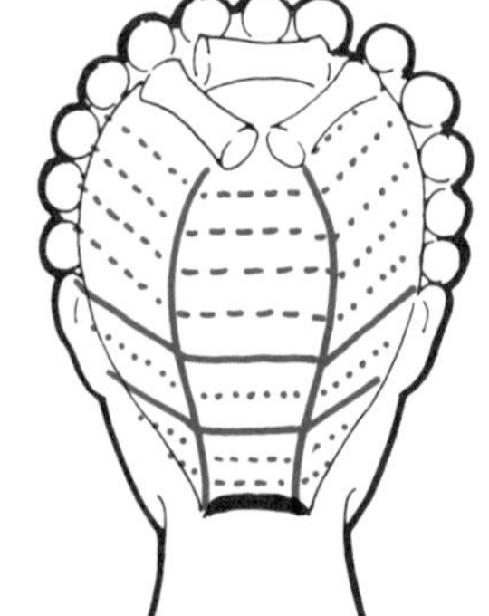

Sectioning diagram

Blocking (sub-sectioning) pattern

Double Halo The **double halo** wrap is usually used for larger size heads.

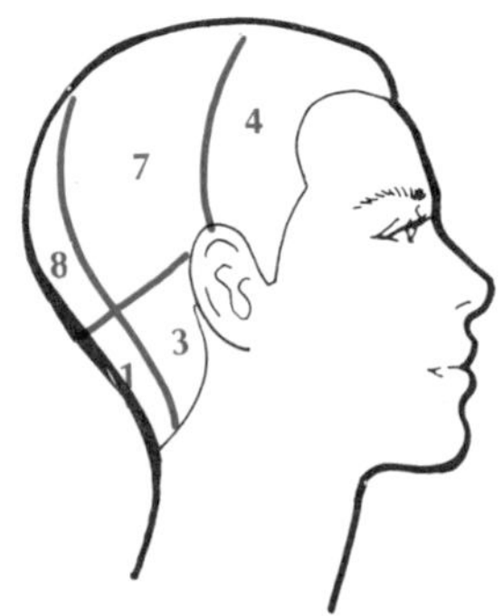

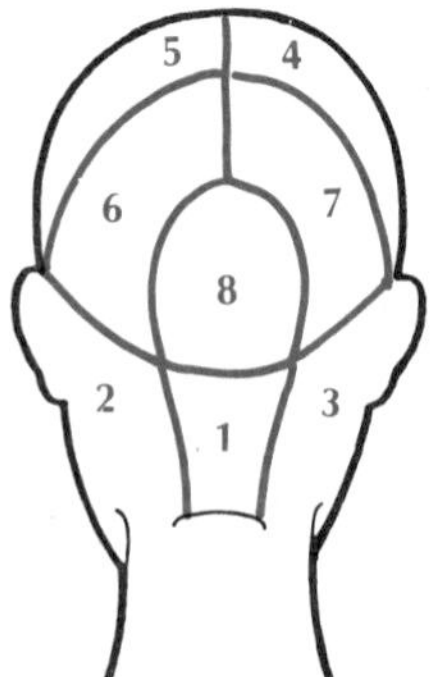

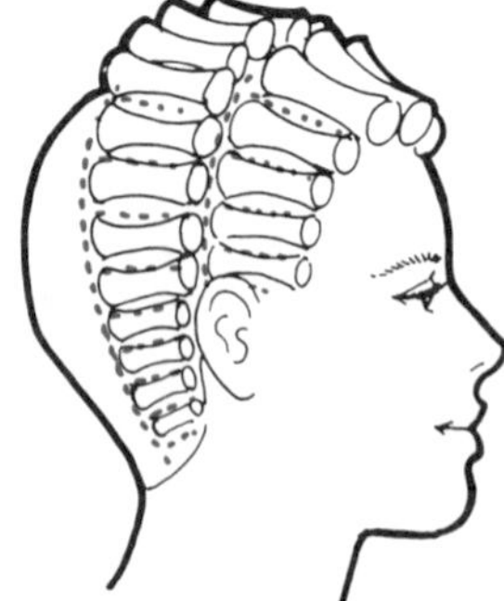

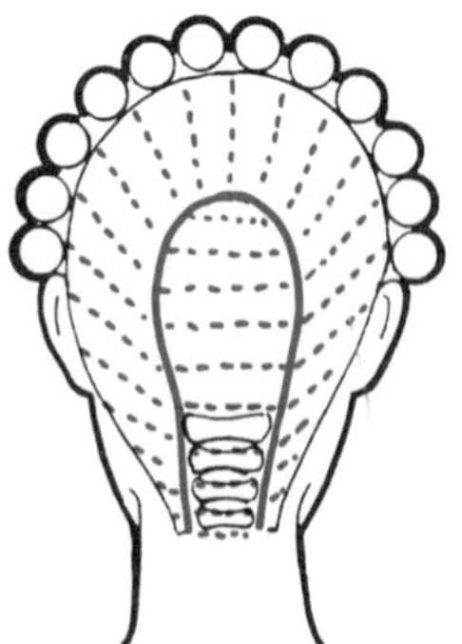

Sectioning diagram

Blocking (sub-sectioning) pattern

Straight Back The **straight back** wrap is used to create a rather soft, full and high style effect, directed off the face.

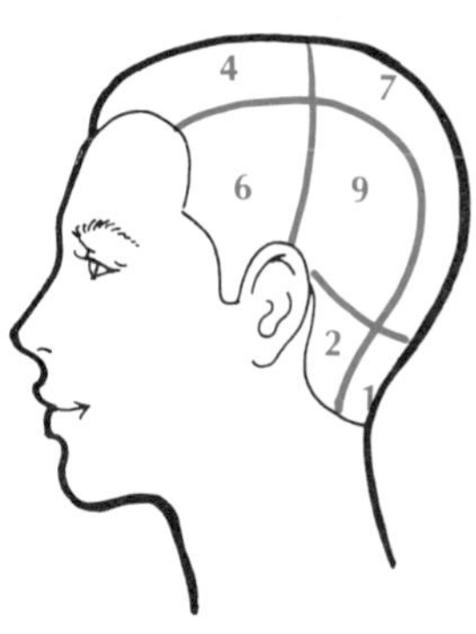

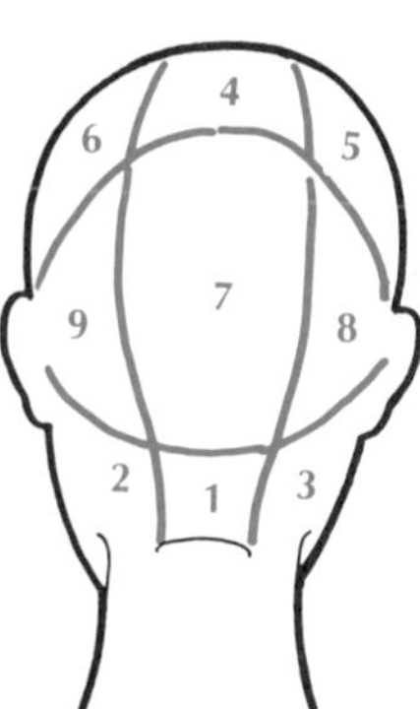

Sectioning diagram

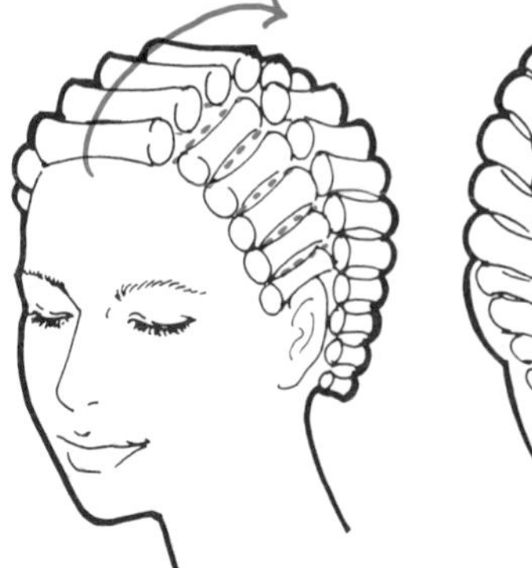

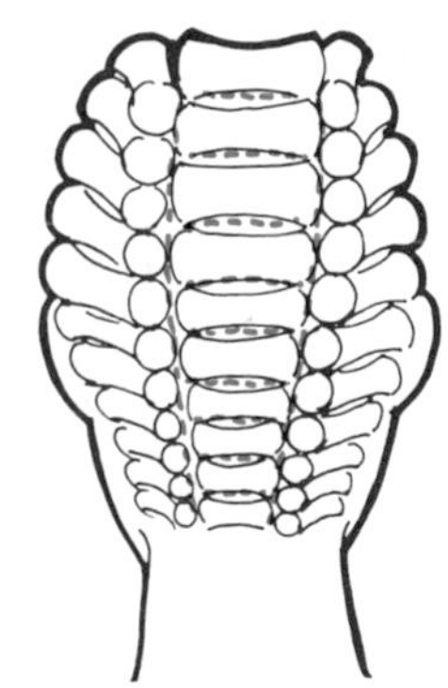

Blocking (sub-sectioning) pattern

Bangs To create bangs on the forehead, the first two top front curls are wrapped in a forward direction.

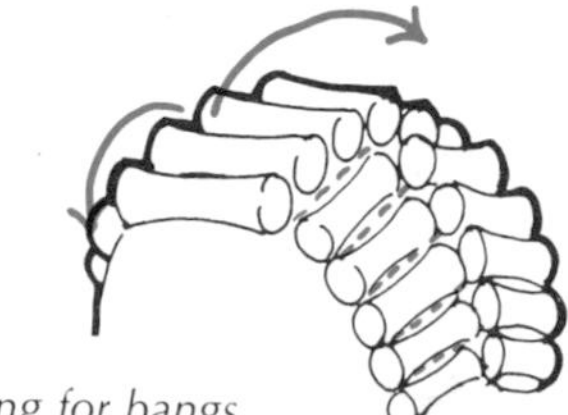

Setting for bangs

Dropped Crown The **dropped crown** wrap is usually used for longer hair and a smooth crown effect.

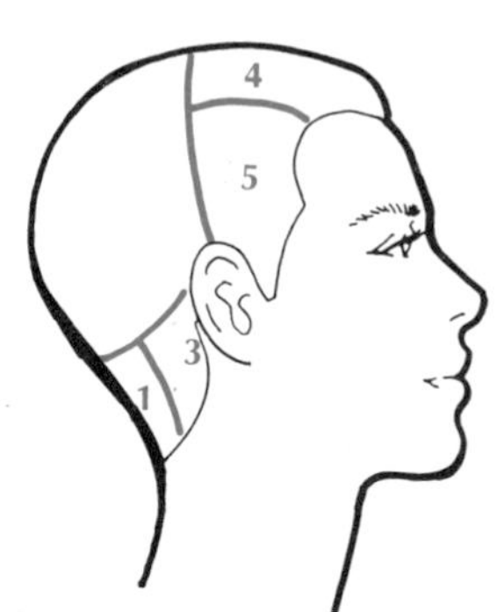

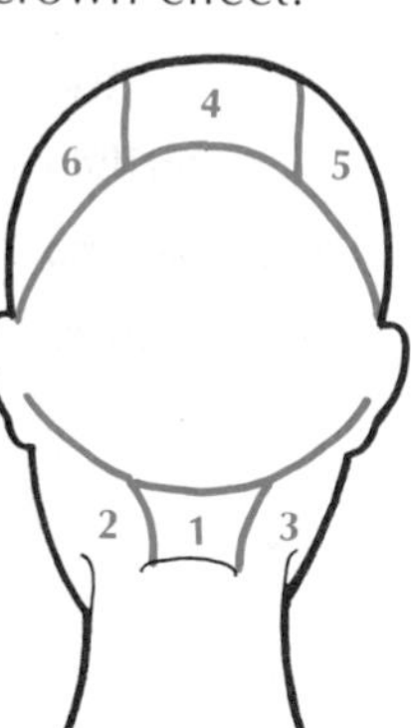

Sectioning diagram

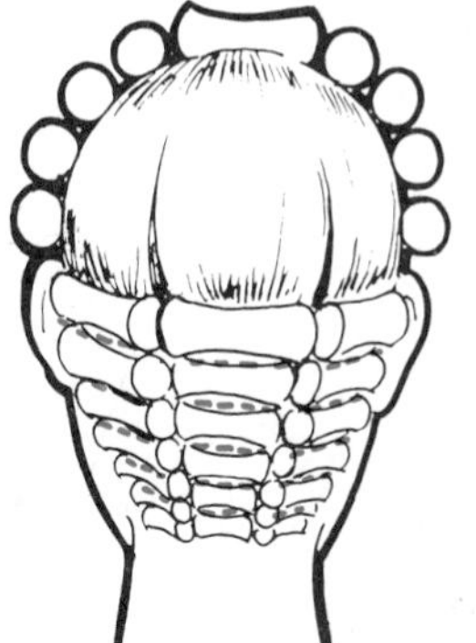

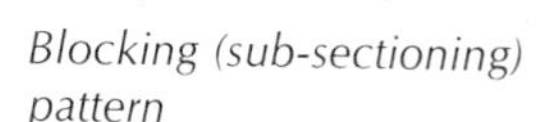

Blocking (sub-sectioning) pattern

Wrapping hair ends of crown area

The hair is sectioned in the same way as for the straight back pattern. However, in the back area that is not numbered, larger hair sections are made, depending on the amount of hair. Only the hair ends are wrapped on larger curling rods, with the rods resting on the smaller rods in the nape area. (Be guided by your instructor.)

Natural Hair Movement Wrap This wrap begins in the crown and continues roller placement in the natural fall or movement of the hair.

Body Waves A body wave is given with extra large straight rods, solely for the purpose of adding slight body or a shallow wave pattern to the hair.

WINDING OR WRAPPING THE HAIR

To form a uniform wave with a strong ridge, wrap the hair smoothly and neatly on each rod without stretching. Hair is not stretched because the penetration of waving lotion causes it to expand. Tight wrapping or stretching interferes with this expansion and prevents penetration of the waving lotion and neutralizer, which can cause hair breakage.

Strand Relation to the Head

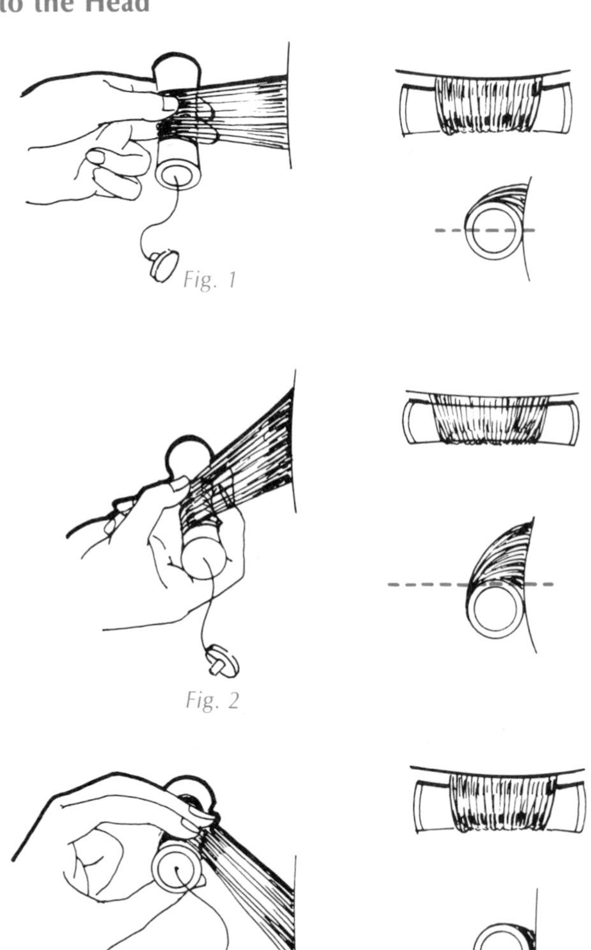
Fig. 1
Fig. 2
Fig. 3

Curl one-half off base. When the strand is held straight out from the head and wound on a curling rod, the curl will rest one-half off base (fig. 1).

The rod rolled in this manner will rest on the base of the rod below it. The weight of the resting rod produces a wave, creating close-to-the-head waves.

Curl off base. When the strand is held in a semi-downward position and wound on a curling rod, the curl will rest off base (fig. 2).

Hair wound in this manner will produce a wave that is closest to the head because the rod above will create an indented wave. The curl will lie close to the scalp, producing close-to-the-head hairstyles.

Curl on base. When the strand is held in a semi-upward position and wound on a curling rod, the curl will rest on base (fig. 3).

Hair wound in this manner will produce waves that are lifted from the head. This is good for coarse textured hair or for hairstyles that require fullness, height and upward movement.

End Papers

Porous end papers are very important aids in the proper wrapping or winding of the hair around rods. Properly used end papers help in the formation of smooth and even curls and waves. They help eliminate the possibility of "fishhooks" and minimize the danger of further damage to the hair ends. They are especially important in controlling the ends while wrapping uneven hair lengths.

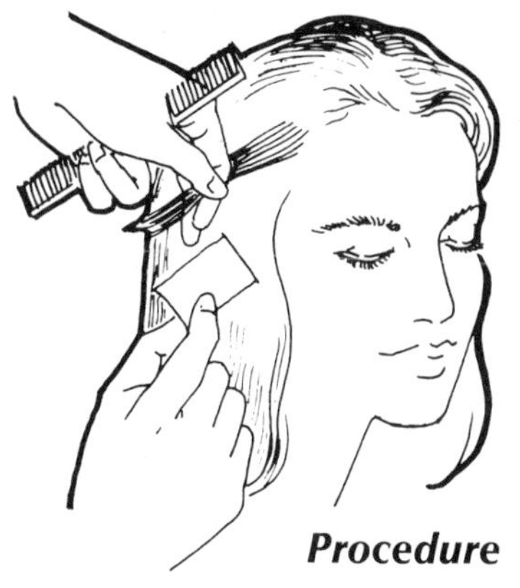

There are three methods of end paper application in general use in permanent waving. The method chosen depends upon the rod type selected and desired results.

1. Double end paper wrap.
2. Single end paper wrap.
3. Book end paper wrap.

Double End Paper Wrap. Depending upon the condition of the hair, wrap with water, pre-wrap solution or processing lotion. Water should be used instead of waving lotion while practicing, until you are proficient in the technique of winding or wrapping the hair.

Procedure A step-by-step procedure for wrapping and fastening an off-base curl is illustrated, using the double end paper wrap method.

Note The blocking (subsection) should not be longer than the length of the rod. If it is, the hair will not wave evenly.

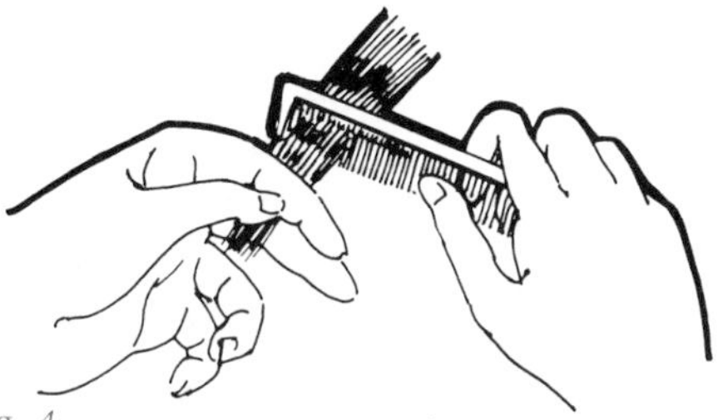

Fig. 4

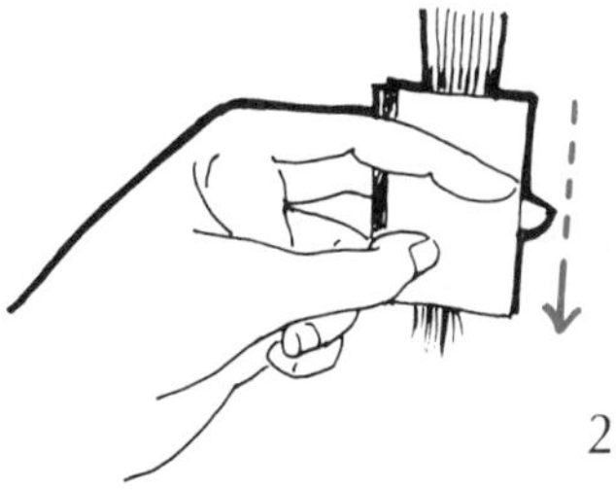

Fig. 5

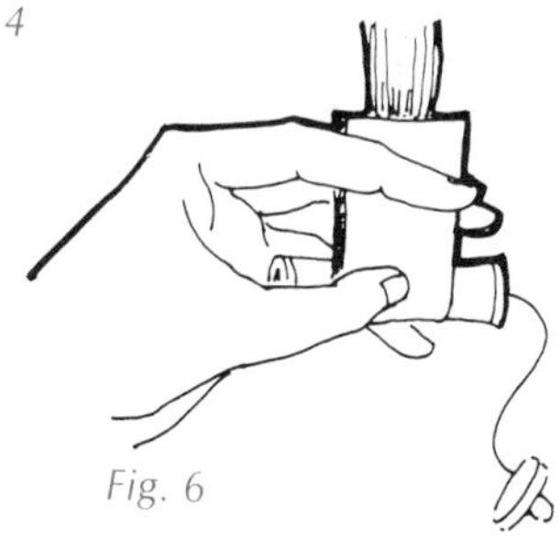

Fig. 6

Fig. 7

1. Part and comb the sub-section until all hair is evenly directed and distributed. Hair should be spread evenly along the length of the rod and the last combing should be on top of the strand with the hair held at a 45° angle (fig. 4).
2. Place one end paper beneath the hair strand and another on top (fig. 5).
3. With the right hand, place the rod under the double end papers, parallel with the hair part. Draw both toward the hair ends (fig. 6).
4. Wind the strand smoothly on the rod to the scalp without stretching (fig. 7).

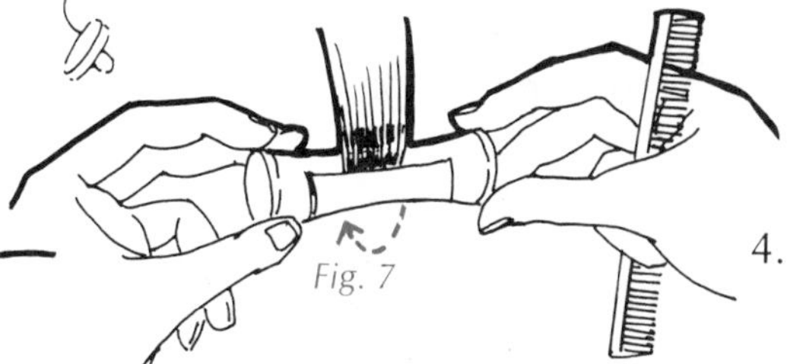

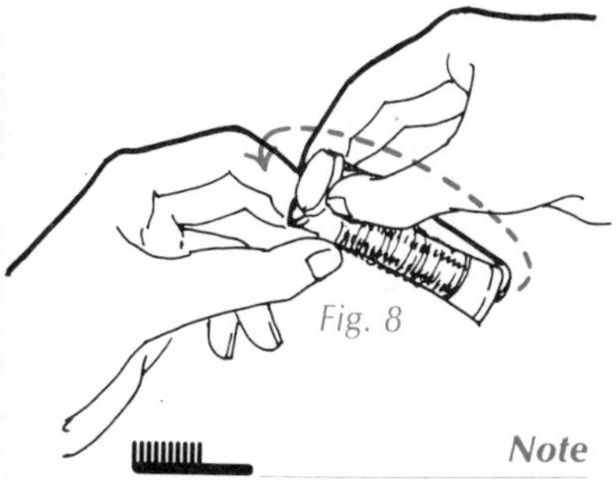

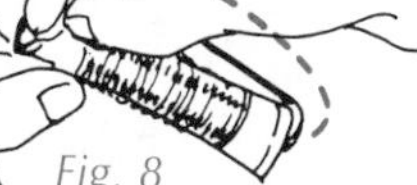

Fig. 8

5. Fasten the band across the top of the rod so as not to have the band resting on the hair nearest to the scalp. This will avoid excess tension (fig. 8).

Note To prevent breakage, the band should not cut into the hair or be twisted against the curl.

Caution: The hair should be wound evenly, much like thread on a spool. Unevenly wrapped hair will not absorb lotion properly, resulting in an undesirable wave.

Other End Paper Wraps

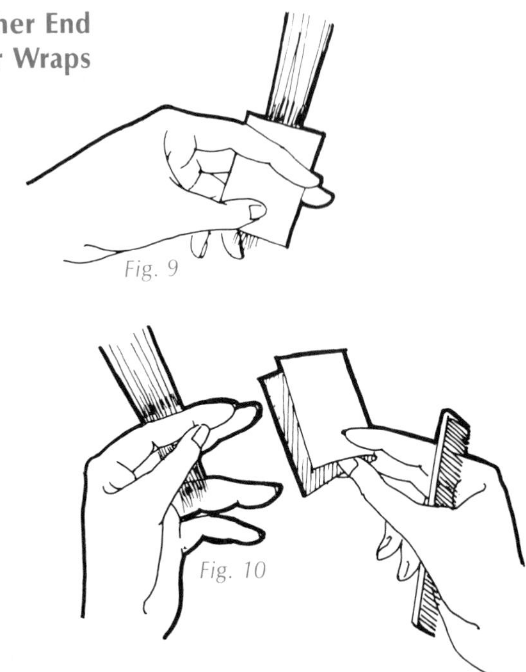

Fig. 9

Fig. 10

The preparation and winding of curls for a single end paper wrap and the book end paper wrap are the same, with the following exceptions:

Single end paper wrap. Place one end of the paper on top and hold it flat between the index and middle fingers to prevent bunching (fig. 9). The hair is wound in the same manner as the double end paper wrap (figs. 6,7, and 8).

Book end wrap. Hold the strand between the middle and index fingers; fold and place the end paper over the strand, forming an envelope (figs. 9 and 10). The winding of the curl is done as in the double-end paper wrap.

Piggyback Wrap

The piggyback method of wrapping is especially suitable for extra long hair. This wrapping technique permits maximum control of the size and tightness of the curl from the scalp to the hair ends. Control of the amount of curl can be exercised by the size of the rods selected. Thus, the use of larger rods will result in a loose, wide wave; small, or medium rods, will give tighter curls. The following is the procedure for wrapping in the piggyback method.

1. Section the head in the usual manner.
2. Select rods of the desired size. To create an equal wave pattern, both rods are the same size; for a tighter curl at the hair ends, use smaller rods.

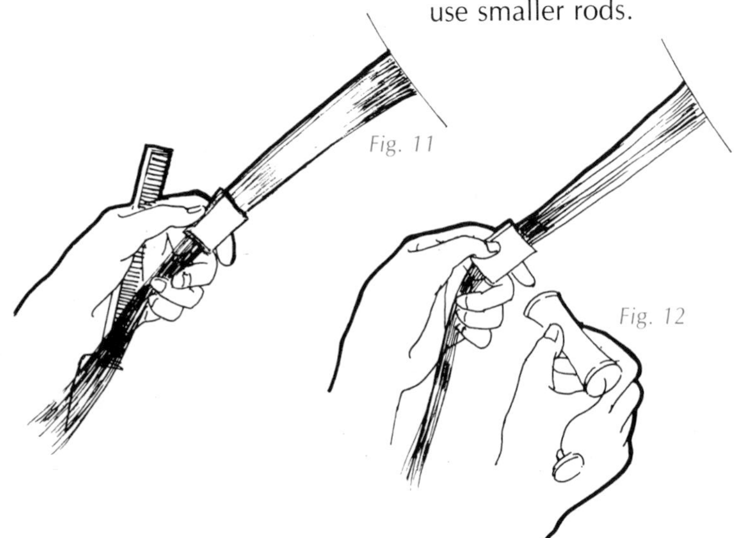

Fig. 11

Fig. 12

3. About halfway up the strand, place porous end papers one on top and one underneath (fig. 11).
4. Start at the midpoint part of the strand. Place the larger rod underneath the hair strand and start wrapping (fig. 12).
5. Roll the rod toward the scalp and, at the same time, control the hair ends by holding them to the side, away from the rod.

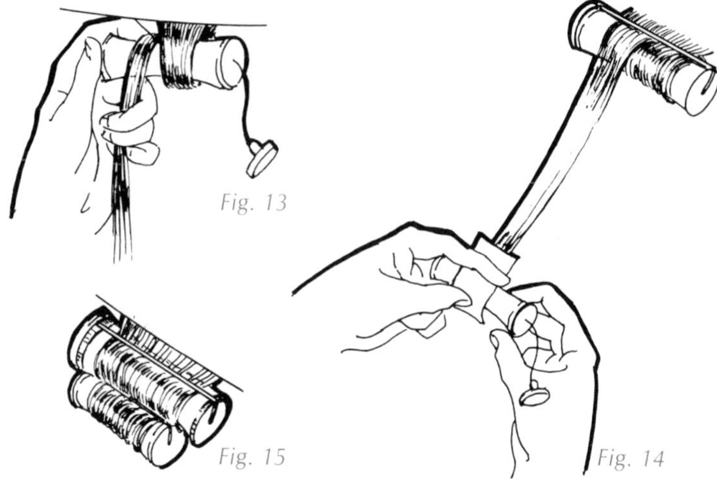

Fig. 13

Fig. 15

Fig. 14

6. Secure the wrapped rod at the scalp, leaving the hair ends (fig. 13).
7. Wrap the hair ends. Place an end paper on the hair strand covering the ends. Using the desired rod size, wrap the hair ends down and under until hair is rolled (fig. 14).
8. Secure the second rod to rest against the first one in a piggyback fashion (fig. 15).
9. To maintain better control over the wrapping and processing, it is advisable to complete the wrapping of each hair strand before proceeding to the next one.
10. Test curls should be taken from the rods at the end because the hair in this area is more resistant since it receives little natural body heat and might require additional processing time.

TEST CURLS

Test curls help to determine in advance how the client's hair will react to the chemical waving process. A test curl gives the cosmetologist information on how to protect the client's hair and how to obtain the best possible results.

Testing enables the cosmetologist to observe the reaction of hair as to:

1. Speed of wave formation.
2. Overall picture of wave formation.
3. Exact time when peak of wave formation has been reached.
4. Resistant waves.

Test curls may be given before or while waving the entire head.

Pre-Permanent Test Curl Method

Pre-permanent test curls should be given if the hair presents any problem, such as damage, poor porosity or poor elasticity. If the client has an illness or if there is any doubt in the cosmetologist's mind concerning the final results, pre-test curls are important.

Procedure

After the hair has been shampooed and towel dried, wrap two or three curls on the upper back of the head. Each curl is given a complete treatment with a different strength waving lotion. The action of the lotion is timed and the curl is examined according to the manufacturer's directions. After neutralizing and rinsing the curls, judge and record the results.

Test Curl-Wave Development Method

This procedure is part of the processing phase of a chemical wave. Each head of hair is different. Conditions also vary on different parts of the head. A client's hair will not always process in the same length of time for each curl. Wave development should be tested:

1. Immediately after the last rod is secured, if wrapping with lotion.
2. Immediately after saturating all rods with lotion.
3. Every three to five minutes until wave formation has occurred. Frequent testing for wave formation will prevent over-processing. Although the manufacturer's directions supply a general guide, the cosmetologist should carefully judge individual curl development.

Procedure

1. Thoroughly blot the waving solution from the curl to be tested.
2. Loosen the rod fastener. (Do not let the hair become loose or unravel on the rod. Hold it firmly with the thumbs touching on the rod.)
3. Unwind the rod 1 1/2 turns, without pulling on the strand. Since the hair is in a softened condition, pulling or stretching it will spoil the test. Permit the hair to relax into a firm "S" wave pattern.
4. Rewind the test curl.

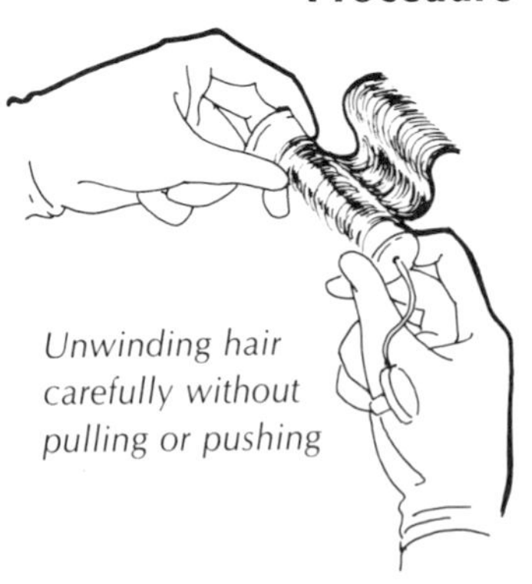

Unwinding hair carefully without pulling or pushing

Continue testing form wave development at regular intervals until the desired wave pattern has been reached. Test on different areas of the head each time. **Do not use the same curl for retesting.**

Safety Precautions

Safety precautions protect the skin and scalp against chemical injury.

1. The cosmetologist must wear protective gloves.
2. For the client's safety, apply protective cream around the hairline, over the ears and across the napeline. Cover with a strip of cotton or neutralizing band before saturating with lotion.
3. If cotton strips or bands become wet with lotion, remove, blot and replace with dry material.
4. If the lotion drips on the skin or scalp, absorb with cotton pledgets saturated with cold water or neutralizer.
5. If the client wears contact lenses, ask that they be removed to avoid damage from lotion.

APPLICATION OF WAVING LOTION

A **plastic bottle** with a nozzle top is the most efficient applicator. It dispenses liquid freely, yet permits good control. There is a minimum loss of lotion. A better distribution is achieved throughout the hair.

Note

Bottles should be absolutely clean before being filled with waving lotion. Be certain that there are no traces of leftover chemicals in the bottle, because they can weaken or spoil the waving lotion.

Protect the client's eyes. If the waving lotion gets into the eyes, rinse immediately with cold water or a preparation recommended by your instructor, then take the client to a doctor. Have the client remove contact lenses before perming.

Applying the Waving Lotion

Pre-wrap wetting or moistening. Following shampooing and towel drying, if required by manufacturer, the hair should be moistened with a weak solution of the waving lotion to facilitate the wrapping procedure. The lotion is applied with a bottle applicator to an entire section at a time. Start about 1/2″ (1.25 cm) from the scalp and extend the lotion to within 1″ (2.5 cm) from the hair ends.

To assure a complete and even distribution, apply the lotion on the top of the section and comb through each section.

Rewetting or saturation. After sub-sectioning and winding the curls over the entire head, the hair is ready for complete saturation. This procedure is important and essential to assure complete penetration and processing of the entire hair shaft.

The lotion is thoroughly applied to each curl, following the same order as that used in the pre-wetting step. It is most important to the success of the permanent that each curl be thoroughly and completely saturated.

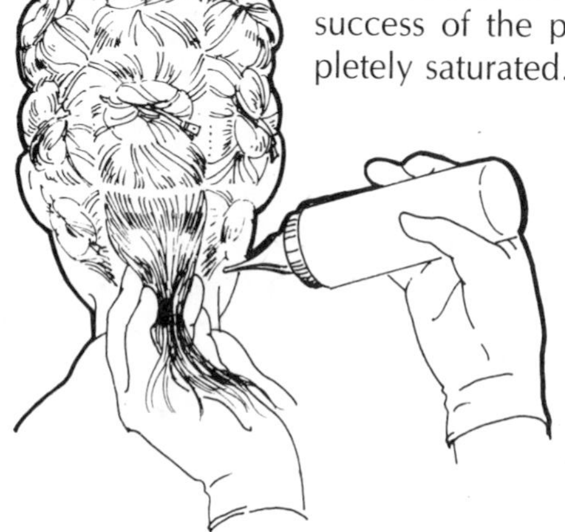

Applying lotion 1/2″ from scalp to about 1″ from the hair ends

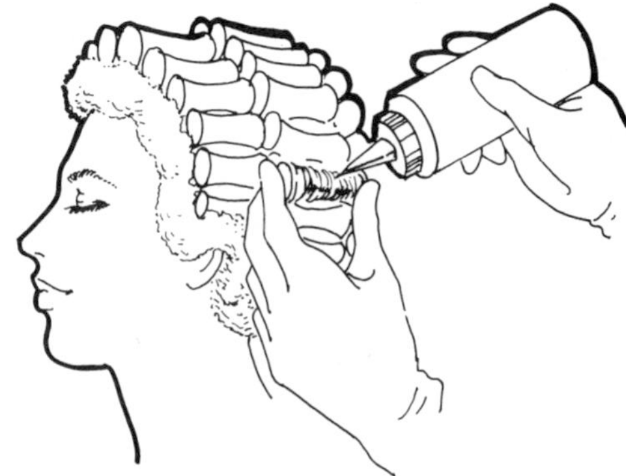

Rewetting or second application of waving lotion

Note Be careful not to disturb the wrapping or the placement of the curls by dragging the nozzle over the hair. Do not leave the client alone while the hair is processing. Do not interrupt the rewet or saturation step. Complete it as quickly as possible.

Processing Time

Processing time is the length of time required for the hair strands to absorb the waving lotion and complete the breaking of the chemical bonds in the hair around the rod. The ability of the hair to absorb moisture may vary from time to time on the same individual, even when the same lotions and procedures are used. A record of the previous processing time is desirable but should be used only as a guide. It is usually safe to anticipate the processing time to be less than that suggested by the manufacturer or a client's previous record card.

The factors affecting processing time are the strength of the lotion, texture, porosity, length and condition of the hair, atmospheric conditions, client's body heat and the working speed of the cosmetologist.

Resaturation step during the processing time. Often, it is necessary to blot and lightly resaturate all the rods a second time during the processing time. This may be due to:

1. Evaporation of the lotion or dryness of the hair
2. Hair poorly saturated by the cosmetologist
3. No wave development after 10 to 12 minutes with an alkaline perm solution
4. Improper selection of solution strength for the client's hair
5. Failure to follow the manufacturer's directions for a specific formula

A reapplication of the lotion will speed processing. Watch the wave development closely, since **negligence can result in hair damage.**

Wave Pattern Formation

The time required to attain the proper depth of the "S" pattern governs the processing time. As the hair is processing, the wave has reached its peak when it forms a well-defined letter "S." The size of the rod used determines the size of the "S" pattern.

The "S" pattern reaches a desirable peak only once. Shortly after the "S" is well formed, the hair becomes **over-processed** and **damaged.**

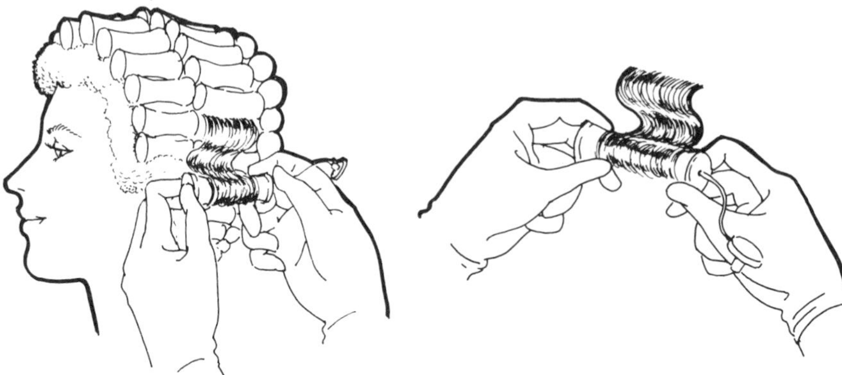

Unwinding hair without pulling or stretching

Processed strand opens up into "S" formation. Rewind the hair carefully.

Different conditions and textures of the hair will form different qualities of wave patterns. Hair of good texture will show a firm, strong pattern, whereas hair that is weak or fine will not produce a well defined "S" pattern. This hair might need the spiral techniques; be guided by your instructor.

Over-Processing

Any lotion that can properly process the hair also can over-process it. Lotion left on the hair too long, beyond the best wave formation point, results in over-processing. Another cause of over-processing is when test curls are not made frequently enough or are improperly judged.

Over-processed hair is easily detected. It is very curly when wet, completely frizzy when dry and refuses to be combed into a suitable wave pattern. The elasticity of the hair has been excessively damaged, and the hair is unable to contract into the wave formation. If the hair feels harsh after being dried the neutralizer might have been left on too long causing the hair to become brittle and too hard.

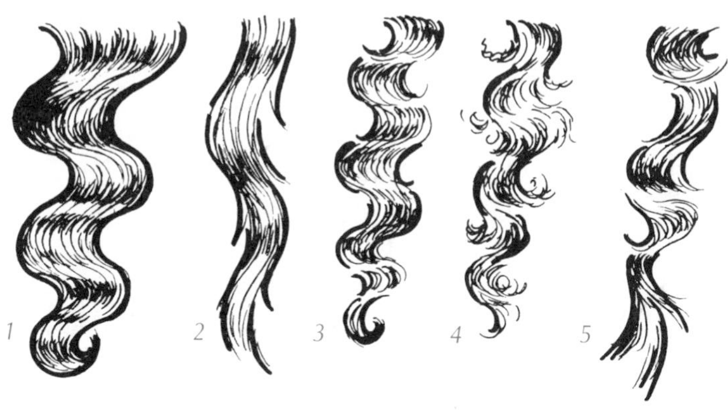

1. A good permanent wave looks like this.

2. Under-processed curl. RESULT: Little or no wave.

3. Over-processed curl. RESULT: Narrow waves when wet, no waves when dry.

4. Porous ends over-processed. RESULT: Frizzy ends.

5. Improper winding; hair ends are wound too tight. RESULT: No wave or curl at the hair ends.

Under-Processing

Under-processing results in a limp, weak wave formation or none at all. The ridges are not well defined and the hair retains little or no wave formation. Under-processed hair should first be given reconditioning treatments. After these treatments, rewrap the hair and apply a milder waving lotion, since the hair has already received some softening. Watch the wave formation closely.

NEUTRALIZATION

The waving lotion produces the curl formation by breaking the disulfide bonds in the cortex into the new alignment. The rods hold the hair in this formation until the bonds are oxidized by neutralization. The neutralizer stops the action of the waving lotion and reforms the chemical bonds.

Preparation

Most manufacturers require thorough rinsing with warm water to remove the waving lotion, followed by careful towel blotting of each curl to remove excess moisture prior to the application of the neutralizer.

To obtain the best results from towel blotting, carefully press the towel with the fingers between each curl. Do not rock or roll the rods while blotting. The hair is in a softened state, any such movement can cause hair breakage.

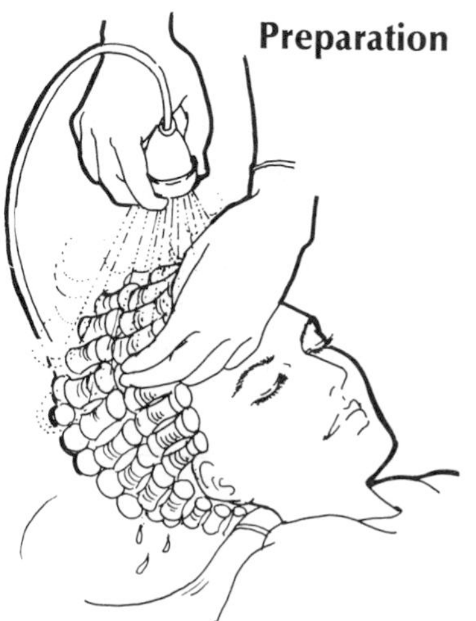

Rinsing waving lotion from the hair

Towel blotting

Method of Neutralization

Neutralizers are packaged in the form of powders, liquids or crystals and must be prepared and applied as directed by the manufacturer immediately before their use.

There are two methods of neutralizer application in general use: Direct or On-the-Rod Method and the Splash-On Method.

Direct or **On-the-Rod Method** (also referred to as the **applicator** or **instant method**) is available in two forms: ready for use and to be prepared.

1. **Ready for use neutralizer:** cut off the tip of the applicator bottle and apply.
2. **Neutralizer to be prepared:** mix it according to the manufacturer's directions, pour into the applicator bottle and apply.

Direct (on-the rod method). Apply neutralizer directly to each curl in the same order as that followed in the application of the waving lotion. Start in the top center of the curl and apply in either direction, then apply at the bottom of the curl, making sure that each curl is thoroughly saturated. Repeat if necessary.

Removing Neutralizer

There are two general methods for removing neutralizers from the hair. (Manufacturer's directions must be followed at all times.)

Method 1. After the neutralizer is thoroughly applied, allow it to remain in the hair according to the manufacturer's directions. Rinse with tepid water followed by a cool water rinse to begin closing the cuticle. Lightly towel blot the hair. Remove the rods carefully and proceed to style the hair.

Method 2. After the neutralizer is thoroughly applied, time according to the manufacturer's directions. Carefully remove the rods without stretching the hair and apply the balance of the neutralizer to the hair ends. Permit an additional minute of neutralizing time, then rinse with cool water. Proceed to style the hair.

Note

It is important that the neutralizing be carefully completed because this step is very important for a successful permanent wave. The hair must be thoroughly and correctly neutralized to rebond it in the curly configuration. Great care must be given to the neutralizer timing because under-neutralization will result in relaxed or no curl and over-neutralization will result in dry, damaged and discolored hair.

COLD WAVING (Alkaline)

Important points to consider when analyzing a client's hair prior to giving a permanent wave are:

1. Strength of waving lotion
2. Proper size rods
3. Blocking and winding the hair
4. Test curls
5. Processing time
6. Neutralization

There are different methods of giving a cold wave. The suggested outline in this section is one of several ways that can be used. However, it can be changed to meet the requirements of your instructor or the manufacturer.

Implements and Materials

Applicators	PW Rods	Combs
Porous end papers	Protective cream	Plastic clips
Cold waving lotion	Cotton or neutralizing bands	Protective gloves
Scissors or razor	Mild shampoo	Record card
Neutralizer	Neck strips and towels	Cotton
Neutralizing bib (opt.)	Acidifying rinse	
Shampoo cape		

Preparation

1. Select and arrange the required materials.
2. Wash and sanitize the hands.
3. Seat the client comfortably. Remove jewelry; adjust towel and shampoo cape.
4. Remove any hairpins and combs from the client's hair.
5. Carefully examine the condition of the scalp and hair. (Check for scalp abrasion.)
6. Seat the client comfortably at the shampoo bowl.

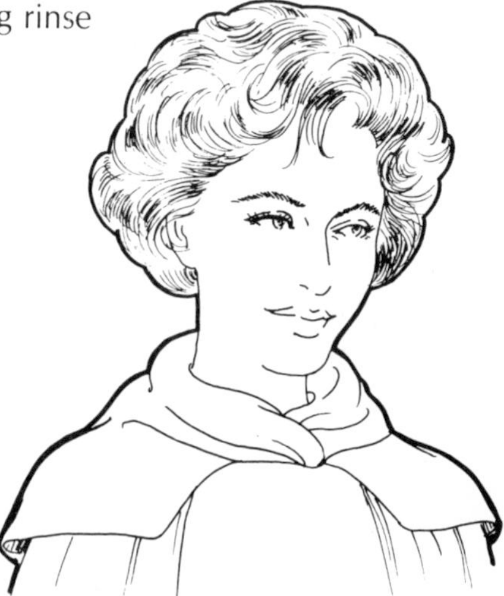

Draping for permanent waving

Draping the Client

There are several ways in which a client may be draped for a cold wave. The comfort of the client, adequate protection of the skin and clothing are important during the entire procedure. One way to drape a client is to place a small folded towel around the neck, fasten the shampoo cape over it and place another towel over the cape. Fasten the towel securely. (Your instructor might recommend another method which is equally correct.)

Note

It is important for the student to remember that there are many correct ways to give a permanent wave. The method recommended in this section is merely one suggested way. Always be guided by your instructor or follow the manufacturer's directions.

Procedure

1. Shape the hair before or after shampoo, as preferred.
2. Shampoo the hair lightly, rinse thoroughly and towel dry.
3. If wrapping is to be done after the application of the cold waving lotion, apply protective cream and cotton strips around the client's hairline and neck. Wear protective gloves or apply protective cream.

If wrapping is to be done with water or after conditioner, no protective cream or gloves are necessary. However, you must **apply protective cream and wear protective gloves before you apply cold waving lotion to the wrapped rods.**

4. Section the hair. Subdivide (block) section and wrap.
5. Apply cold waving lotion as recommended by the manufacturer.
6. **Test curl immediately** after saturating the hair with cold waving lotion. Take frequent test curls on different areas of the head.
7. Process the hair for the required time. If rewetting the curls is necessary, blot the rods and apply the lotion in the same order originally followed. Protect the client with fresh cotton strips around the hairline and neck whenever the cotton becomes dampened by lotion.
8. Remove waving lotion by blotting or rinsing according to the manufacturer's directions.
9. Blot excess moisture from the hair wound on rods. Do not rock or roll the rods while blotting. Because the hair is in a softened state, any movement can cause hair breakage.
10. Thoroughly apply neutralizer and time as directed to re-form the sulfur bonds.
11. Rinse with tepid water, followed by a cool water rinse. Lightly towel blot.
12. Unwind and remove the rods carefully.
13. Apply the neutralizer again if required.
14. Rinse the hair again, with cool water, if required. Apply the finishing rinse, then rinse.
15. Apply a normalizing rinse to begin closing the cuticle and to return the hair to its normal acid state.
16. Towel dry and style the hair.

Important Reminders

A normalizing or acid rinse applied after the permanent wave will protect the curl and facilitate the styling of the hair. If the manufacturer has included a special rinse with the product, its use will prevent excessive stretching while combing and will counteract any alkaline residue. If used, setting lotion should be of a light consistency. **Avoid excess tension in styling the hair.**

Caution

Do not use excess heat when drying the hair. When handling soft, fine, limp or damaged hair, it is very important to use as little tension as possible.

Cleanup

1. Discard used supplies
2. Cleanse and sanitize implements
3. Wash and sanitize hands
4. Complete the perm record card

BODY (PERMANENT) WAVING

A body (permanent) wave gives the hair softer, wider waves. It is given when a strong curl or wave effect is not desired.

A body wave gives a holding action to the hairstyle and permits the style to last longer from one shampoo to another.

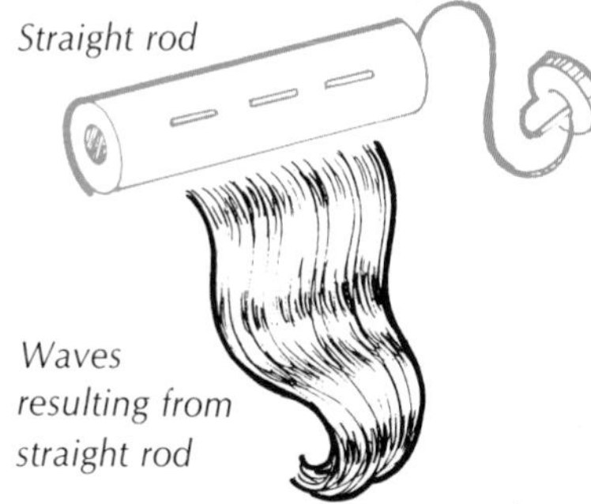

Curling rods. For a body (permanent) wave, use straight rods to give uniform curl formation over the entire strand.

Processing and Neutralizing

Processing and neutralizing closely follow the procedure for a conventional cold wave.

Each manufacturer has its own formula; therefore, it is important to follow instructions exactly.

Advantages

The body (permanent) wave has a number of advantages:

1. The large rods make it possible to produce natural looking waves.
2. The waves created are wide and long lasting.
3. The set or style holds for a longer period of time.
4. It adds body, resilience and manageability to the hair ends. This gives the hair adaptability to many styles and styling techniques.
5. The strong, wide waves relax very slowly and, therefore, the body wave lasts a long time.

HEAT PERMANENT WAVING

Neutral and Acid-Balanced Lotions

Neutral permanent waving products have a pH range of 7.0 to 7.9. Acid-balanced permanent waving products have a pH range of 4.5 to 6.5.

Advantages

1. There is no harsh alkali to damage the hair or skin.
2. There is no swelling of the hair, minimizing damage and breakage.
3. Most of these waving lotions are activated only when heat is applied, thus giving the cosmetologist greater control.
4. No ammonia is used and, therefore, no color is removed from tinted hair.
5. Since no ammonia is used, there is no offensive odor.
6. Since there is greater control, there is less possibility of overprocessing.
7. Soft and natural-looking waves are produced.

Disadvantages

1. Curls are not as tight as in the conventional thio (alkaline) wave.
2. Curls tend to relax sooner than with the cold thio (alkaline) wave.
3. Due to the pH range of these lotions, they are slow to penetrate into the cortex, thus increasing processing time. To overcome this, heat is usually applied.

Objectives of Heat Application

1. To speed up the penetration of the neutral or acid-balanced lotion into the cortex.
2. To increase the processing rate of the lotion within the hair.

Methods of Applying Heat

Manufacturers have developed a number for methods of applying the necessary heat to the hair.

1. Pre-heated hair dryer method
2. Heated clamp method
3. Thermal cap method
4. Chemical heat method
5. Self-heating method

Pre-Heated Hair Dryer Method

The pre-heated hair dryer method is very similar to the heated clamp method. The major difference is in the technique used to apply heat.

The hair is saturated with the permanent wave lotion and wound on rods. The hair is then covered with a thin plastic cap to concentrate the heat and to prevent heat loss. The client is then placed under a pre-heated dryer. Processing begins as soon as the heat is applied.

When the required length of time has elapsed, the plastic cap is removed and the hair rinsed and neutralized in the usual manner.

The pre-heated dryer method has the same three control features as found in the heated clamp method.

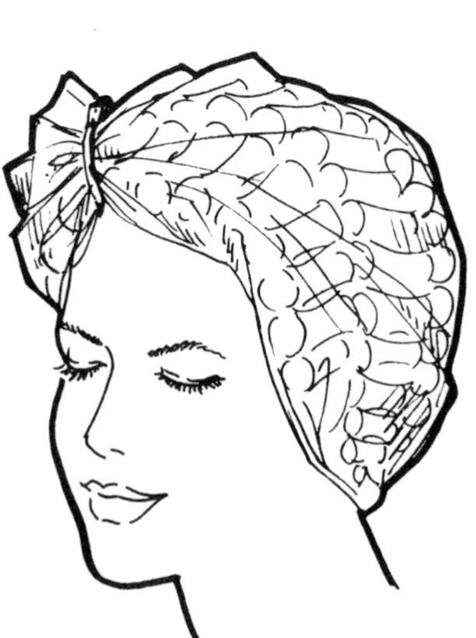

Applying processing cap

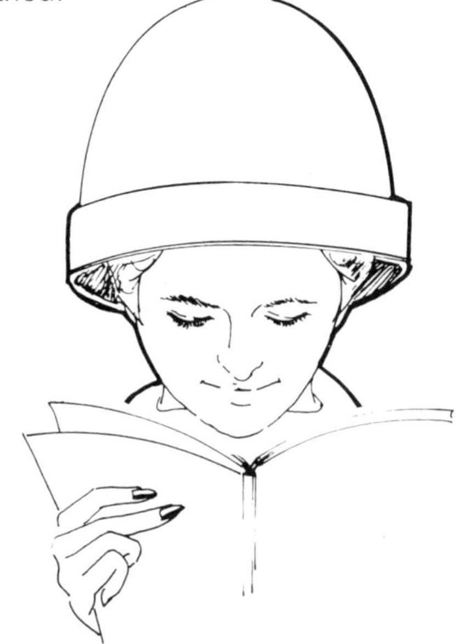

Putting client under pre-heated dryer

Heated Clamp Method

This technique of acid-balanced permanent waving involves the use of heated clamps applied directly to the hair.

The hair is completely wound on rods and thoroughly saturated with the permanent waving solution. During this period, the proper number of clamps is being heated for immediate use. After the hair is saturated with lotion and wound on the rods, a pre-heated clamp is placed on each curl. Processing begins as soon as the heat is applied.

After the hair has been processed for a pre-determined time, the clamps are removed and the hair is rinsed and neutralized in the usual manner.

There are three special control features in the heated clamp method:

1. The temperature of the rods is strictly controlled.
2. The processing does not start until the heat is applied.
3. All curls are processed for exactly the same length of time.

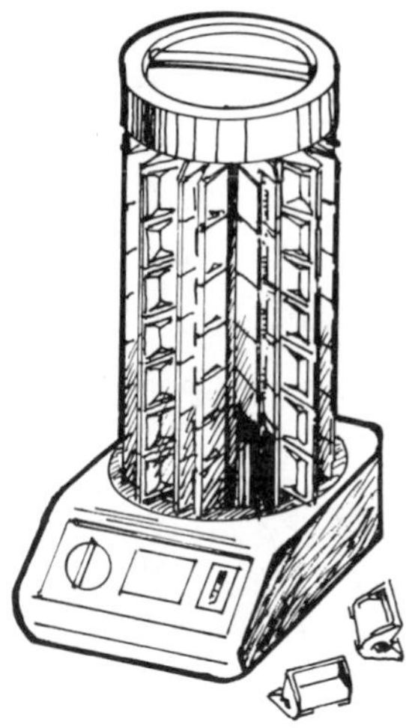

Permanent wave machine

Processing Hair with Thermal Cap

A thermal cap is frequently used to process a heat-activated formula. It is pre-heated at about the middle of the wrapping step, then placed on the head immediately after the preliminary test curl.

Cover curls first with a plastic covering.

The cap-processing technique can be substituted with the use of a dryer or heat lamp. The test-curling technique is used by most types of thermal processing unless directions indicate different procedures.

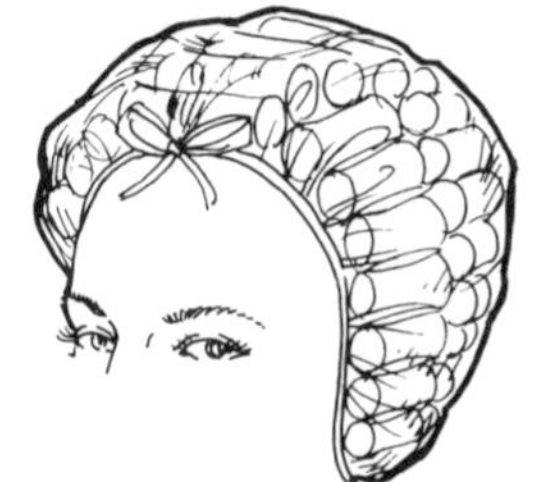

Chemical Heat Method

This method uses chemicals that are mixed together to create heat. Heat is generated by a chemical reaction produced by mixing another chemical with the waving solution.

This reaction slightly swells the hair temporarily and causes it to become warm. The moderate heat generated mildly accelerates the waving action.

Self-Heating Method

This method is used to generate heat by the self-heating technique. The hair is saturated with lotion and wound on rods. A plastic cap is carefully applied to cover the hair and is sealed airtight during processing. Body heat produces enough heat to process the hair.

However, this method has been found to be too slow and uncertain to be effective for professional service.

Neutralizers

The application of the neutralizer for neutral and acid-balanced permanent waving is very similar to the techniques used for the alkaline permanents. However, manufacturer's directions vary somewhat with different products.

Because each manufacturer has its own formula and special features related to its products, it is essential that the manufacturer's instructions be followed carefully.

PERMANENT WAVING FOR MEN

Permanent waving techniques are substantially the same for both men and women.

1. The same chemicals are used.
2. The winding procedures are the same.
3. The placement and fastening of the permanent wave rods are the same.
4. The same processing and neutralizing procedures are followed.

The only differences between permanent waving on female clients and male clients are found in the styling patterns.

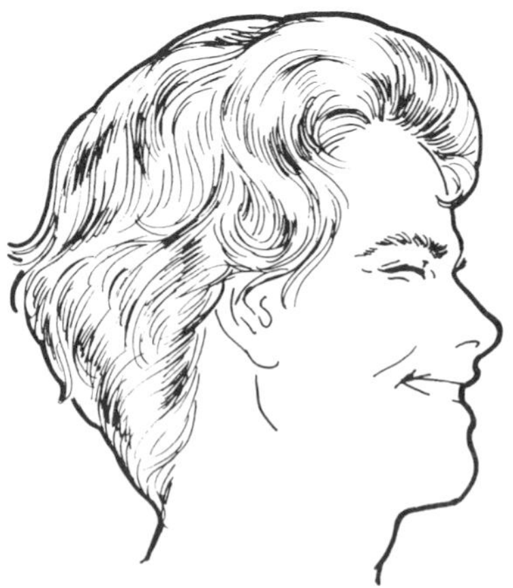
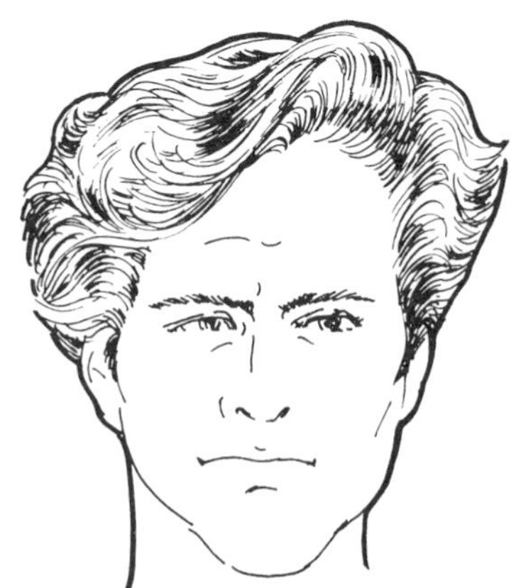
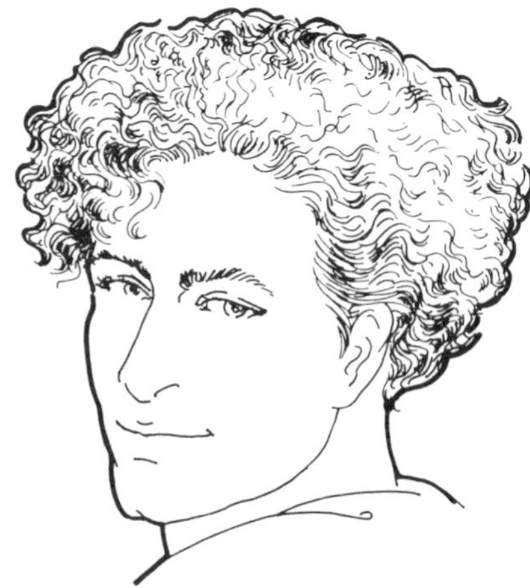

Permanent waving in popular men's hairstyles

Note

Permanent waving is one of the most common services requested of a cosmetologist. Proficiency in the techniques outlined in this chapter can only be achieved by constant practice and by taking painstaking care of all details.

Release Statement

A release statement is used for permanent waving, hair relaxing or any other type of chemical service. It relieves the salon owner to some extent from responsibility for accidents or damages.

Permanent wave release form

RELEASE FORM

Client's Name.......................... Address...........................

Condition of Hair:...

Permanent Wave: Kind..................... Given by ....

I fully understand that the permanent wave treatment that I have requested and am about to receive is ordinarily harmless to normal hair, but may damage my hair because of its present condition.
In view of this, I accept full responsibility for any possible damage that may result, directly or indirectly, to my hair.

Signature of Client...

Witnessed by........................... Date............................

Permanent Wave Record

A record of each permanent wave must be kept for each client. It is referred to each time the person is given a permanent. It contains all essential information and helps eliminate guesswork. The following is a typical form of permanent wave card.

Permanent wave record card

PERMANENT WAVE RECORD

Name .... Tel. ....

Address .... City .... State ....

DESCRIPTION OF HAIR

Form	Length	Texture		Porosity	
☐ straight	☐ short	☐ coarse	☐ soft	☐ very porous	☐ less porous
☐ wavy	☐ medium	☐ medium	☐ silky	☐ moderately porous	☐ least porous
☐ curly	☐ long	☐ fine	☐ wiry	☐ normal	☐ resistant

Condition:
☐ virgin ☐ rewave ☐ dry ☐ oily ☐ bleached

Tinted with ....

Previously waved with .... system

☐ Original sample of hair enclosed ☐ not enclosed

TYPE OF PERMANENT WAVE
☐ cold ☐ heat ☐ body wave ☐ other ....

No. of curls .... Lotion .... Strength ....

Results:
☐ good ☐ poor ☐ too tight ☐ too loose ☐ sample of finished P.W. enclosed
☐ sample not enclosed

Date	Operator	Date	Operator
....	....	....	....
....	....	....	....
....	....	....	....

REMINDERS AND HINTS ON PERMANENT WAVING

For the protection of both the client and the cosmetologist, the following rules should be observed:

1. When giving a permanent wave, always follow the manufacturer's directions.
2. Examine the scalp for abrasions and lesions.
3. Analyze the hair before every permanent wave.
4. Obtain information concerning the client's permanent wave history.
5. Protect the client's clothing by proper draping.
6. Have the client remove glasses or contacts, earrings and neck jewelry.
7. Select a mild shampoo and apply it without irritating the scalp.
8. Eliminate hair brushing or massaging before a permanent wave.
9. Use protective cream around the client's hairline and neck, if necessary.
10. Protect the client's face and neck with cotton strips or neutralizing band during processing.
11. Protect your hands with gloves or protective cream.

12. Use clean applicator bottles for all solutions. Use glass or plastic measuring cups and bowls. Do not use metallic cups or bowls.
13. When in doubt, take pre-permanent test curls.
14. Subsection the hair evenly. Uneven blockings produce uneven waves.
15. Select the proper size rods and correct waving lotion for the hair.
16. Do not stretch the hair when wrapping or stretch the bands over the curls; hair breakage can result.
17. When applying waving lotion, be sure the curls are thoroughly saturated.
18. Keep lotion from dripping on the scalp and skin. Remove lotion by blotting with cotton saturated with cold water and apply neutralizer.
19. Remove cotton strips or neutralizing bands from the face and neck if saturated with waving lotion. If the neck towel gets wet with lotion, remove it immediately.
20. If waving lotion gets into the client's eyes, wash immediately with cold water or be guided by your instructor. Take the client to a doctor.
21. Do not leave the client alone while the hair is processing.
22. Test wave formation frequently during processing.
23. Neutralize the hair thoroughly as directed by the manufacturer.
24. Remove lotion from the floor as soon as possible. Follow timing directions of the manufacturer. Avoid over-wetting.
25. Do not give a permanent to a client that has experienced an allergic reaction during a previous permanent wave.
26. Do not allow the client to sit in a draft, or near an air conditioner.
27. Complete the record card carefully and accurately.

SPECIAL PROBLEMS

Reconditioning Treatments

Dry, brittle, damaged or over-porous hair should be given reconditioning treatments. However, avoid any treatment requiring massage or heat just prior to a cold wave. Such treatment could create a sensitive scalp.

Special Permanent Wave Fillers

Over-porous or damaged hair must be pre-conditioned before the application of waving lotion. Special fillers with contain protein are available that recondition the hair and equalize its porosity. Some fillers also contain lanolin or essential oils that help to protect the hair against the harshness of the waving lotion.

Aftercare

Reconditioning treatments also have a place in the aftercare of a permanent wave and between permanents.

The aftercare of the permanent wave helps to keep the hair in the best possible condition. It includes regular hair care, as follows:

1. Shampoo the hair with mild shampoo and rinse.
2. Use the appropriate hair conditioner as directed by the manufacturer.
3. Comb and brush the hair daily. Use the type of brush best suited to the hair. Avoid excessive brushing or combing in the opposite direction.
4. Suggest that the client have the hair trimmed and styled at regular intervals, to maintain the hairstyle.

Waving Tinted or Lightened Hair

Special precautions are recommended when waving tinted or lightened hair, such as:

1. Shampooing the hair with a mild shampoo before waving
2. Wrapping the hair with a special conditioner, as required for damaged hair
3. Using a special permanent waving lotion according to directions
4. Giving test curls, using a milder waving solution and a shorter processing time than is used for normal hair
5. Giving an acid perm which is milder than an alkaline cold wave

Hair Tinted with Metallic Dye

Hair tinted with a metallic dye must first be treated with a dye remover to avoid hair discoloration or breakage. Do not wave the hair if the test curls break or discolor. This type of discoloration is very difficult to remove.

Curl Reduction

Sometimes a client is unhappy with the hair after a permanent wave because the hair appears to be too curly. If the hair is fine in texture, do not suggest curl reduction until after two or three shampoos. This type of hair relaxes to a greater extent than normal or coarse hair. Usually, after the second shampoo, the hair has relaxed enough to be satisfactory.

If the hair's texture is normal or coarse, curl reduction may be given either immediately following neutralization or after a few days.

Cold waving lotion may be used to relax the curl as needed. Carefully comb it through the hair to widen and loosen the wave. Rinse the hair when sufficiently relaxed, towel blot and neutralize.

Be sure to analyze the hair carefully before application to avoid damaging hair. **Be guided by your instructor.**

Caution

Do not attempt curl reduction in hair that has been over-processed. Such a treatment will further damage the hair.

Permanent Waving Hair with Partial Permanent

Previously permanently waved hair should be given a reconditioning treatment. Leave the conditioning agent over the old permanent and cover this hair with non-porous end papers. Then proceed with the usual permanent wave routine.

This is only one way of waving this type of hair. Your instructor's method is equally correct.

REVIEW QUESTIONS

Permanent Waving

1. *What is the history of permanent waving?*
2. *What is the purpose of cold waving?*
3. *What is the importance of the pre-permanent shampoo?*
4. *What are the steps involved in permanent waving?*
5. *Name the categories of scalp and hair analysis and give at least one method for testing each.*
6. *What is the importance of the pre-permanent shampoo?*
7. *How are the proper size rods selected to achieve the desired curl effect?*
8. *What chemicals are available for the lotion and neutralizer in modern permanent waving?*
9. *What is the importance of sectioning and blocking?*
10. *What are the five different patterns for sectioning and blocking?*
11. *In what positions may the hair be wrapped in relation to its base? What effect is achieved by each base position?*
12. *Why are test curls necessary and what is the correct technique for taking them?*
13. *How is lotion correctly applied?*
14. *Why is proper neutralization important to the success of the permanent wave?*
15. *What are the differences in the procedure for heat permanent waving?*
16. *What are the advantages and disadvantages of heat permanent waving?*
17. *What are some considerations when permanent waving a man's hair?*
18. *What are the items of importance to be included in the record card?*
19. *What are at least five safety precautions designed to protect the client during the permanent wave procedure?*

Chapter 15

HAIR COLORING

LEARNING OBJECTIVES

The student successfully mastering this chapter will be able to:

1. *Explain the principles of color theory and relate their importance to hair coloring.*
2. *List the classifications of hair color, explain their activity on the hair and give examples of their use.*
3. *Demonstrate the correct preparation for hair coloring including consultation and strand test procedures.*
4. *Demonstrate the procedure(s) for the application of temporary color.*
5. *Discuss client needs that are well suited to semi-permanent color.*
6. *Perform the entire single process tint procedure.*
7. *Explain the differences in the procedure for a tint retouch.*
8. *List at least 12 safety precautions during hair coloring procedures.*
9. *Explain the uses of hair lighteners and give examples when each type of lightener would be preferred.*
10. *Relate the activity of hydrogen peroxide in hair coloring.*
11. *Outline the procedure for lightening virgin hair.*
12. *Demonstrate methods to achieve special effects highlighting.*

13. *List preventive and corrective steps to avoid hair coloring problems.*
14. *Explain the procedure for a tint back.*

Hair coloring (tinting) is both the science and art of changing the color of hair. Hair coloring involves the addition of an artificial color to the natural pigment in the hair or the addition of color to lightened hair. (The terms "tinting" and "coloring" are used interchangeably in this text.)

Hair lightening involves the partial or total removal of the natural pigment or artificial color from the hair.

Skills in hair coloring and hair lightening can be accomplished by continuous practice and study. They can become profitable sources of income in the salon because they represent **repeat business**. The client who has tinted hair usually returns for retouching at regular intervals. Satisfactory service will encourage a return to the same salon.

The principal reasons for coloring or lightening hair are to:

1. Restore gray hair to its natural shade
2. Change the natural shade of hair to a more attractive color
3. Restore hair to its natural color
4. Create decorative effects
5. Enhance or create highlights

Typical clients are:

1. Men and women with gray hair
2. Men and women who think a change of hair color would be attractive
3. Women and men who want to maintain a youthful appearance

The successful cosmetologist must know:

1. Structure of the hair and scalp
2. Proper selection and application of coloring and lightening products
3. Chemical reactions of tints and lighteners

COLOR THEORY

It is important that you understand the theory of **color pigment** before you begin applying hair coloring products to clients. It is only through knowledge of color theory that you can think your way through color problems to the correct color formulation for each situation.

Primary Colors

For pigment, all color is created with the **primary colors**, red, yellow and blue. A primary color is one that is not derived from a mixture. All colors are created by combining these three primary colors in varying proportions.

Each primary color has its unique characteristics. Red adds warmth and richness; yellow adds lightness and brightness; blue adds depth and darkness.

Secondary Colors

Secondary colors are made by combining two primaries. Red and yellow mixed create orange; yellow and blue mixed form green; blue and red mixed form purple, or violet.

Tertiary Colors

Tertiary colors result from the combination of a primary color and its adjacent secondary color. Red and orange, for example, mix to form red-orange.

Tertiary colors often must be considered when a client's hair color has an off-color cast and when creating the formula for toners.

Complementary Colors

Complementary colors are extremely important to the colorist because they determine the cause of a color problem and indicate the solution. Complementary colors are pairs of colors located opposite each other on the color wheel. They are always composed of a primary and a secondary color. The complementary pair always consists of all three primary colors. Looking at the color wheel, you can see that the complement of the color red is green. Green is composed of blue and yellow, so all three primaries—red, blue and yellow—are present in the complementary pair.

When the colors that make up a complementary pair are placed side by side, they accent each other. When mixed together, however, they make a shade of brown. So, red and green side by side are holiday bright; but red and green mixed together make a neutral brown.

In any color correction problem, it is important to consider complements and ensure that all three primaries are present in the final color result.

Concentration

Concentration reflects the amount of black present. Black is an even mixture of all primary colors. Concentration in a hair color formula will indicate the amount of **deposit** of color that can be expected.

Colors that have a lower amount of concentration (black) will produce more **lift** or lightening of the natural hair color. Color manufacturers arrange colors into different levels so that you can anticipate their concentration. Manufacturers provide materials to explain the level systems they use, and your instructor can assist you in determining the correct level of color to achieve the result you desire.

CLASSIFICATIONS OF HAIR COLORING

Hair coloring is the application of artificial color to the hair. Hair coloring falls into three main categories: **temporary, semi-permanent** and **permanent**. The professional colorist must know how each group acts on the hair and how hair porosity and the addition of heat affects each category of hair color.

Temporary Hair Coloring

WATER OR COLOR RINSES

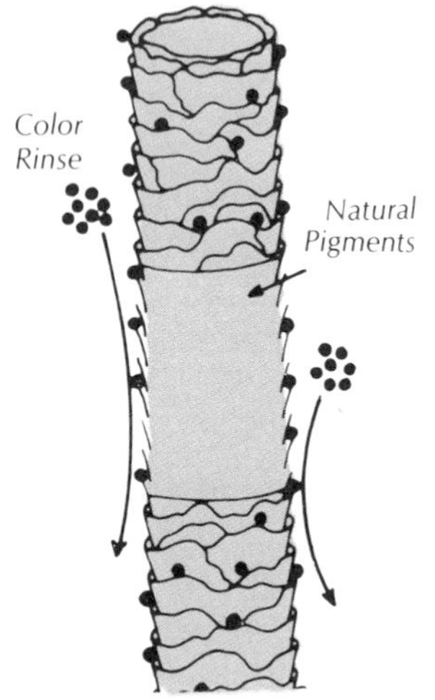

Temporary hair coloring is designed to last on the hair from shampoo to shampoo. Excessively porous hair can cause this type of hair coloring to last longer, fading with each shampoo. A patch test is not necessary for this type of hair color. Temporary color can only deposit pigment, it cannot lift.

1. **Color rinses** are prepared rinses used either to highlight or add color to the hair. These rinses contain certified colors and remain on the hair until the next shampoo. Color rinses are now available as creams and gels and have been added to lightweight setting agents in the form of mousses, and the like.
2. **Highlighting color shampoos** combine the action of a color rinse with that of a shampoo. These shampoos give highlights and add color tones to the hair.
3. **Crayons and mascara** are temporary colors used for makeup. They are available in many shades and are usually compounded with synthetic waxes. They are generally used to add color to eyebrows and lashes.
4. **Hair color sprays** are applied to dry hair from aerosol containers, usually for special or party effects.

Semi-Permanent Hair Coloring

Semi-permanent hair coloring agents are formulated to last from four to six shampoos. They penetrate into the cuticle layer and, on overporous hair can penetrate into the cortex for a more longer lasting effect. They are applied without peroxide, so they do not change the basic structure of the hair. The addition of heat, however, can sometimes transform this type of hair color into a permanent one. Be guided by the information supplied by the manufacturer and your instructor's directions.

SEMI-PERMANENT COLOR

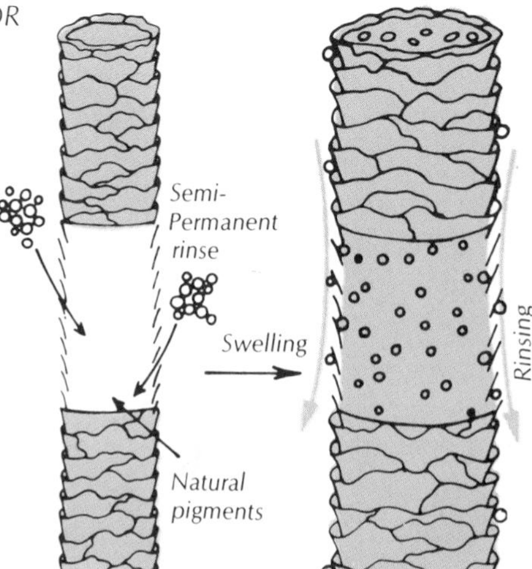

Semi-permanent color penetrates the cuticle slightly. Molecules are gradually shampooed from the hair.

Semi-permanent colors are designed to add color to the hair. They can be used in the following ways:

1. Cover or blend partially gray hair without affecting its natural color. Most semi-permanent colors are designed to cover hair that is 10% or less gray.
2. Enhance or blend partially gray hair without affecting its natural color. This can be done successfully on almost any percentage of gray, depending upon the desired color.

3. Highlight and enhance the color tones of the hair. Semi-permanent colors can be used to add golden or red highlights and to deepen the color of the hair. This type of color is especially effective on ethnic clients and those whose natural hair color is too light or too drab for their complexions.
4. Serve as a non-peroxide toner for pre-lightened hair. Due to the porosity of the hair, the toner will be permanent.

Most semi-permanent hair colors require a patch test, because most contain aniline derivative agents. The following illustrations indicate how this type of hair coloring works on the hair shaft.

Permanent Hair Coloring

Permanent hair colorings are designed to penetrate the cuticle and deposit molecules into the cortex. Due to the penetration and the addition of peroxide, these colors can both lift and deposit.

ACTION OF HAIR TINTS

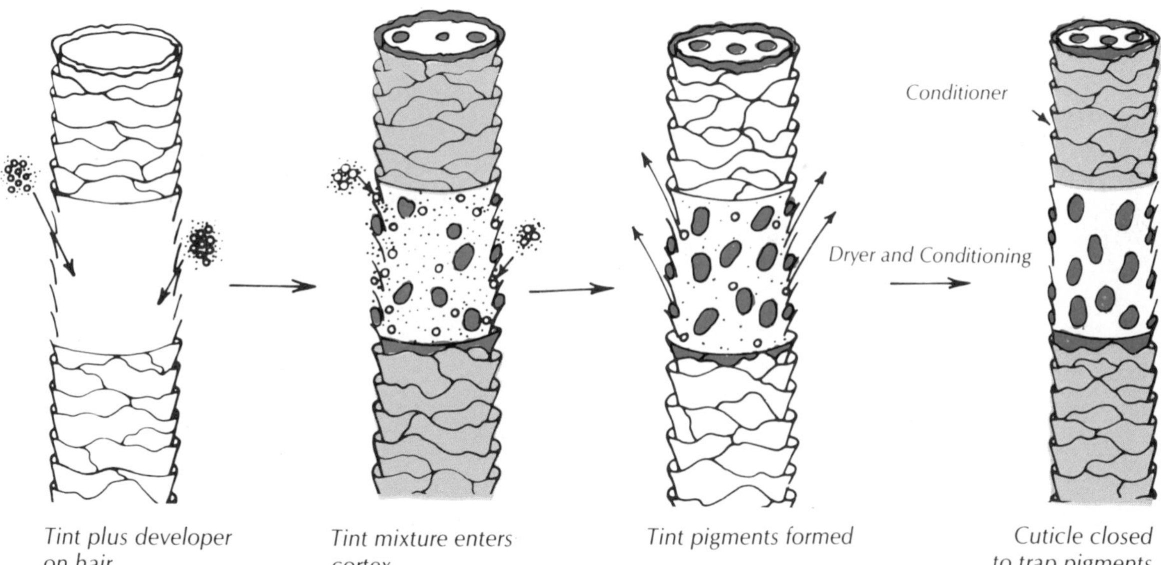

Tint plus developer on hair — Tint mixture enters cortex — Tint pigments formed — Cuticle closed to trap pigments

1. **Aniline derivative tints** are also known as penetrating tints, synthetic organic tints, peroxide or oxidation tints and are commonly called "tints" in the industry. Tints can both lift and deposit, and have the widest variety of colors available. Toners also fit into the category of aniline derivative tints, but can only deposit tones to pre-lightened hair. A patch test is required for all permanent color that is based on aniline derivatives.
2. **Pure vegetable tints.** In the past, indigo, camomile, sage and Egyptian henna were used for hair coloring. They deposited a coating on the hair. Today, only henna is still used professionally, although other ingredients are added to it to produce non-red shades. It is important that the person receiving vegetable tints is

not also a permanent wave client. Current day vegetable products not only coat the hair but also have a certain degree of penetration. They can prevent absorption of permanent wave lotion, cause uneven curl, damage and even breakage.

3. **Metallic or mineral dyes**, such as lead acetate or silver nitrate, are the **progressive type** known as **color restorers**. They form a metallic coating over the hair shaft, making it unsatisfactory for permanent waving, hair lightening or tinting. Successive applications are made until the proper shade has developed. Metallic dyes are *not* professional colors and should be avoided.
4. **Compound dyes**, such as compound henna, are combinations of vegetable dyes with certain metallic salts and other dyestuffs. The metallic salts fix the color. Compound dyes coat the hair shaft and make the hair unfit for permanent waving, lightening or tinting. They are also not used professionally.

Metallic and compound dyes are never used professionally. However, people do buy and apply such products to their hair at home. Therefore, the hair colorist must be able to recognize and understand their effects. Such coloring agents must be removed and the hair reconditioned prior to any other chemical service. Hair treated with a metallic or any other coating dye appears to be dry and dull. It is generally harsh and brittle to the touch. These colorings usually fade to unnatural tones. Silver dyes have a greenish cast, and leave a purple color; those containing copper turn red.

Test for Metallic Salts and Coating Dyes

1. In a glass container, mix one ounce (30 ml) of 20 volume (6%) peroxide and 20 drops of ammonia.
2. Cut a strand of the client's hair, bind with tape and immerse in the solution for 30 minutes.
3. Remove, dry and observe the strand.

Hair dyed with lead will lighten immediately.

Hair treated with silver will have no reaction at all. This indicates that other chemicals will not be successful because they cannot penetrate the coating.

Hair treated with copper will start to boil and will pull apart easily. This hair would be severely damaged or destroyed if other chemicals were applied.

Hair treated with a coating dye will either not change color or will lighten in spots. This hair will not receive chemical services evenly, and the length of time necessary for penetration might very well damage the hair.

Removing Coatings from the Hair

Specialized shampoos, preparations designed to remove metallics and non-peroxide dye solvents can assist in the removal of metallic and coating dyes from the hair. Follow the manufacturer's directions and retest to ensure the coating is removed. The most effective guarantee of future successful services is to remove the hair by cutting.

ANILINE DERIVATIVE TINTS

The aniline derivative tints are the most widely used in hair coloring. These tints remain in the hair until they are removed by chemical means or until the hair grows out. The coloring penetrates through the cuticle into the cortex, then binds into a complex molecule that is permanent.

An aniline derivative tint contains, as its essential ingredient, **para-phenylene-diamine**, or a related chemical compound. With this type of preparation, it is possible to duplicate the various shades of human hair without a loss of condition or sheen. These tints can be applied successfully over permanently waved and chemically relaxed hair.

Aniline derivative tints are sold in bottles or in tubes. The stock of tints should be kept fresh, because they deteriorate on standing.

Aniline derivative tints must be mixed with hydrogen peroxide to achieve lift and deposit colors. The peroxide causes a chemical reaction known as **oxidation**. This reaction begins as soon as the two compounds are mixed together, so the mixed tint must always be used **immediately**.

Timing of the applied tint depends upon the product and the volume of peroxide selected. Consult the manufacturer's directions and your instructor for assistance. A strand test should always be taken to ensure satisfactory results.

Allergy

Allergy to aniline derivative tints is an unpredictable condition. Some clients may be sensitive and others may suddenly develop a sensitivity after years of use. To identify such individuals, the U.S. Federal Food, Drug, and Cosmetic Act prescribes that a **patch** or **predisposition test** be given 24 hours prior to each application of an aniline derivative tint or toner.

Caution Aniline derivative tints must never be used on the eyelashes or eyebrows. To do so may cause blindness.

Patch Test

The patch or predisposition test must be given 24 hours before each tinting or toner treatment. The tint used for the skin test must be of the same formula as that used for the hair coloring service.

Procedure

1. Select the test area, either behind the ear or the inner fold of the elbow.
2. Cleanse an area about the size of a quarter.
3. Dry the area.
4. Prepare the test solution according to the manufacturer's directions.
5. Apply to the test area with a sterile cotton swab.
6. Leave the area undisturbed for 24 hours.
7. Examine the test area.
8. Note the results on the client's record card.

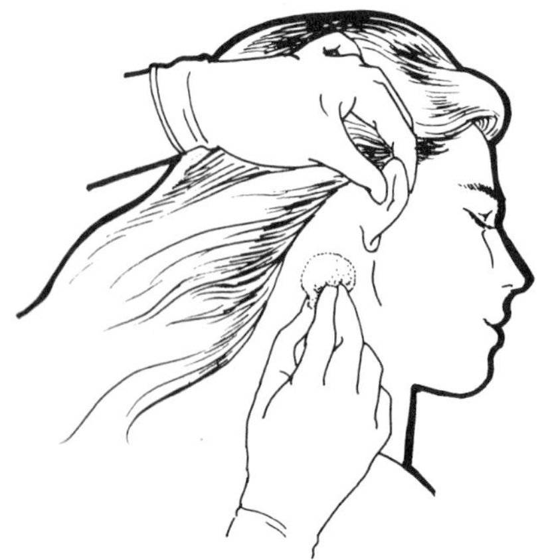
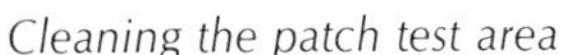

Cleaning the patch test area

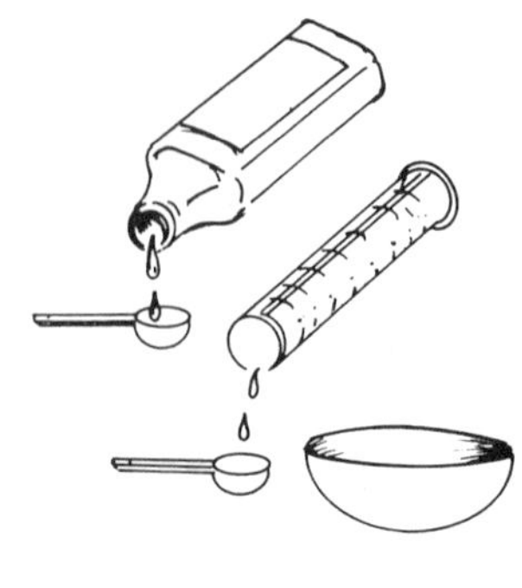

Mixing tint and peroxide

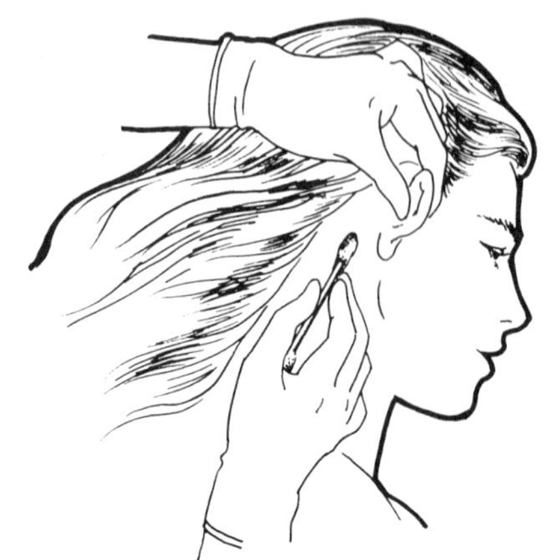

Applying tint mixture

A **negative skin test** will show no sign of inflammation and an aniline tint may be safely applied.

A **positive skin test** is recognized by the presence of redness, swelling, burning, itching and blisters. A client with such symptoms is allergic and **under no circumstances should receive an aniline derivative tint**. Application of an aniline derivative tint in this instance could result in a serious reaction for the client and a malpractice suit for the hair colorist.

Examining Scalp and Hair

Carefully examine the scalp and hair to determine if it is safe to use a hair coloring product and whether any special hair problems exist.

The results of such an examination may indicate the need for any of the following:

1. Reconditioning treatments
2. Color removal
3. Removal of metallic coloring
4. Postponement of service due to breakage, and the like

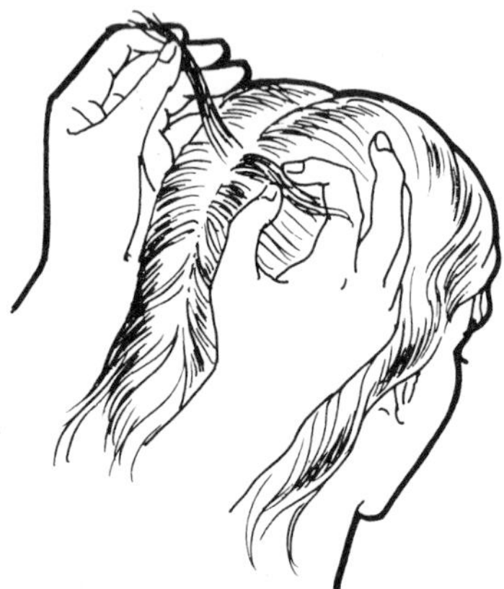

Examining the scalp and hair

An aniline derivative tint **should not** be used if the following conditions are noted:

1. Positive skin test
2. Scalp irritations or eruptions
3. Contagious scalp or hair disorders
4. Presence of metallic or compound dyes

If the scalp and hair are in healthy condition, observe carefully and record the data on the client's record card.

PREPARATION FOR HAIR COLORING CONSULTATION

Consultation is one of the most important steps in the hair coloring service. The finest formulation combined with the most talented application will still result in color failure if it is not what the client wants.

Always record the consultation on the **client's record card**. Perform the consultation in a well-lit room, preferably with natural lighting. If this is not possible, arrange lighting so that it is incandescent in front of the client (around the mirror) and fluorescent behind the colorist (ceiling fixtures). Full color fluorescent lights are also available.

When talking with the client, consider what colors will suit the skin tones and how those tones might be changing with maturity. Also consider the personality and make sure that the color desired will not clash. Pay close attention to the described lifestyle so you do not select a coloring procedure that requires a great deal of care for a very active person. Check that the person is willing to use a good quality shampoo at home that will not strip the color and conditioners that will maintain the condition of the hair.

The following chart will help you in your selection. Remember that each person is unique and consult with your instructor.

Hair Color Selection Chart

SKIN TONE	EYE COLOR	HAIR COLOR OPTIONS
Warm, Yellow-red Undertones such as:		
Ivory, Peaches & Cream, Creamy beige, Light golden brown, Cafe au lait, Tawny, Coppery, Deep golden brown, Golden-red brown (red)	Blue, Blue-green, Green, Topaz, Amber, Cinnamon, Coffee bean	Golden highlights Golden with red highlights, Golden brown, Honey brown, Chestnut, Copper, Auburn, Mahogany, Warm tones of gray, Warm tones of white
Cool, Blue-Red Undertones such as:		
Alabaster, Rosey pink, Rose beige, Light pearl, Light olive, Dark olive (green), Gray-brown (light to dark), Dark brown, Ebony Slate	Light blue, Gray blue, Gray green, Blue green, Deep blue, Deep green (medium to dark), Black	Plum, Burgundy, highlights, Ash Platinum blonde, Ash brown (medium to dark), Dark brown, Black, Salt and Pepper, Pure white

Tint colors are usually divided into four groups:

1. Shades with no red are classified as **ash** (drab).
2. Shades with yellow are in the **gold** series. The gold series can also have warm shades that contain red.

3. Shades with red are the **very warm** or **red** series.
4. Shades with blue are classified as the **cool** series.

Many manufacturers include this information in their numbering system.

Basic Rules for Color Selection

1. Make sure the client's hair is **clean** and **dry**.
2. Look through the hair. To see depth as well as highlights, raise the hair by pushing it up with the hands against the scalp.
3. Analyze the depth present in the hair. Does the client want to go lighter or darker?
4. Analyze the depth of the desired color. Add or subtract from the natural color to determine the level of color necessary.
5. What are the natural highlights? What highlights does the client want? Select the color within the level that will supply those highlights or determine what primary additive should be used.
6. Know the properties of the product you are using. Consult the manufacturer's information on each color when applied to light, medium, dark hair and so on.
7. Analyze the condition of the hair, especially its porosity. Does the hair need to be conditioned prior to the service so the color will be true and will not fade?

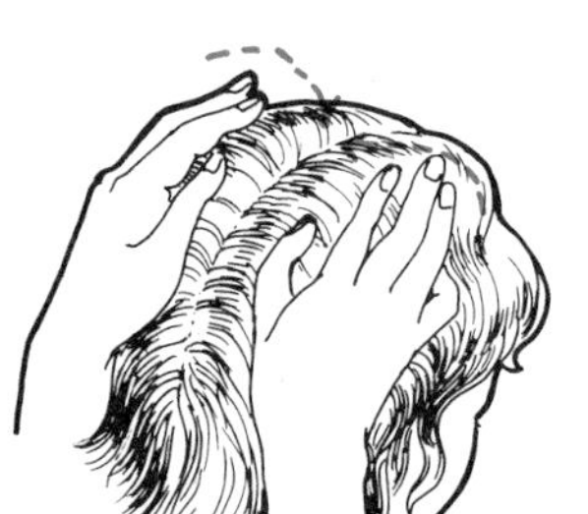

Checking hair color

Strand Test to Confirm Color Selection

Before applying any tint, strand test to confirm your selection. You will learn the following information:

1. Whether the proper color selection was made
2. Timing to achieve desired results
3. If further pre-conditioning treatments are needed
4. If it is necessary to apply a filler

Strand Test Procedure

1. Mix 1/2 tsp. of color with peroxide according to the manufacturer's directions.
2. Apply mixture to 1/2" section, usually in the crown area of the head.

NOTE It is important that the hair has received all pre-treatments necessary according to your analysis before the strand test is given so that the results will be true.

3. Process with or without heat, keeping careful records of timing on the client's record card.
4. Rinse the strand, towel dry and examine the results. Adjust the formula, timing or pre-conditioning necessary and proceed with tinting on the entire head.
5. If results are unsatisfactory, perform the strand test again.

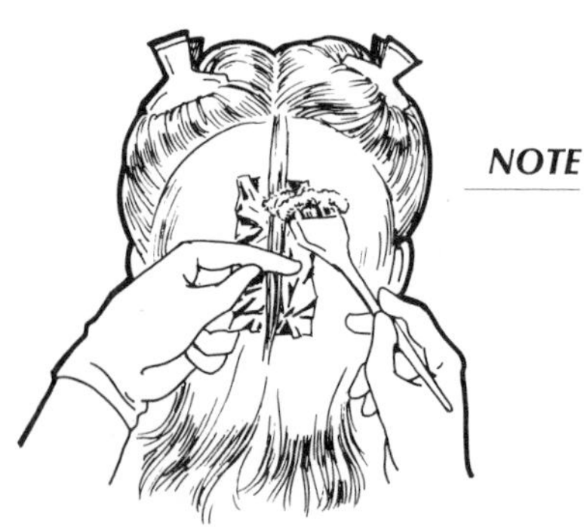

Applying color to the strand test

Follow Working Plan in Tinting

For successful hair coloring services, the technician must follow a definite procedure. A system makes for the greatest efficiency and the most satisfactory results. Without such a plan, the work will take longer, results will be uneven and mistakes will be made.

A working plan includes the materials and supplies needed for the tinting service and a thorough knowledge of the product to be used.

Keep a permanent record of each client's color service.

Keeping Hair Color Records

It is of the utmost importance to keep an accurate record so that any difficulties encountered in one service can be avoided in the next. **A complete record** should be kept containing all analysis notes, strand test and whole head results, timing and suggestions for the next service.

HAIR COLOR RECORD

Name .... Tel. ....

Address .... City..................................

Patch Test: Negative ☐ Positive ☐ Date..................................

DESCRIPTION OF HAIR

Form	**Length**	**Texture**	**Porosity**	
☐ straight	☐ short	☐ coarse	☐ very porous	☐ resistant
☐ wavy	☐ medium	☐ medium	☐ porous	☐ very resistant
☐ curly	☐ long	☐ fine	☐ normal	☐ perm. waved

Condition

☐ normal ☐ dry ☐ oily ☐ faded ☐ streaked ....% grey

Previously lightened with .... for ....(time)

Previously tinted with .... for ....(time)

☐ original sample enclosed ☐ not enclosed

CORRECTIVE TREATMENTS

Color filler used .... Corrective treatments with ....

HAIR TINTING PROCESS

whole head .... retouch .... inches (cm) shade desired ....

Formula: color .... lightener ....

Results:

☐ good ☐ poor ☐ too light ☐ too dark ☐ streaked

Date	Operator	Price	Date	Operator	Price

Release Statement A release statement is used for chemical services. It releases the school or salon owner from responsibility for accidents or damages and is required for some malpractice insurance.

SAMPLE RELEASE

Client's Name...................................... Address ....

Condition of Hair: ....

Hair Coloring: Kind .... Given by ....

I fully understand that the hair coloring treatment that I have requested and am about to receive is ordinarily harmless to normal hair, but may damage my hair because of its present condition.

In view of this, I accept full responsibility for any possible damage that may result, directly or indirectly, to my hair.

Signature of Client ....

Witnessed by... Date ....

TEMPORARY COLORS

A temporary color coats the cuticle of the hair with a film of color pigment. Since the color remains on the cuticle and does not penetrate into the cortex, it lasts only from shampoo to shampoo. Excessive porosity can allow temporary color to penetrate, however, making it last much longer. Temporary colors usually contain certified colors, that have been approved by the FDA for use in cosmetics.

Temporary colors can be used for the following advantages:

1. Bring out highlights in the hair
2. Temporarily restore faded hair to its natural color
3. Neutralize the yellowish tinge in white or gray hair
4. Tone down overlightened hair
5. Temporarily add color to the hair without changing its condition
6. Perform hair coloring without a required skin test

Temporary hair colorings also have several disadvantages:

1. Color is of short duration and must be applied after every shampoo
2. Coating is thin and might not cover hair evenly
3. Color can rub off on pillows, collars and the like and might run with perspiration or other moisture
4. Can only add color, it cannot lift
5. May result in staining if the hair is porous or if a dark color is used on very light hair

However, for the clients who want to highlight the color of their hair or glamorize gray hair, a temporary color is very helpful. Temporary colors come in various shades: blonde, brown, black, red, silver and slate. They are applied easily and are valuable as an introduction to hair coloring.